Pragmatics in Dementia Discourse

Pragmatics in Dementia Discourse

Edited by

Boyd H. Davis and Jacqueline Guendouzi

CAMBRIDGE
SCHOLARS
PUBLISHING

Pragmatics in Dementia Discourse,
Edited by Boyd H. Davis and Jacqueline Guendouzi

This book first published 2013

Cambridge Scholars Publishing

12 Back Chapman Street, Newcastle upon Tyne, NE6 2XX, UK

British Library Cataloguing in Publication Data
A catalogue record for this book is available from the British Library

ISBN (10): 1-4438-5167-1, ISBN (13): 978-1-4438-5167-1

TABLE OF CONTENTS

ACKNOWLEDGMENTS

We gratefully acknowledge our colleagues who were kind enough to critique these chapters prior to our submitting the manuscript to the press, while absolving them of any remaining errors or lacunae:

Michelle Bourgeois (Ohio State University), Tami Howe (University of Canterbury), Filip Loncke (University of Virginia), Laura Murray (Indiana University), Rebecca Roeder (University of North Carolina – Charlotte), Meghan Savage (Southeastern Louisiana University)

The *Carolinas Conversation Collection*: The project described was supported by Grant Number G08LM009624 from the National Library of Medicine. The content is solely the responsibility of the authors and does not necessarily represent the official views of the National Library Of Medicine or the National Institutes of Health.

PREFACE

The dementias whose discourse is discussed in this collection include Dementia with Lewy bodies and Parkinson disease dementia, as well as dementia of the Alzheimer's type (DAT). The magnitude of dementia and the impact on the global community is immense. Perhaps some statistical information about DAT will aid in making our case for the compelling need to look at pragmatics in dementia discourse. The most common form of dementia, DAT, affects more than five million citizens in the US: one in eight people aged 65 and older have Alzheimer's disease. Dementia is the sixth leading cause of death in the US and costs billions of dollars annually in care (*AlzFacts and Figures 2012*). According to the World Health Organization (http://www.who.int), DAT affects an estimated thirty-five million people worldwide, with prevalence particularly high in developed countries. Persons diagnosed with dementia of the Alzheimer's type (DAT) may live many years after diagnosis; care is most often given by family members who do not have specific training in dementia care or in communication. Attitudes toward DAT vary: in many cultures throughout the world, dementia is regarded as a part of old age and is frequently stigmatized.

A major challenge in any kind of health discourse is that within the majority of the studies focused on language in medical or clinical settings, pragmatics constructs are seldom the explicit or exclusive focus, though they may be a part of the larger discussion:

> Instead, pragmatics is more typically embedded within studies combining a variety of theoretical approaches from discourse, sociolinguistics, conversation analysis (CA) and ethnography….We have not yet seen a confluence of studies of health discourse focusing exclusively on areas within the domain of pragmatics such as speech acts, inference and intended meaning, politeness theory, or relevance theory (Davis 2010, 381).

This collection, ***Pragmatics in Dementia Discourse,*** is intended to bridge that gap.

Pragmatics in Dementia Discourse is a comprehensive contribution to the literature, applying several classical traditions within pragmatics research. This collection illustrates the applicability of pragmatic and discourse research methods to the analysis of communication in persons with dementia. More specifically, this collection highlights for the reader the value of studying pragmatics in discourse as a way of revealing the nuances of disordered language and social skills in neurodegenerative disorders such as dementia. Individuals with dementia present with complex disorders of language including challenges with retaining knowledge of words and concepts but also using language structure and rules to create linkages among words and ideas in order to communicate meaning. In addition to disruption of discrete language processes, persons with dementia may have challenges recognizing social contexts and engaging in appropriate social interactions. As a result of these changes to communication, care providers and interlocutors of persons with dementia face substantial challenges in conveying and interpreting information. Also these changes create challenges in establishing and maintaining relationships between an individual with dementia and other members of his/her environment. As the disease progresses, the unimpaired conversation partner bears an increasing share of the communication burden. Moreover, because of these communication challenges, the individual with dementia may progressively develop a compromised sense of personhood as they lose their 'voice' and the ability to convey their 'story'. However, few comprehensive sources exist to guide conversation partners, clinicians, and researchers, in understanding of the complex aspects of language and discourse production, particularly as affected by pragmatics.

Those aspects of dementia, which most deeply impact friends and family members, are the increase in problems with short-term memory, language production, and language comprehension that affect monologue and dialogue. At the same time, conversation, whether one-on-one or in small groups, is the most frequently recommended socio-behavioral or non-pharmaceutical intervention for individuals with dementia. Without an understanding of preserved discourse abilities in dementia and which aspects of language can be used to support conversation and interaction, formal care providers, therapists, and family members are left with few resources to assist the person with dementia. Over the past decade, impelled by earlier sociolinguistics studies, linguists and affiliated researchers on dementia discourse have initiated work on usage, contexts, politeness/im-politeness, meaning and intention in language production and interaction. The proposed collection grew from presentations at the First Annual Conference of the American Pragmatics Association (Charlotte, NC, 2012), augmented by additional chapters by valued colleagues who were unable to attend the conference. Among other purposes, these chapters are intended to serve as a starting point for further dialogue and research around pragmatics in dementia discourse. They are intended to inform and inspire care partners, clinicians, and researchers in supporting those living with communication disorders in dementia.

Chapter one, by Jacqueline Guendouzi and Boyd Davis, is "Dementia discourse and pragmatics: Varied viewpoints." The authors explore differences between how linguists and clinicians (i.e. speech language pathologists) draw on different aspects of pragmatics when investigating dementia discourse. They highlight key studies in communications disorders, speech pathology and linguistics, tracing interactions among the disciplines and their gradual implementation of a range of pragmatics approaches.

Chapter two, "So what's your name? Relevance in dementia," by Jacqueline Guendouzi, focuses on how relevance theory (Sperber and Wilson 1995) can be used to explore characteristics in the management of conversations involving people with dementia (PWD). Relevance theory suggests interlocutors interpret inferences in a way that, all things being equal, alights on the best interpretation for the current context, specific speech event, the particular participants, and the verbal message as interpreted within the local context of the conversation itself. Thus, relevance theory suggests that interlocutors focus their attention on factors that are relevant to the situation at hand in order to draw the appropriate illocutionary inference. This is a process that requires interlocutors to engage several cognitive systems such as working memory, the ability to inhibit competing information, access to long term memory items, and recognition of the identity and role of the other interlocutor. In the context of dementia some or all of these processing mechanisms are compromised. In particular, attention, inhibition and working memory may be severely affected in people with dementia and thus affect their ability to draw accurate inferences. This chapter examines interactions between a researcher and a group of PWD who attended a day center for people with mild to moderate dementia. Analyses focus on the interaction between cognitive mechanisms and interactional resources to consider whether the apparent dependence on non-novel language by speakers with dementia is a volitional compensatory strategy or reflexive artifact of constrained cognitive processing resources, and whether the use of non-novel constructions hindered or enhanced the conversations.

Chapter three, "Positioning and membership categorization in monoracial and interracial interactions of persons with dementia" is by Charlene Pope. She begins by pointing out how the use of language positions both speaker and their conversational partner in identities past, present and projected, as they perceive and categorize their social identities and group memberships in the immediate shared world and the worlds they have known. For persons with Alzheimer's disease, memories and ways of knowing may fade, but social and cultural conditioning continue to appear in the talk of social interaction. Using Levinson's overview of links between pragmatics and conversation analysis, acts of positioning associated with social identity are compared in a series of dialogues between Black and White persons with Alzheimer's disease and non-cognitively impaired same-race and differing-race conversational partners. The findings show that multiple social identities present beyond the variations that appear in same-race and differing race pairs, and suggest how people with Alzheimer' s disease mobilize speaking resources. Particular practices specific to monoracial and biracial interactions suggest how intercultural pragmatics might identify markers of sociocultural contexts, power, and distance, beyond issues of sequencing and turn-taking usually analyzed in conversation analysis

Chapter four, "'Aw, so, how's your day going?': Ways that persons with dementia keep their conversational partner involved" is by Boyd Davis, Margaret Maclagan and Julie Wright. Their multimodal analysis of the communication repertoire of a person with dementia uses interpersonal pragmatics to explore a person with dementia's preserved ability to manipulate pauses, filled pauses, extenders and formulaic utterances. Interpersonal pragmatics deals with the role of language in relational work, specifically how 'social actors use language to form relationships in situ' (Locher & Graham 2010:1), making it a good framework for the examination of key features in discourse between persons with dementia (PWD) and their unimpaired interlocutors. The progression of dementia curtails verbal communication in several ways: the ability to access words and story components diminishes, as does the ability to process conversation and respond to others. However, the PWD wants to communicate, and to be seen as responsive, even competent. With some speakers, repetition of stories and story fragments becomes a shorthand way of signaling memory and emotion (Davis 2011; Schiff et al 2006); with others, extenders, pauses and filled pauses, the *um*s and *er*s of conversation, allow a PWD to involve the conversation partner in completing a sentence or a story (Fox Tree and Schrock 2002; Davis & Maclagan 2009; Maclagan, Davis & Lunsford 2008). Many PWD draw on a repertoire that includes extenders, pauses and formulaic utterances: here, the authors look at their association with head nods and gestures in video-recordings of "Maureen Littlejohn."

Chapter five, by Alison Wray, is titled "Mislaying compassion: linguistic triggers for inadequate care-giving in Alzheimer's disease care." She proposes that caregivers can find themselves in an emotionally perilous environment, because, on account of the pragmatics of communication, they are cornered into a choice between equally undesirable responses to the repetitive language produced by a person with Alzheimer's disease. There is a strong imperative in communication to assume that one's interlocutor intends to be meaningful and relevant, but this assumption is difficult to sustain if questions or statements are repeated in a manner that exceeds the typical rules of interaction. Interpreting the repetition as necessary entails that the speaker has not been attending adequately to the previous conversation. The natural inference is that the other party—the caregiver—is not being treated with respect, and this is likely to instill responses such as hurt and anger. Wray suggests that this may be one explanation of the lack of compassion frequently reported as a problem in the care sector. Yet caregivers know that the repetition is caused by the disease. However, allowing for the linguistic behavior not to be an insult requires the caregiver to release the speaker from the standard rules of pragmatics. Since these rules are perceived to be universal in human interaction, the speaker must then fall outside of the definition of 'a human interacting', which is an uncomfortable and potentially risky situation for him or her. Wray suggests that caregiver stress may be partly due to the constant need to manage this dilemma.

Chapter six, "Discourse in Lewy Body Spectrum Disorder," is by Angela Roberts and J.B. Orange. They present a comprehensive overview of the literature relating to discourse and pragmatic deficits in Lewy body spectrum disorders (i.e., Parkinson disease, Parkinson disease dementia, and dementia with Lewy bodies). They review the literature from both monologic and interactional discourse paradigms. The cognitive impairments associated with LBSD have a substantial effect on the quality of life and the communication of individuals with LBSD and their caregivers. Individuals with LBSD present with cognitive-linguistic impairments such as difficulty finding words and difficulty comprehending and producing complex syntactic forms. A growing area of research over the last decade has demonstrated the presence of cognitive-linguistic deficits that contribute to pragmatic problems such as impaired theory of mind, disrupted metaphor comprehension, compromised ability to decode emotional cues, and diminished comprehension of irony. What is less known, however, is the profile of pragmatic deficits during discourse in individuals with LBSD. Exploring these competencies is critical for increasing our understanding of Parkinson's disease and LBSD disorders, and for developing strategies/interventions for optimizing social communication

Chapter seven, "Challenges and opportunities of group conversations: The day care center as a communication milieu," by Camilla Lindholm, examines how unimpaired conversation partners can be challenged by faulty communication; yet draw on other practices to maintain their ability and willingness to converse. Regardless of the interactional challenges created by the group situations (involving parallel discussions, overlapping talk, and participants' varying capabilities of functioning in group settings), the group is demonstrated to be a potential resource – the individual can achieve help both from the health care personnel and from the other elderly participants. Lindholm's study identifies pragmatics problems for interlocutors who must carry the greater responsibility for conversation maintenance with persons who have dementia.

Chapter eight is a "Summary of an Online Roundtable," by Orange and Davis, who pull together what authors identified as desirable next steps in research on pragmatics in dementia discourse, from an online hour-long audio conference call after the authors had circulated chapters among themselves.

Chapter nine, by Robert Schrauf, is "Epilogue: Reading Compromised and Preserved Cognition Into and Out of Conversational Data." This chapter draws on data from the various contributors to address the mutual enrichments of pragmatics and cognitive gerontology/cognitive neuropsychology in understanding the language of persons with dementia. On the one hand, moving from *cognition to conversation*, the chapter asks: how might we interpret the conversational data of persons with Alzheimer's in light of the signature cognitive deficits of the disease—severely diminished working memory, impaired executive function, problematic lexical retrieval and degenerating semantic organization—and of preserved abilities in language functioning—such as, for example, syntactic processing and turn-taking? This question starts from cognitive abilities as identified, articulated, and operationalized in cognitive gerontology and the neuropsychology of Alzheimer's disease and looks for ways of understanding Alzheimer's speech. On the other hand, moving from *conversation to cognition*, we might ask: what cognitive competencies are presupposed by the real-time, naturally-occurring, communicative performances of persons with Alzheimer's disease? This question starts from a pragmatic analysis of actual conversation and seeks to identify (and perhaps construct) candidate cognitive abilities that likely undergird performance. Different pragmatic theories (e.g. relevance theory, emergent pragmatics, interpersonal pragmatics, etc.) lend themselves to either side of this equation, and these reflections serve to formulate new questions for both pragmatic and cognitive approaches to communication in dementia.

CHAPTER ONE

DEMENTIA DISCOURSE AND PRAGMATICS

JACQUELINE GUENDOUZI
SOUTHEASTERN LOUISIANA UNIVERSITY
AND BOYD DAVIS
UNC CHARLOTTE

Introduction

Dementia, particularly Alzheimer's disease, is currently one of the most widely publicized disease syndromes, and continues to puzzle researchers. A diagnosis of dementia in a living person identifies multiple cognitive deficits affecting language and memory which interfere with and may prevent that person's ability to function independently at work or during usual activities, which "represent a decline from previous levels of functioning and performing; and are not explained by delirium or major psychiatric disorder" (McKhann et al 2011, 263). In 1906, Alois Alzheimer gave his name to the syndrome; subsequently thirteen cases of Alzheimer's disease were reported between 1907-11, and "by 1920 physicians had integrated this new disease category, which seemed to link specific organic changes in the brain to clinical symptoms, into medical thinking (Holstein 1997, 1). We can see the exponential growth of interest in dementia, and particularly Alzheimer's dementia, by checking the number of articles registered in PubMed, the biomedical literature index published by the National Center for Biotechnology Information (NCBI), a division of the National Library of Medicine (NLM) at the National Institutes of Health (NIH). Between 1906 and 1913, only one article was cited in the index. In 1974, PubMed contained citations to 17 articles; in 1984, it cited 423 articles including caregiver concerns. In 1994, the year that former President Ronald Reagan announced his condition, there were 2061 citations; ten years later, in 2006, the number had more than doubled, at 4436 for the single year. For 2012 until 1 April 2013, 9942 citations are listed in the database.

In his 1989 study of the rise of what he calls the Alzheimer Disease movement, Patrick Fox, notes that heightened public awareness has moved the disease "from an obscure, rarely applied medical diagnosis to its characterization as the fourth or fifth leading cause of death in the United States in little more than 12 years" (1989, 58). A few years later Herskovits (1995, 147) echoed Fox's findings expanding the analysis to consider why so much interest could arise so quickly. "The current Alzheimer's construct emerged from the recent sociocultural and political-economic context in the United States", a context in which fear of the loss of self had moved to the forefront, and the experience of aging and "senility" had become "monstrous" (*Ibid.* 59).

As it is through language that memory and family ties are expressed, it is, perhaps, in language use by persons with dementia (PWD) that unimpaired persons find the most grievous and even startling changes. As dementia increases, PWD have greater difficulty first in retrieving words, then phrases; they substitute words or use semantically empty placeholders, making their communication seem vague. They gradually increase repetition of word, phrase or story, but decrease in their ability to manage conversation or introduce topics. As Biernacki (2007, 94) notes, damage to their episodic memory linking times, places and events means that "While specific events from long ago may be remembered, increasingly more and more support from others is required to sustain even these memories." Family members often feel that their loved ones have lost themselves, and that they as family members have lost those with dementia, since PWD can no longer show in their language use that they can access memories that include themselves and their family members. Indeed, as discussed by Herskovits (1995,152), "The overwhelmingly dominant pernicious effect of the current Alzheimer's construct is the dehumanization or debasement of 'self'."

Using a social constructionist approach, Sabat (2008, 87-88)) posits that people have three selves: Self 1, which is the expression of personal identity ("I", "me"); Self 2, which "is comprised of a person's physical and mental attributes, past and present, along with the person's beliefs (political, ethical, religious, etc.) and beliefs about his or her attributes"; and Self 3, a person's social persona. Each of these is retained by PWD, says Sabat: the way PWD are positioned by others ("he always forgets to do that") or learn to position themselves ("I don't always know how to do that") are part of why PWD are seen as persons who are losing selfhood.

We follow Ballenger's claim that dementia and the fear of loss of self is emblematic of our time and our place, concluding with him (2007, 153) that

> Alzheimer's disease is deeply troubling both because of what it does to people who have it and because people with this disease remind us so pointedly of our own difficulties in creating and maintaining selfhood. We need to find ways to listen to and appreciate the experience of people with dementia…because we need to bear witness to their struggle as a shared experience.

Bourgeois and Hickey (2009, 2) credit Bayles and Kaszniak (1987) with being the first speech-language clinicians to document "cognitive-linguistic deficits and skills" which could be used to develop support and intervention for persons with dementia. However, as we will see below, a continuing emphasis by speech-language researchers on the clinical and biomedical aspects of language in dementia typically exclude psychosocial contexts for language use, analysis and interpretation, an exclusion that is only recently beginning to change. In the discussion below, we identify issues and movements in different disciplines and their construct of dementia discourse.

This collection of essays presents a series of studies about the pragmatics of dementia discourse in order to build a bridge between researchers who are more clinical in their approach and researchers who are more focused on the embodiment of that language use within sociocultural contexts. Accordingly, in what follows, we highlight issues and constructs from different disciplinary perspectives. By looking through the lens of pragmatics, we are able to look at comprehension and production from the perspective of language interaction and language use. In drawing from a range of pragmatic theories, our collection adopts a viewpoint that looks not at language deficits but at retained linguistic competencies by persons with a chronic and debilitating condition. As in an earlier collection (Davis 2005, xv), the chapters provide data-rich language examples that augment and enhance findings from clinical testing, and support the analysis of how "language in aging interacts with identity, social practices, and intergenerational issues."

How is the term pragmatics applied and understood in Communication Disorders?

Clinical Linguistics & Speech-language pathology

In the field of communication disorders, the term *pragmatics* typically refers to the ability (or lack *thereof*) of populations with acquired or developmental disorders such as autism spectrum disorders (ASD) or traumatic brain injury (TBI) to use language appropriately in specific social contexts. Researchers in this field have sought to describe pragmatic deficits, and construct reliable measures to assess a client's pragmatic skills (e.g. Penn 1988). Any communication disorder, including those that are not necessarily the result of a cognitive deficit (e.g. stuttering or voice disorders) may result in some level of unintelligibility or a disruption in the communication process, therefore, a search of the literature in this field will yield articles relating to a wide range of communication disorders. However, disorders such as ASD and TBI appear to be the focus of much of the research relating to the social use of language. This is due to the fact, that people with these particular disorders are likely to manifest noticeable problems in social interaction. Dementia can be included in this group although, as a literature search of the *ComDisDome* and *Psychlit* databases revealed, there were fewer studies pertaining to dementia and pragmatics than the previously mentioned disorders. For example, a literature search using the following keywords, "pragmatics", "communication disorders", "dementia", "autism", and the phrase the "social use of language" in the *ComDisDome* database yielded fifty five articles, four related to dementia, seventeen related to other acquired disorders (predominantly TBI), and thirty four related to developmental disorders, particularly ASD and specific language impairment.

Communication disorders as a discipline draws on many other academic fields, such as neurology, clinical linguistics, education, psychology and speech-language pathology (SLP). However, much of the work relating to pragmatics and communication disorders has emerged from research in SLP and clinical linguistics. At this point, it is useful to separate and explain some of the differences in the background and approaches of clinical linguistics and speech-language pathology (SLP) to the areas of pragmatics and social interaction.

Clinical linguistics

Clinical linguists are typically researchers who have gone through an academic program of general linguistics and then subsequently apply their skills to the area of communication disorders. In Europe the field of clinical linguistics is a field in its own right stemming from the seminal work of David Crystal (1981) and the formation of International Clinical Linguistics and Phonetics (ICPLA) organization. Many of researchers in the field of clinical linguistics do not have professional certification to practice speech-language therapy but acquire, through their research, a basic knowledge of the terminology and medical background of the particular area of communication disorders under scrutiny. However, clinical linguists may be less knowledgeable about the assessment and therapy practices associated with the particular disorder they investigate.

In some contexts, particularly in Europe, there has been an attempt to bridge this gap with the establishment of a graduate program in the field of clinical linguistics that involves institutions located in several countries. Indeed, it is the case in the United Kingdom (as dictated by the Royal College of Speech Therapists) that classes covering linguistics and phonetics have to be taught by faculty with a background in linguistics. There are, however, clinical linguists who subsequent to their linguistics degrees go on to study and acquire certification in speech-language pathology. However, because of their background, research carried out by clinical linguists may draw more closely on traditional theories of linguistics or pragmatics when analyzing language samples. For example, Ryder and Leinonen (2011) have applied Relevance Theory (see chapter two) to analyze and better understand at what point children with, and without, language impairment acquire the ability to make inferences.

Investigations of pragmatic difficulties have also drawn on conversational analysis and interactional sociolinguistics to examine the use turn-taking and cohesive devices in children with ASD and specific language impairment (Bishop, Chan, Adams, Hartley, and Weir 2000). The use of direct and indirect speech acts has been used in a psycholinguistic approach to pragmatic disorders in adults with acquired disorders (e.g. Airenti, Bara, and Columbetti 1993; Bara, Bosco, and Bucciarelli 1999). More recently Bara has put forward a theory of cognitive pragmatics to examine mental states such as 'belief and intention' (2011, 443) in both developmental and acquired contexts. Work in ASD (Barnes and Baron-Cohen 2011) and TBI often includes a greater degree of reference to pragmatic theories such as theory of mind, systemic functional linguistics and interactional sociolinguistics (e.g. Body, Perkins, and McDonald

1999; Lundgren and Brownell 2011; McDonald and Pearce, Pearce 1999; Togher 2011). In addition, there has been a move to apply specific pragmatic theories such as politeness theory (Guendouzi and Pate, forthcoming) to conversational data involving PWD.

Speech-language pathology

The interest in pragmatics in the field of SLP emerged from the study of developmental disorders (e.g. autism and specific language impairment), and acquired disorders such as TBI, a condition in which pragmatic skills may be noticeably affected (Togher 2011). Initially SLP research rather than start with a particular pragmatic theory or research question described the pragmatic deficits found in such disorders. Although, aphasia does not produce pragmatic deficits in the manner noted in TBI, the person with aphasia may be unable to carry out a conversation thus a pragmatic problem arises from deficits in other areas of language production. Aphasia research, in particular, has drawn on interactional sociolinguistics and conversational analysis to explore interactions involving people with aphasia to develop conversational partner training programs (e.g. Hickey, Bourgeois, and Olswang 2004; Kagan, Black, Duchan, Simmons-Mackie and Square 2001)

It is important to note that the academic training of SLPs requires studying and acquiring competency in a wide range of both academic and professional skills. As noted above, SLP students in Europe are more likely to undertake discrete courses that specifically examine pragmatics and social interaction. In the USA, and countries that follow a liberal arts system of education, communication disorders programs tend to embed pragmatics across a range of courses in undergraduate studies, and the extent to which the topic is covered varies considerably across programs. At the graduate level, the focus is on clinical assessment and applications for intervention and pragmatics as a topic is typically discussed in core courses on specific disorders. The first author's experience in teaching on SLP programs suggests pragmatics is often perceived by students as a discrete skill or component of language that is studied alongside, but is different from, phonology, syntax, and semantics. Thus, they are sometimes unaware of the growing perspective that pragmatics is an emergent property of both the neuro-typical person and the person with a language disorder (Perkins 2007) rather than a disorder in its own right. This may mean that SLP students at the undergraduate and master's level will have some familiarity with Grice's maxims, but no experience in how those maxims may play out in interactions. This minimal presentation of

Grice's work is also seen in texts that are used in SLP education (e.g. Bliss 2003) where it is suggested Grice's maxims can be used as therapy tool. SLP students are also less familiar with key terms from pragmatics such as implicature (a speaker's intentions) and inference (meanings that the listener draws or infers from a speaker's utterances). However, the above comments are not a criticism of countries who train their SLP students in this manner. Rather they are made to clarify the different research approaches taken by clinical linguists, particularly those trained outside of the USA, and researchers who were trained in programs of communication disorders.

A further issue is the growing body of knowledge that SLPs (across the globe) need to acquire in order to gain certification. Indeed, to obtain ASHA (American Speech-Hearing Association) accreditation, an SLP training program must provide knowledge in the following subject areas: acquired and developmental disorders, swallowing disorders, hearing disorders, hearing screenings, aural rehabilitation, speech sciences, professional issues, assessment and management of child disorders, assessment and management of adult communication disorders, phonetics, the grammatical structure of language, neuro-anatomy, cultural diversity, and bilingualism. Furthermore, in this age of growing technology, it is necessary to remain cognizant of new developments in augmentative and alternative communication devices. Professional issues should include (among other things) topics such as medical billing, participating in Individual Education Assessments (IEPs), understanding a particular education authority's criteria for providing services, and counseling of clients and their families. It is no wonder that researchers coming from this academic background may not have had the opportunity (much less the time) to take specialized courses that cover pragmatic theories in any detail, or understand the role that philosophy, social psychology, and anthropology have had to play in the development and application of pragmatic theories.

Pragmatics in the clinical linguistics literature

Clinical pragmatics, as a sub-discipline emerged from an interest in understanding how people with communication disorders interact beyond clinical contexts in everyday situations. Although, clinical linguists have applied methods and theories from both interactional sociolinguistics and pragmatics to their data there are few comprehensive texts addressing or outlining the parameters of this area of communication disorders. Here we will review the three major texts (Cummings 2009; Müller 2000; Perkins 2007) that have attempted to delineate this area of study.

Clinical language studies is typically known as the field of clinical linguistics and phonetics to demarcate the divide between studies that are examining syntax and semantics and studies that focus more on actual speech production (e.g. articulation, fluency etc). The primary organization (and journal) founded in Europe in response to David Crystal's work (1981) is known as The International Clinical Linguistics and Phonetics Association (ICPLA). Its members have been responsible for products such as extensions to the International Phonetic Alphabet symbols (ExtIPA) that more accurately describe or denote sound distortions and voice quality (VoQs). In her introduction to this area Müller noted that clinical linguistics and phonetics as a 'distinct discipline of study' (2000, 1) faces two tasks; the first is the application of linguistic methods and theories to clinical data with a goal to informing assessment and intervention. The second task is using the results from such studies to extend and better inform the theoretical basis of this area of communication studies. Müller also raised the question of whether clinical pragmatics should be considered as a sub-discipline of clinical linguistics or an "independent discipline in its own right" (2000,1). Clinical linguistics as a discipline initially focused on refining phonetic description for disordered speech and systematic profiling of grammatical deficits (e.g., Crystal, Fletcher, and Garman 1976). Clinical pragmatics has emerged in a more ad hoc way, in particular through single-subject descriptive qualitative studies of individuals diagnosed with developmental disorders (Perkins 2000) and acquired disorders such as dementia (Guendouzi & Muller 2001). Individuals with these disorders may not have noticeable grammatical of phonological deficits but instead present with problems in the social use of language. Originally these were referred to as "Semantic-Pragmatic Disorders" (McTear & Conti-Ramsden 1991) but more recently researchers have separated these terms to signal the fact that a pragmatic disorder does not necessarily mean a semantic or grammatical deficit. Indeed, in the case of Asperger's Syndrome, semantic and grammatical abilities are not typically affected rather the individual has problems using language appropriately in social contexts.

Müller's edited collection includes chapters that cover a wide range of topics (e.g., pragmatic assessment, the relationship of cognition to pragmatic disorders etc.) and some chapters do draw on pragmatic theories (e.g., Theory of Mind) to explore particular aspects of the communication disorders. However, this text was an introduction to a field that is still (even now) in the process of establishing itself as a sub-discipline within the field of clinical linguistics.

Cummings' book (2009) is a more comprehensive attempt to provide a description of clinical pragmatics. It begins by providing an overview of the main theories that underpin the study of language use (e.g. speech acts, implicature, discourse, etc) and then subsequently describes the populations (developmental and acquired) that frequently manifest with pragmatic problems. In a review of Cumming's text, Perkins points to the fact that clinical pragmatics is an area of study 'renowned for its lack of coherence, inconsistent terminology, and proliferation of assessment and intervention procedures' (2011, 1). As he notes, the production of such a work is an "ambitious undertaking" (2011, 1) in a field that lacks systematic application of theory, methods, and terminology. Cummings' text attempts to reconcile some of these problems by providing an overview of pragmatic theories, and a detailed survey of both developmental and acquired pragmatic deficits, a review of pragmatic protocols, and a discussion of whether pragmatic theories (e.g. theory of mind, relevance theory) can answer some of the pragmatic problems that arise in individuals with communication disorders. However, as Perkins notes "the nature and scope of pragmatics have proved difficult to pin down" and in the clinical literature 'there is little consistency in the way the term is used' (2011, 2). Cummings appears critical of other interpretations of the term clinical pragmatics, and suggests that "concepts such as speech acts and implicature [...] are core pragmatic notions" (Cummings 2009, 2). She suggests that conversational management (e.g. turn-taking) draws on competences that aid with the generation and recovery of implicatures. Yet she ultimately tends to define pragmatics in unspecific general terms, suggesting pragmatics is the "use of language to achieve communicative purposes" (Cummings 2009, 6).

A further problem with Cummings' interpretation of clinical pragmatics is the exclusion of nonverbal behavior, a phenomenon that she suggests is an "error" (2009, 218). Thus for Cummings, pragmatics is an "exclusively linguistic phenomenon" (Perkins 2011, 3). In the case of people with dementia, as will be shown in chapter three (Davis, Maclagan and Wright), excluding the non-verbal and paralinguistic aspects of communication from a study would limit the potential interpretations of the PWD's communicative intentions. Indeed, monitoring people with dementia's use of face expressions or gestures is crucial to successful interactions and, although there is little research evidence for the efficacy of her work, monitoring non-verbal behaviors has formed the basis of the clinical success of much of Naomi Feil's validation therapy (1993).

Traditionally, formal pragmatics focused on the linguistic aspects of speaker utterances but applied linguists working in the field of pragmatics have long been aware that non-verbal aspects of communication are an important factor in interpreting a communicative message. Even within the realms of mainstream pragmatic theory, non-verbal behaviors are part of the discussion, for example, Wilson and Sperber (2002) note that if a guest at a party, touches or gestures towards his/her empty glass it may indicate the message she wants another drink. As Perkins notes, Cummings' book has many merits and is essential reading for those who wish to gain greater knowledge of both communication disorders and clinical pragmatics. However, Cummings' text is just one account of this field of study and should be "consumed as part of a balanced diet' (Perkins 2011, 5).

Perkins own text (2010), on the other hand, explores (amongst other things) how we define what constitutes a pragmatic impairment. Perkins has long argued (2000) for pragmatic impairment to be considered an emergent phenomenon of conversation that results from interactions with other domains of cognition. Stainton, taking up Perkin's discussion, raises the question of "what properly speaking is a pragmatic impairment'"(2011, 86), and he further suggests that currently, this is a question which is "doubtful we can even come close to answering". Stainton notes the lack of agreement in the academic discussion surrounding this topic, and like Perkins, he also raises the issue of confusion in relation to "crosstalk in the literature" (2011, 86). Both Perkins' and Cummings' books are a good starting point for those who wish to familiarize themselves with some of the current perspectives from clinical pragmatics, and although there are differences in Perkins' and Cummings' approaches, there are some common themes that reflect the current state of affairs in clinical pragmatics as a specific field of study.

The following points appear to be some of the issues that need addressing in order to arrive at a "coherent overall picture" (Stainton 2011, 86) and move the study of clinical pragmatics forward within the field of communication disorders:

(a) Lack of a common use of terminology
(b) Lack of agreement as to what constitutes a pragmatic impairment
(c) Lack of agreement as to what features of communication should be included in pragmatic research
(d) Lack of application of theory to data analyses (e.g. neo-Gricean approaches, politeness theory, or relevance theory)

The term pragmatics in the SLP literature

A search for books relating to pragmatics in the SLP literature will typically yield either the books mentioned above, or texts that are focused on social skills therapy. The term pragmatics in SLP has become synonymous with the phrase "social skills" and indeed, this is often a therapy goal for clinicians when carrying out interventions. SLP students often note in clinical reports that they are going to work with their client on "pragmatics" or "social skills" in order to improve the client's ability to carry out conversations and interact with others in a variety of a contexts (school, workplace, home etc.). In one sense, for clinicians this is the obvious endpoint for application of their pragmatic knowledge. However, consider the following (factual) example, a SLP student working with a high functioning autistic adolescent decided on that the clinical goal for the semester would be to teach the boy Grice's maxims (literally). The boy was videotaped interacting in several contexts and was then asked to review the videotapes and note at what points in the interaction he had broken any of the four maxims. It is not hard to imagine that if he attempted to generalize this new behavioral skill into his school environment by pointing out when his peers broke the maxims he might appear even less socially acceptable to his peers. It is not difficult to see how this situation came about, both the student and his clinical instructor had, in this case, learnt the term pragmatics not from a course on linguistics or pragmatics but from its' embedded use as a synonym for social skills in discussions within courses on child development or specific disorders.

Texts such as Bliss (2003) that cover pragmatics may focus on basic speech act theory and Grice's maxims. Students thus often assume that Grice studied actual conversational data and identified four rules that can be taught to clients so they can learn to carry out conversations in an appropriate manner. There is minimal discussion of *implicature* versus *inference*, or the difference between v*iolating* versus *flouting* the maxims. It is a crucial point in pragmatics to understand that all individuals regularly flout Grice's maxims to attend to face needs, politeness, or be sarcastic, whereas a person with ASD may accidently violate the maxims. Thus, researchers who come from an SLP background may have no initial grounding in the specific theories (e.g. relevance theory or politeness) that underpin pragmatics, nor are they aware of the academic debates associated with this area of communication (see Guendouzi, forthcoming for a more extensive review of this issue). As the literature search revealed, much of the work in SLP research uses the term pragmatics in the context of single-subject studies where the focus of analysis is describing the themes in the social skills of a particular client. Such studies do incorporate the use of methods associated with discourse analysis or conversational analysis (Sacks, Schegloff, and Jefferson, 1974) to analyze specific units of interactional behavior but often they do not specifically relate findings to pragmatic theories. There are some exceptions Hays, Niven, Godfrey, and Linscott (2004), for instance, assessed the Pragmatic Profile Impairment in Communication (PPIC), an instrument grounded in Gricean principles of co-operation and conversational maxims. The goal of the study was to assess the PPIC's reliability and validity rather than consider how it reflected the pragmatic theory but it is refreshing to note the authors did start with Grice's theory to ground their research. In addition, theoretical approaches to research in ASD have considered social deficits in relation to Theory of Mind (Baron-Cohen, 1995) and Weak Central Coherence Theory (Frith, 1989).

A further issue to consider when comparing the approach taken by SLP research is the fact that assessment of communication disorders requires a process of differential diagnosis. In the case of dementia and/or aphasia this requires the therapist to conduct separate assessments targeting specific areas of communication (e.g. comprehension, word naming, pragmatics etc.) and cognition (e.g. memory, attention). This is necessary for making clinical decisions on therapy goals, thus, the nature of assessment creates an approach that is compartmentalized into specific areas (e.g. memory, comprehension, production, and pragmatic social skills). This diagnostic process traditionally results in a perspective that tends to treat these aspects of communication as separate modules. Although, a participation model of treatment is the approach is more likely to be taught in educational contexts, recent focus discussions by the author with clinicians in the field suggested that although they preferred the participation model, time considerations and health insurance billing requirements often resulted in the use of more traditional approaches to both diagnostics and therapy.

Problems in applying theory: The case of implicature and inference in dementia

Speaker implicature and listener inference are two important points of discussion in the field of theoretical pragmatics; indeed much of the work in early pragmatics focused on potential interpretations of sentences or utterances. This is not surprising given that pragmatics emerged from more formal semantics and logic in the philosophy of language and focused on propositional meaning (e.g. the work of W.V. Quine 1960).

However, pragmatics differed from formal semantic approaches by considering language in terms of form versus function (such as Speech Act Theory associated with J. L. Austin 1961/1971, and J. R. Searle 1969) and conversational implicature (Grice 1989). For example, consider the exchange below.

Extract 1

1. Mark: what's for dinner?
2. Jan: I'm sat here watching this show but there's bread on the counter and ham and cheese in fridge

Grammatically, the form of Mark's utterance is an interrogative that contains a semantic proposition relating to which items of food are available for dinner. Jan's utterance is two statements containing three semantic propositions relating to her current location, occupation and what items of food the fridge contains. Most first language speakers of English, however, could infer several potential implicatures or pragmatic paraphrases for these utterances. Mark's question could imply any of the following, (a) *are you going to cook dinner now,* (b) *isn't it time you got dinner ready,* (c) *I'm hungry*, or perhaps *(d) Pay me some attention.* Jan's response suggests she has interpreted Mark's question as a request for her to prepare his dinner. Her response contains implicatures that might include, (a) *I'm comfortable, don't disturb me*, (b) *I'm not getting you dinner,* (c) *you can get it yourself,* or even (d) *don't be lazy.* If the listener (or researcher) has access to ethnographic information about the participants and their relationship to each other, it is not hard to draw these particular inferences even when the speakers use indirect speech acts. Furthermore, in the case of a research studies that collect conversational data from neuro-typical speakers, a researcher can return to the participants and ask them what they were implying in a particular utterance. It is also possible for a researcher to show a video recording of an interaction to actual participants and ask how they interpreted a particular behaviors or comments. This would not be the case in the context of people with dementia.

However, now consider the following extract among four people with dementia (PWD) seated around a table in a rehabilitation daycare center. Prior to this exchange, all four PWD had been given a cup of coffee and two cookies on individual plates.

Extract 2

1. Angie: do you want some of this **cookie** (taking a cookie from her own plate)
2. Jill: do I want **cookies?** (looking at her plate where there is only one cookie)
3. Angie: ask **the boss** (nods towards a care assistant stood nearby)
4. Theresa: they know whose **boss** I don't take it (laughs and reaches across for a cookie)
5. Jill (reaching for her glasses that are near Paul's arm) I need **my glasses** (pointing to a magazine)
6. Paul: (puts Jill's glasses in his pocket) these are my **glasses!** I brought them from **home**
7. Jill: are **my glasses home**?
8. Angie: he is a nice looking **boy** (points to a student volunteer)
9. Jill: oh that one he is **that boy**

In this interaction the contributions to the conversation appear to be triggered by environmental cues (e.g. objects that are on the table and people in the room) or by constructing a (seemingly) coherent topic line from the prior speaker's utterance. To infer a speaker's implicature or a listener's inference in the context of this interaction is purely speculative on the part of the analyst, but we could suggest the following three observations,

(1) that (albeit triggered by environmental cues) an uninterrupted conversational exchange takes place,
(2) that the interlocutors respond to the contribution of others,
(3) that the participants appear to respond in a manner that is centered around particular topics (highlighted in extract 2 above).

It is possible using methods associated with conversational analysis to describe and isolate conversational moves such as question-answer sequences and note whether the person with dementia used particular linguistic features (e.g. minimal responses) in his or her discourse but can the data offer any useful conclusions relating to specific pragmatic theories from this extract? Certainly, it is possible to suggest that what is unfolds here supports some of the claims of politeness theory (Brown and Levinson, 1987). That is, the speakers appear to adhere to a cooperative principle and fulfill the social obligation of reciprocity. However, in relation to indirect speech acts, it is more difficult to draw inferences about speaker intentions and listener interpretations. The exchange begins with a question from Angie asking Jill if she would like a cookie. Jill responds with another question (line 2) which could imply she is unsure whether Angie is asking her whether she wants a cookie, or she is unsure whether she does want another cookie. Angie (line 3) then tells Jill to 'ask the boss' and looked towards the care assistant *but* is Angie implying Jill should ask the care assistant for some cookies or ask the care assistant whether she (Jill) wants a cookie. Theresa's remark appears to be self-directed, but is she implying she is the boss, or is she implying she is not a person who can "bossed" around? The second clause could imply Theresa does not let people boss her around or, alternately, that she does not take other people's cookies. The latter is possible because during coffee-time there is often some "accidental" taking of other people's cookies or cups, and as reflected in "the glasses incident" occasional disputes over the ownership of items on the table.

The first author was a participant-observer during this interaction and her interpretation, at the time, was that Angie had asked her question as a politeness move. This assumption was based on several months of ethnographic observations where she noted in field notes that Angie typically opened conversations with this type of remark (e.g., would you like some cookie? can I get you some coffee?). However, Jill's facial expression suggested genuine confusion but this could have been for one of two reasons (a) she was unsure whether she wanted cookies, or (b) she was unable to access the appropriate words to respond and repeated Angie's utterance. Thus, her response may have been a reflexive conversational move prompted by the words Angie uttered; words that were still activated in Jill's working memory (Guendouzi and Pate, in press). Similarly, Theresa's comment (line 4) might have been prompted Angie's comment informing Jill to ask the boss (line 3). There are explanations for the exchanges in this data that might rely on considering the PWD's deficits in cognitive processing therefore it is a difficult task to interpret the interaction in terms of speaker intentions or listener interpretation (and indeed analyst's inferences).

The data above reflects some of the problems involved when analyzing and interpreting conversations involving people with dementia; therefore, it is not surprising that researchers often describe their data using methods associated with conversational analysis but are less likely to attempt to ground it in pragmatic theory. If, as was suggested above, applying the cornerstone of pragmatic theory (i.e. implicature) to disordered data is problematic, it is no wonder that researchers in communication disorders do not to go beyond identifying discursive features that appear to affect the individual's pragmatic competence. However, applying inferential models of communication to dementia data can reveal insights on how conversations with people with dementia differ from conversations involving only neuro-typical interlocutors. If, as relevance theory (see Chapter Two) suggests, humans have an innate faculty or module for interpreting (or unpacking) implicatures, then interlocutors become accustomed to managing their interactions by searching for (or ruling out) other potential non-literal meanings. That is, we tend in everyday conversations to expect a degree of implicature rather than literal meanings. Conversations, such as the one above (extract 2), may prove difficult for both interlocutors and researchers to interpret. In contrast to conversations involving neuro-typical interlocutors, the utterance in this case may literally mean what the form signifies. Relevance theory suggests that we are hard-wired to seek implicatures and thus socially conditioned to manage our conversations this way. If this is true, the above interaction suggests that the issue of form versus function is blurred in the context of dementia (for both listener and analyst). A neuro-typical interlocutor's normal conversational habits, of seeking implied rather than literal meanings, may add to the problems encountered when interacting with PWD. Indeed, clinicians may need to look beyond literal interpretations and consider the various possible implicatures that might be present in an utterance.

Barriers to bridging the divide

Before considering the divide between mainstream linguistics and communication disorders a second divide needs bridging; the fact that there is, at times, an uneasy relationship between clinical linguistics and SLP. Clinical linguists often comment that SLP researchers do not understand or apply the theory, and SLP researchers in turn, often comment that clinical linguists are too theoretical and not practical enough in their application of theory. This is an artifact of the career paths of both professions. Clinical linguists are predominantly academic teachers and researchers, whereas SLP researchers may be involved in academic research and teaching, but also choose (or in some institutions are required) to carry out clinical practice or supervision. SLP researchers ultimately strive to apply and/or disseminate their findings to clinical practice in order to enable clinicians in the field to help improve the quality of life for PWD. Clinical linguists seek to effect clinical practice and illuminate theory through their analyses of clinical data, but often their work is more observational rather than experiential. That is they do not have the experience of being a clinician and in some cases do not carry out data collection or observational studies, rather they analyze data in collaboration with clinicians who carry out the interaction or who have collected the data. A question arising is whether these different research approaches matter and what can be done to bridge this divide?

One obvious solution to the above question is more collaboration across disciplines in the areas of both research and teaching. There is a need for students and researchers to experience greater exposure to work from other disciplines that might inform their own studies. However, despite constant calls for such collaboration, researchers from particular fields still tend work within the boundaries of their own discipline. If we consider what is at stake in interdisciplinary research, this is not surprising. What does it take to engage in interdisciplinary research? First, one has to step out of one's comfort zone in relation to theoretical background knowledge, and accept alternate explanations or methods of analyzing data. Second, this involves allowing others to (re) interpret one's data or inferences about conclusions. Third, the researcher has to accept that particular models of theories are not a "theory of everything", that is they are not complete descriptions of the mechanisms that explain (a) how language operates in everyday contexts, or (b) how the individual's own language processing network works. In addition, as noted above, logistical requirements of tenure and promotion often mean that it is imperative for the researcher to publish and present their work within their own academic community, so they may be more reluctant to cross academic boundaries early in their career. For example, SLPs need to publish within accepted field-specific journals (e.g. the *Journal of Speech Language & Hearing Research*) and likewise for clinical linguists, social psychologists, mainstream linguists, nurses, etc. Although, this is not true for all researchers it is the case in some academic departments and institutions in order to gain tenure and promotion.

The obstacles mentioned above are, however, worth overcoming, particularly in the case of examples of data collected from people who do not represent the neuro-typical language user. It is true to say much of the discussion of theories in pragmatics in the past has been exemplified through examples of hypothetical language exchanges. Although, applied pragmatics researchers do translate the theories to real world contexts, typically, such research involves "normal" interlocutors. Pragmatic theories have, as of yet, not been applied in a systematic way to populations who have communication disorders.

Articles addressing "pragmatics" within the field of SLP do utilize methods drawn from conversational analysis in order to describe and better understand the interactions of particular populations, assess the efficacy of pragmatic profiles, or to carry out evidence-based case studies. However, it could be argued that, it is not possible to derive "evidence" from a case study (reviewer's comment) because CA is in fact methodological framework for describing conversations rather than actually analyzing outcomes or explicating theories of pragmatics. Conclusions in such studies are often dependent on the extent of the researcher's knowledge of the theories (and academic disciplines) from which both CA and DA emerged. Thus, some studies, although offering excellent descriptive accounts of the interactions may fall short in answering the "so what" question that clinicians often seek, or help academic theorists understand how analyses of everyday conversations might reflect the strengths and weakness of a particular theory (e.g. relevance theory's notion of an innate inferencing mechanism).

A personal anecdote at the time of writing can help illuminate this point. An SLP researcher who needed some input interpreting clinical interactions recently contacted the second author, a clinical linguist. Rather than analyzing the segments of the interactions that incorporated the clinical activities, he was interested in the opening segments of the interactions involving the small-talk between the clinicians and their clients. He had noted generally that there appeared to be a considerable amount of small-talk occurring and thought it important to examine this aspect of their communication. However, he had not previously been exposed to sociolinguistic theories relating to this area but a literature search in turned up a clinical linguistic article that explored small-talk in people with aphasia. The article referred to areas of pragmatic and sociolinguistic theory but did not fully explain the theories because (it was assumed) the audience of the journal would be familiar with such literature. It was serendipitous that he contacted the second author because, although he was unaware of the fact, she had in the past worked with some of the researchers cited in the article and was, therefore, able to (a) explain the theories and (b) suggest some directions for him to proceed in exploring his data. In this case, it was coincidental that a personal relationship led to a useful research connection and this does not always occur frequently. However, it illustrates the need to reach out beyond one's own research paradigm and concede a certain level of academic naivete in order to move forward in new directions.

How is pragmatics currently applied in linguistics to the study of dementia discourse?

Several threads are interwoven in the development of pragmatics in dementia discourse: researchers profit from familiarity with the uses or "flavors" of pragmatics across areas within linguistics such as anthropological linguistics, psycholinguistics and sociolinguistics, and allied fields such as conversation and discourse analysis, philosophy, communication studies and communication disorders, as discussed above, and more recently, cognitive science, neuropragmatics, which examines potential connections between neuronal architecture and speaker meaning (see, for example, Bara et al. 1997), and cognitive pragmatics. The degree to which an area or field emphasizes one or more pragmatics constructs and takes a theoretical stance differs, and while this is partly due to the flexibility of pragmatics as an approach incorporating several theories, it is also due to competing interests and emphases developing since the mid-twentieth century.

In the 1970s, often in opposition to Chomsky's theories, one can chart the rise of psycholinguistics, of sociolinguistics, of work keyed to speech act theory and philosophy of ordinary language, of language in natural contexts as opposed to laboratory situations, of explorations in the analysis of conversation, and of work with speech errors and signed languages. Each of these will intertwine with the development of various pragmatic approaches. As for the phenomenon of discourse by the cognitively impaired, until the mid 1990s it has primarily been studied as the production and comprehension of language in the aphasias, and divided by the extent to which language deficits are the focus as opposed to retention of competencies. Within each field and sub-field, other dichotomies emerge, often keyed to how researchers have viewed distinctions between competence and performance, or have looked instead at the construct of communicative competence.

While we cannot presume to offer a full historiographical account of the rise of pragmatics, we can offer a series of highlights and historical tendencies. For instance, a number of sources for 20th-century pragmatics have been identified by Nerlich (1993) and Nerlich and Clarke (1994; 1996); they focus on language use in interaction in German, American and British work leading up to the 1950s, "the eve before the institutionalization of pragmatics as a serious topic in linguistic research" (Funk 1997). They identify foundational traditions in pragmatics as speech acts, Peircian approaches to pragmatics, and the German critical theory movement (1994, 442). However, the application of pragmatics to aphasia and other cognitively impaired language use is but minimally mentioned.

To trace the growth of interest in the pragmatics of dementia discourse is to some extent an examination of the intersections between brain and language and language and cognition. Levelt (2012) begins his masterful history of psycholinguistics by discussing language study toward the end of the 18th century and throughout the 19th century: early researchers were focused on the aphasias because of what could be revealed about language and the brain, drawing on discoveries by Broca and Wernicke. As Levelt notes (2012, 336) , the classic study of aphasia by Roman Jakobson in the first half of the twentieth century (1941) – "a work of genius" - has had a sizeable impact on both linguistic theory and language disorders, particularly as he worked to refine phonological theory.

Fromkin (1993,148) commented in a discussion of modularity in the brain, that Jakobson "was the first linguist to apply linguistic theory to aphasia research, following up on the insights of de Courtenay in 1885 and Saussure in 1879 who had expressed the belief that a study of language pathology could contribute to linguistics." However, Jakobson's subsequent impact on aphasia studies has partly come about through the analysis, rebuttal and current reexamination of his regression hypothesis (RH), which in simplest form states that the order of attrition of language features is the mirror image of their original acquisition (the last learned features of a language will be the first forgotten or "lost"). Subsequent research has severely questioned the full hypothesis (Caramazza and Zurif 1978); a less strong version of this hypothesis has been proposed (Caramazza 1994; Keijzer 2007). Interestingly, several researchers have suggested that the weak form is worth investigating in terms of dementia (see Kemper 2006). More recently, attention to the RH has arisen through the cognitive turn in pragmatics, discussed below, although often still focused primarily on the aphasias: Joanette and Ansaldo (2000,108) comment that the pragmatic aspects of language—the intentionality of the speaker and the utterance's appropriateness in its context—have only recently been included in theories of language. It is now well known and accepted that pragmatics is an integral component of language, not an add-on (e.g., Gibbs, 1999). Chomsky (Stemmer, 1999) himself states that ". . . 'pragmatics' must be a central component of any general linguistic theory that aims to be comprehensive".

Pragmatics of one sort or another has been focused to some extent on the study of aphasia, as discussed above. Dementia, particularly Alzheimer's dementia, has only recently become part of the larger conversation about language and the brain and was preceded, in the U.S., by a focus on speech errors, or slips of the tongue. For example, Fromkin, in her (1971, 27) study of speech errors and anomalous language, noted that speech error study could show relationships between Chomsky's notions of competence and performance. She moved to draw from Freud, who "questioned 'whether the mechanisms of this (speech) disturbance cannot also suggest the probable laws of the formation of speech' ([I924; 1938:71). It is to that general question that this paper [Fromkin's] is directed."

In her 1981 review of Irigaray's earlier *Le langage des déments* (Irigaray 1973), Obler drew on the studies included in Caramazza and Zurif to recommend instead that researchers consider comparing the language of children with the language of persons with dementia as opposed to aphasia, commenting:

> To the extent that similarities are documented, we may learn about cognitive underpinnings of language: to the extent that linguistic dissimilarities are documented in the face of similar cognitive states we should learn about life-span development of language. Furthermore, in the process of devising tests of the regression hypothesis, we may hope to gain insight into the interaction of language and cognition (1981: 385).

Language in dementia became a focus for clinical and linguistic analyses, beginning in the 1990s. Looking at communicative competence, Ripich and her colleagues (1998; 1991; 2000) exemplify the turn to examine discourse, cohesion and conversational skills beginning in the 1980s, drawing directly on linguistics, discourse analysis and conversation analysis methodologies. Extended analyses of specific language features, and of topic, narrative and conversation in Alzheimer's dementia were appearing (see, for example, Bayles and Kazniak 1987), and comparisons to aphasia were being drawn (see, for example, Obler et al 1985). Pragmatics was still discussed, however, primarily in clinical studies. In 1994, Sabat published a review of recent research in phonology, semantics and pragmatics in the language of dementia, asserting that "many of the extant methodological approaches and interpretations are questionable and that they also may lead either directly or indirectly to the creation of negative stereotypes concerning the communicative abilities of A.D. sufferers" (1994, 331). In that same year, however, an interactional emphasis began for dementia discourse, with the appearance of Hamilton's *Conversations with an Alzheimer's patient.*

Both Hamilton's study, and that by Ramanathan, which soon followed (Ramanathan 1997), used data that was naturally occurring, as opposed to being collected as part of clinical testing, and emphasized interaction.

Each systematically reviewed asymmetry of power in the relations between interlocutors, examining perceptions by PWD of the situation and task, with a later discussion by Ramanathan (1995) contrasting the role of conversation taking place in institutional as opposed to home settings. In essence, both studies worked to identify the communicative competence of the person with dementia, and established the importance of context, including the role of the unimpaired speaker. In essence, these studies by Hamilton and Ramanathan looked at language production and language interaction by and with persons with dementia in a social context, which fed a growing emphasis in clinical linguistics on discourse (Guendouzi and Müller, 2005), an anthology of discussions of retained competencies from multiple theoretical perspectives (Davis 2005) and the development of a web portal including several hundred conversations with PWD (Pope and Davis 2011).

A search of the literature since Sabat's 1994 update used *Ovid/Medline* and *Linguistics and Language Behavior Abstracts* with these search terms: (a) the field name plus pragmatics plus dementia, such as *anthropology* and *pragmatics* and *dementia,* and (b) specific pragmatics constructs plus *dementia.* Manual searches of *Brain and Language* and the *Journal of Pragmatics* were also conducted. Studies of dementia discourse were often embedded in discussions of language and aging. Hamilton (2003, 569) comments that the 1980s and 1990s were replete with studies of language and aging from a multiplicity of disciplinary perspectives; deBot and van der Hoeven (2011) offer a cognitive overview including the rising interest in neuroscience; they comment that more work has been done from the psycholinguistic perspective, and call for a "more social/sociological perspective" (124).

Building on earlier studies of elderly discourse, which began to incorporate the analysis of politeness and facework (Spiers 1998) as well as descriptions of production and screening and evaluation of interventions, current studies since the mid-1990's include the following constructs, though they do not always specifically refer to their work as rooted in pragmatics:

- Studies of naturally-occurring conversation in dementia: pauses, discourse markers, repairs, topic management, and the impact of formulaic or rehearsed sequences (e.g. Davis and Maclagan 2009; Orange 1996; Mentis 1995);
- Studies of narrative by persons with dementia: narrative analysis as "small stories" vs canonical Labovian format; story boundaries;

identity; unshared contexts and confabulation (e.g, Hamilton 2008; Backhaus 2011; Davis 2010);

- Studies with a new emphasis on coherence, focusing primarily on memory, informativeness, and communication interventions (e.g. Burke, 1997; Williams et al 2009);
- Continuing studies of social interaction in dementia add power and social behaviors to studies of identity (e.g. .Martin 2013; Kontos 2006).

Where pragmatics may be taking center stage in the study of dementia discourse is in the burgeoning field of cognitive pragmatics. Like psycholinguistics, the study of pragmatics and dementia has taken a cognitive turn. According to Field (2011, 473), there are two traditions in current psycholinguistics. The first draws from cognitive science, "evidence-led," and including brain imaging; the second is more concerned with theory used to interpret samples of language. From the perspective of clinical linguistics, seen as part of applied linguistics, Perkins and Howard (2011, 110) call attention to the differences between behavioral and medical models for language pathology and note the growth of ethnographic studies, seen as "contextualized social action" (114) and work with conversational interaction. These different traditions can be seen in the current provocative discussions in cognitive pragmatics, as seen, for example, in a special journal issue with articles discussing points raised by Bara (2011, 444):

> The central point is to define the stages in the acquisition of pragmatic competence, from the first few seconds of birth to adulthood. . . . A valid theory should be able to correlate with the neurosciences, predicting how communicative capacities may decline with age, or suffer damage as a consequence of given pathologies that may be general — as in Alzheimer's disease — or focal — as is the case with brain injury."

Other specialists responded, asking for extended work about how people act to cooperate across cognitive disabilities (Carassa and Columbetti 2012), the refinement of theorizing in pragmatics (Cummings 2012), greater theoretical rigor (Jaszczolt 2012) and in resolving inconsistencies and contradictions in cognitive pragmatic theory (Yokoyama 2012). The debate continues.

Bridging the divide: a tentative first step

This chapter has intended to achieve two objectives, first, to consider how pragmatic theory has been applied in both the field of communication disorders and in mainstream general linguistics, and second to address the need for creating a bridge between mainstream theoretical pragmatics and applied research in communication disorders. This does not mean we are suggesting that all linguists should be conversant in all areas of SLP and *vice-versa* but perhaps SLPs would benefit by exposure to politeness/im-politeness theory and relevance theory in order to modify and better ground their case studies and linguists might find that clinical data can inform, extend, or validate some of the theories. Finally, there is a need for a bridge wide enough to encourage true interdisciplinary research. That is, researchers should actively seek to look beyond their own realm and explore what other disciplines and research approaches can add to a fascinating area of language and communication studies.

References

Austin, John. 1961; 1971. *How to do things with words*. Oxford: Oxford University Press.

Backhaus, Peter, ed. 2011. *Communication in elderly care. Cross-Cultural Perspectives*. London, New York: Continuum.

Ballenger, Jesse. 2006. *Self, senility, and Alzheimer's disease in modern America*. Baltimore, MD: Johns Hopkins University Press.

Bara, Bruno. 2011. Cognitive pragmatics: The mental processes of communication. *InterculturalPragmatics* 8, 443-485.

Bara, Bruno, Maurizio Tirassa and Marina Zettin. 1997. Neuropragmatics: Neuropsychological constraints on formal theories of dialogue. *Brain and Language* 59, 7-49.

Baron-Cohen, Simon. 1995. *Mindblindness: an essay on autism and theory of mind*. Boston: MIT Press/Bradford Books.

Bayles, Kathryn and Alfred Kaszniak. 1987. Communication and cognition in normal aging and dementia. Austin, TX: Pro-Ed.

Bourgeois, Michelle and Ellen Hickey. *Dementia: From diagnosis to management: A functional approach*. NY: Psychology Press Taylor and Francis Group.

Brown, Penelope and Steven Levinson. 1987. *Politeness: Some universals in language usage*. Cambridge: Cambridge University Press.

Burke, Deborah and Donald Mackay. Memory, language and ageing. *Philosophical Transactions of the Royal Society B: Biological Sciences* 352, 1845-1856.

Caramazza, A. 1994. Parallels and divergences in the acquisition and dissolution of language. *Philosophical Transactions: Biological Sciences* Vol 346, No. 1315, 121-27.

Caramazza, Albert and Edgar Zurif, eds. 1978. *Language acquisition and language breakdown: Parallels and divergencies.* Johns Hopkins University Press

Crystal, David. 1981. *Clinical Linguistics.* Vienna: Springer-Verlag

Crystal, David, Paul Fletcher and Michael Garman. 1976. *The grammatical analysis of language disability.* London: Arnold.

Cummings, Louise, 2009. *Clinical Pragmatics.* Cambridge: Cambridge University Press.

Cummings, Louise. 2012. Theorising in pragmatics: Commentary on Bara's *Cognitive pragmatics: The Mental Processes of Communication* MIT Press, 2010. *Journal of Intercultural pragmatics* 9, 113-120.

Davis, Boyd. Ed., 2005. *Alzheimer talk, text and context.* NY: Palgrave.

—. 2010. Intentional stance and Lucinda Greystone: Embodied memory in conversational reminiscence by a speaker with Alzheimer's disease. In *Language, Body and Health*, edited by Paul McPherron and Vai Ramanathan. NY/The Hague, deGruyter.

Davis, Boyd, and Maclagan, M. 2009. Examining pauses in Alzheimer's discourse. *American Journal of Alzheimer's Disease and Other Dementias* 24, 141-54.

De Bot, K. & Bert. Weltens. 1991. Recapitulation, regression, and language loss. In *First language attrition.* Edited by Herbert Seliger and Robert Vago, 31-52. Cambridge, Cambridge University Press.

De Bot, Kees and Nienke van der Hoeven. 2011. Language and ageing. In *Routledge Handbook of Applied Linguistics*, edited by James Simpson, 124-137. Abingdon, Oxford: Routledge.

Feil, Naomi. 1993. *The Validation Breakthrough: Simple Techniques for Communicating with People with Alzheimmer's-Type Dementia.* Baltimore: Health Professions Press.

Field, John. 2011. Psycholinguistics. In *Routledge Handbook of Applied Linguistics*, edited by James Simpson, 472-486. Oxford: Routledge

Fox, Patrick. 1989. From senility to Alzheimer's disease: The rise of the Alzheimer's disease movement. *Milbank Quarterly* 67, 58-92.

Frith, Uta. 1989. *Autism: Explaining the enigma* .Oxford: Blackwell.

Fromkin, Vicki. 1971. The non-anomalous nature of anomalous utterances. *Language* 47, 27-52.

—. 1993. What studies of the brain can tell us about language if anything and vice versa. *Proceedings of the Nineteenth Annual Meeting of the Berkeley Linguistics Society: General Session and Parasession on Semantic Typology and Semantic Universals* 1993,143-158. Available through http://elanguage.net

Grice, Herbert.P. 1975. Logic and Conversation. In P. Cole & J. Morgan Eds., *Syntax and Semantics, 3: Speech Acts*. New York: Academic Press.

Guendouzi, Jackie. and Nicole Muller. 2006. *Discourse approaches to dementia*. Lawrence Erlbaum Associates.

Guendouzi, Jackie. and Anna Pate. forthcoming. Interactional and cognitive resources in the presentation of Self: A Perspective from Politeness Theory. In Robert. Schrauf and Nicole. Muller eds. *Dialogue and dementia: Cognitive and communicative Resources for Engagement.* Oxford: Blackwell

Hamilton, Heidi. 1994. *Conversations with an Alzheimer's patient.* Oxford: Oxford University Press.

—. 2003. Discourse and aging. In *Handbook of Discourse Analysis*, edited by Deborah Schiffrin, Heidi Hamilton & Deborah Tannen , 568-589. NY: Routledge.

—. 2008. Language and dementia: sociolinguistic aspects. *Annual Review of Applied Linguistics* 28, 91-110.

Hickey, Ellen, Bourgeois, Michelle, and Olswang, Lesley. 2004. Effects of training volunteers to converse with nursing home residents with aphasia. *Aphasiology,* 18, 625-637.

Holstein, Martha. 1997. Alzheimer's disease and senile dementia, 1885-1920: An interpretive history of disease negotiation. *Journal of Aging Studies* 11, 1-13

Irigaray, Luce. 1973. *Le langage de déments*. The Hague: Mouton.

Joanette, Yves and Ana Ansaldo, A. 2000. The ineluctable and interdependent evolution of the concepts of language and aphasia. *Brain and Language*, 71, 106-109.

Kagan, Aura., Black, Sandra., Duchan, Judith., Simmons-Mackie, Nina., and Square, Paula. 2001.Training volunteers as conversation partners using "supported conversation for adults with aphasia" (SCA): A controlled trial. *Journal of Speech, Language and Hearing Research,* 44, 624-638.

Kemper, S. 2006. Language in adulthood. In *Lifespan cognition: Mechanisms of change,* edited by Ellen Bialystok and Fergus Craik Eds. Oxford: Oxford University Press.

Kontos Pia. 2006. Embodied selfhood: An ethnographic exploration of Alzheimer's disease. In *Thinking about dementia: Culture, loss, and the anthropology of senility,* edited by Lawrence Cohen and Annette Liebling, 195–217. New Brunswick, NJ: Rutgers University Press.

Martin, Wendy, Pia Kontos, and Richard Ward. 2013.Embodiment and dementia. [Introduction to Special Issue]. *Dementia* 12, 283-87.

McKhann, Guy, David Knopman, Howard Chertkow, Bradley Hyman et al. 2011. The diagnosis of dementia due to Alzheimer's disease: Recommendations from the National Institute on Aging– Alzheimer's Association workgroups on diagnosing Alzheimer's disease. *Alzheimer's & Dementia* 7, 263-269.

McTear, Michael and Gina Conti-Ramsden. 1991. *Profiling pragmatic disability in children: Assessment an intervention.* London: Whurr.

Mentis, Michelle, Jan Briggs-Whittaker and GD Gramigna. 1995. Discourse topic management in senile dementia of the Alzheimer's type. *Journal of Speech and Hearing Research* 38, 1054-66.

Müller, Nicole. 2000. *Pragmatics in speech and language pathology: studies in clinical applications.* Amsterdam: John Benjamins.

Nicholas, M. Loraine Obler, and Martin Albert. 1985. Empty speech in Alzheimer's disease and fluent aphasia. *Journal of Speech and Hearing Research* 28, 405-510.

Obler, Loraine. 1981. Review, *Le langage des déments*, by Luce Irigaray. The Hague: Mouton, 1973. *Brain and Language* 12, 375-86.

Orange, JB, Rosemary Lubinski, and Donald Higginbotham. 1996. Conversational repair by individuals with dementia of the Alzheimer's type. *Journal of Speech and Hearing Research* 39, 881-95.

Penn, Claire. 1988. The profiling of syntax and pragmatics in aphasia. *Clinical Linguistics & Phonetics,* 2, 179-208.

Perkins, Michael. 2007. *Pragmatic impairment.* Cambridge: Cambridge University Press.

—. 2011. Book Review: Cummings' Clinical Pragmatics. *Aphasiology* i*First*, 1–5.

Pope, Charlene and Boyd Davis. Finding a balance: the CCC corpus. *Corpus Linguistics and Linguistic Theory* 7, 143-61.

Quine, Willard. 1960. *Word and Object.* Boston: MIT Press.

Ramanathan, Vai. 1997. *Alzheimer discourse: Some sociolinguistic dimensions.* Mahwah NJ: Lawrence Erlbaum.

Ripich, Danielle, Diane Vertes, Peter Whitehouse, Sarah Fulton and Barbara Ekelman. 1991. Turn-taking and speech act patterns in the discourse of senile dementia of the Alzheimer's type patients. *Brain and Language*, 40, 330-343.

Ripich, Danielle, and Brenda Terrell. 1988, Patterns of discourse cohesion and coherence in Alzheimer's disease. *Journal of Speech and Hearing Disorders* 53, 8–15.

Ripich, Danielle, Brian Carpenter and Elaine Ziol. 2000. Conversational cohesion patterns in men and women with Alzheimer's disease: a longitudinal study. *International Journal of Language and Communication Disorders* 35, 49-64.

Sabat, Steven. 1994. Language function in Alzheimer's disease: A critical review of selected literature. *Language & Communication* 14, 31-51.

—. 2008. Positioning and conflict involving a person with dementia: A case study. In *Global conflict resolution through positioning theory*. Edited by Fathali Moghaddam, Rom Harré, and Naomi Lee, 81-93. NY: Springer.

Sacks, Harvey, Emmanuel Schegloff and Gail Jefferson. 1974. A simplest systematic for the organization of turn taking in conversation. *Language* 50, 696-735.

Searle, John. 1969. *Speech Acts*. Cambridge: Cambridge University Press.

Spiers, Judith. 1998. The use of face work and politeness theory. *Qualitative Health Research* 8, 25-47.

Stainton, Robert. 2010. Pragmatic Impairments. *International Review of Pragmatics* 3, 85–97.

Vonk, Frank. 1997 [Review] Brigitte Nerlich & David D. Clarke. *Language, action and context: The early history of pragmatics in Europe and America*, 1780-1930. *Henry Sweet SocietyBulletin*, 29, 48-52.

Williams, Kristine, Ruth Herman, Byron Gajweski and Kristel Wilson. 2009. Elderspeak communication: Impact on dementia care. *American Journal of Alzheimer's Disease and Other Dementias* 24, 11-20.

Wilson, Deirdre and Dan Sperber. 2002. Relevance theory. In *Handbook of Pragmatics*, edited by Laurence Horn and Gregory Ward, 249-90. Oxford: Blackwell.

CHAPTER TWO

'SO WHAT'S YOUR NAME?': RELEVANCE IN DEMENTIA

JACQUELINE GUENDOUZI
SOUTHEASTERN LOUISIANA UNIVERSITY

Introduction

As noted in chapter one, the aim of this text is to provide a bridge between researchers who work in mainstream pragmatics and researchers in communication disorders who examine their data from the perspective of pragmatic function. Given the potential range of disciplines amongst the target audience, it is likely that some readers are unfamiliar with pragmatic theories such as Relevance Theory (Sperber and Wilson 1986; 2002; Wilson and Sperber 2002), and equally, some readers may be less knowledgeable about the field of communication disorders. Therefore this chapter will first, describe the areas of communication and cognition affected in dementia, second, outline the basic inferential model (Grice 1975) and Relevance Theory (RT), and third, discuss the application of RT to interactions involving people with dementia (PWD).

Dementia, Communication and Cognition

Dementia is a progressively degenerating disease that affects cognitive faculties across multiple domains (e.g. memory, attention and inhibition), physiological functions (e.g. continence and balance), behaviors (e.g. affect, mood, etc.), and communication (e.g. semantics and pragmatics). There are several forms of this disease including Alzheimer's disease, Pick's disease (Fronto-temporal dementia), Huntington's disease, Parkinson's disease, multi-infarct (vascular) dementia, and Lewy Body disease. Each type of dementia has its own unique features but a common characteristic is memory impairment and, in particular, the decreased ability to learn or retain new information. In the case of Pick's disease, memory loss is less noticeable in the initial stages although recent studies suggest a greater involvement of semantic memory loss than previously indicated (Hornberger and Piguet 2012). Unlike some forms of aphasia that can remain stable in relation to language and communication deficits, dementia is a degenerating disease that results in "an ever-changing presentation of symptoms" (Bourgeois 2002, 132).

Research has linked communication deficits in dementia to the PWD's decline in cognitive abilities (Bayles, Tomoeda and Trosset 1992; Bourgeois 2002). PWD presents with deficits in the areas of semantics and pragmatics. In addition, knowledge of factual events, words, concepts and symbols is significantly impaired resulting in a number of communication deficits. Semantic deficits include word finding, naming, semantic paraphasias (selecting the wrong word), comprehension, empty speech, non-specific or ambiguous reference, and neologisms. Pragmatic deficits include topic drift, inappropriate responses, repetition, off-topic comments, talking too much, comprehension, and talking too loud (Santo Pietro and Ostuni 1997). As the dementia progresses, the PWD may become increasingly uncommunicative and in the later stages may become verbally unresponsive. Semantics and pragmatics do not function as separate modules of language, and indeed, the pragmatic deficits noted in dementia are a result of the interaction between cognitive and semantic deficits in relation to communicative requirements of specific social situations (Ripich 1994).

Cognitive faculties that support conversation are crucial factors in the communicative process. Listeners must go through a multi-stage process that involves (1) focusing attention on a speaker's utterance, (2) retaining the utterance in their working memory, (3) processing the propositional content, (4) considering the relevance of the utterance to the current situation, and (5) extracting any potential implicature that may be inherent in the utterance. In addition, a listener needs to inhibit any associated representations that may be activated in his/her semantic network by the process of spreading activation (Guendouzi and Pate, forthcoming; Shelley-Tremblay 2011). Interlocutors are thus always engaged in an active ongoing process of assessing potential inputs (e.g., verbal and non-verbal stimuli, social context, participants, etc.) and making decisions about which information is relevant for the task-at-hand. Some of this processing (e.g., perception) takes place automatically and does not involve overt cognitive effort. However, listeners also need to focus their attention on specific aspects of the incoming stimuli, assess their importance, and then consciously make decisions about the potential meanings of an interlocutor's utterance. Thus, conversations involve a behavioral performance that results from an interaction between language and cognitive systems that are adapted "online" in response to a particular context. Engaging in conversations does not just require the ability to focus attention on what is important, but also on the ability to inhibit inputs that are not relevant, or are taken for granted in the situation at hand and therefore require less processing effort. For example, when interacting with others, a speaker typically knows where he/she is located and why he/she is in that location; therefore, it is not necessary for interlocutors to allocate extensive communicative or cognitive resources to establish or monitor information that is normally a *given* variable in the context. For PWD however, this is not necessarily the case and a fixation on clarifying where they are, for example, may interfere with their ability to process other communicative inputs and impede their ability to recover meanings, and in particular implied meanings that require inference.

The Inferential Model of Pragmatics

Grice's inferential model of communication (1989) was proposed as an alternative to the classical code model. The classical model posits that speakers encode their messages into a signal, which is then decoded by a listener using a matching (or identical) code. This process implies that competent language users should (typically) be able to unpack messages based on their knowledge of the language in question. In contrast, the inferential model suggests a speaker provides evidence of a particular meaning and the listener must then infer the implied meaning based on the evidence the speaker has provided. Grice's central claim was that recognition and expression of intentions are key features of human communication. In the case of conversations the primary mode of communication is verbal utterances, that is, the message is linguistically encoded. However, the meaning inferred by the listener depends on both the linguistic content and other evidence that may accompany the utterance (e.g. nonverbal behaviors, participant roles, the situational context, etc.).

Grice (1989) claimed that listeners have expectations based on the evidence in the current situation and this guides them to the most likely interpretation of a speaker's utterance. In order for everyday communication to proceed in a fluid and coherent manner, these expectations must lead to inferences that can be generalized across interactions. Based on the evidence provided, members of a speech community will typically extract the same inferences from particular utterances. Grice further suggested that speakers fulfill a cooperative principle by observing four maxims, Quality (truthfulness), Quantity (informativeness), Relation (relevance), and Manner (clarity). The maxims were an attempt to provide a basic framework for the "ideal" conversation, thus the maxims were not "rules" but a means to examine the structure and dynamics of everyday conversations. Thus, by observing these maxims speakers encode the appropriate amount (quantity) of truthful information (quality) relevant to the context in a way that is both socially acceptable and clear (manner). Grice did however point out that speakers may unintentionally violate the maxims (e.g., a person with autism spectrum disorder might take a figurative comment such as "at the end of the day" literally) or they can deliberately flout the maxims (e.g., in the case of sarcasm one might deliberately say the opposite of what one believes to be true). Indeed, in everyday conversations it is likely that we frequently both violate and flout these maxims.

Although Grice's discussion of speaker meaning focused on examples involving verbal utterances, he also noted that listeners made use of non-verbal signals (e.g., gesture, facial expression, etc.), paralinguistic information (e.g. intonation, etc.), and prior knowledge (e.g shared public or personal history) to draw inferences. As was noted in chapter one, some pragmatic scholars have paid less attention to the importance of non-verbal inputs (e.g. Cummings 2007), but as Wilson and Sperber (2002) suggest, both verbal and non-verbal features of an interaction are essential to the interpretation of speaker implicatures and listener inferences. Indeed, researcher generated inferences of conversational data involving PWD are often (necessarily) based on non-verbal and paralinguistic features of an interaction rather than the actual words uttered. Thus, the main goal of Grice's inferential model of pragmatics is to understand and explain how a hearer infers a speaker's meaning relative to the evidence provided, or to put it in other words, it is how listeners decide what is relevant.

Relevance Theory

Grice (1989) suggested that listeners generally choose an interpretation that (based on the four maxims) meets their expectations of the cooperative principle. The cooperative principle is not a prescriptive command rather it suggests that interlocutors in a conversation operate under the premise that all parties should make their contributions to a conversation in a manner that is as informative as is required for the context of the exchange in order to be mutually understood. Although RT shares the intuitions of Grice's model regarding listener expectations, it questions several other aspects of Grice's inferential model (Wilson and Sperber, 2002). In particular, RT questions the need for the four maxims, the cooperative principle, or the notion of deliberate maxim violation. Thus, the central argument of RT centers on the issue of expectations raised by an utterance. As Wilson and Sperber suggest, if the expectations raised by an utterance are 'precise enough and predictable enough' (2002, 250) the hearer will interpret the speaker's utterance as it was intended. The goal of RT then is to 'explain in cognitively realistic terms what these expectations of relevance amount to and how they might contribute to an empirically plausible account of comprehension' (Wilson and Sperber 2002, 250).

The basic tenets of RT suggest that relevance is 'a property of inputs to cognitive processes' (Van der Henst and Sperber 2004, 141), that is, the inputs include both external stimuli (e.g. utterances) and internal stimuli (e.g. memories or previously stored information). Listeners assess stimuli by the degree of their relevance, and as a result, many inputs are competing for the individual's processing resources, therefore focused attention will be directed to the inputs that appear 'relevant enough to deserve attention' (Van der Henst and Sperber 2004, 142). In cases where inputs have an equal amount of cognitive effect, attention is likely given to the inputs that require less processing effort. Thus Sperber and Wilson's theory characterizes relevance in terms of both the *effect* and the *effort* required to process an input; they suggest the less processing effort required, the greater the effect. That is, the greater the positive effect of an input, the greater the relevance, and conversely, the greater the cognitive effort required to process an input, the lower the relevance of the input (Van der Henst and Sperber 2004).

Relevance theory claims that an innate, universal tendency to maximize relevance is the product of human evolution. Given this spontaneous tendency, Van der Henst and Sperber (2004)) suggest that it is 'possible to predict to some extent to which available stimuli people will pay attention and how they will process them' (2004, 143). Van der Henst and Sperber also note that there 'is a wealth of evidence in the experimental study of attention and memory' (2004, 143) that might be re-analyzed to see if it supports the Principle of Relevance. They admit that this task is not within the scope of their expertise, but note the challenge is to find evidence specific enough to support RT's Cognitive Principle (CP) rather than explore the CP in the manner of more familiar psychological approaches. Although Sperber and Wilson's reticence to comment about RT in relation to experimental cognitive research is understandable, when positing a cognitive theory, researchers should consider both traditional psycholinguistic approaches and current cognitive neuroscience research. Perhaps it is now time to explore the interface between pragmatics and psycholinguistics and a good starting point is to consider conversational data to assess whether the interactions show evidence for the principles and claims of RT.

Ven der Henst and Sperber (2004) note that researchers have extensively explored a principle that suggests interlocutors maximize the relevance of inputs to not only to predict (or interpret) other's intentions but also to influence them. Human communication involves not just the comprehension of propositional meaning but also the attribution of mental states and beliefs to others. This aspect of communication often referred to as Theory of Mind (Baron Cohen, Leslie, and Frith 1985) is essential for understanding implied meaning. That is, it is necessary to understand that although other people may share your ideas, beliefs or mental states, they may also have different beliefs about the world and different interpretations of a speaker's implicatures. Implicature is a term coined by Grice and adopted by the field of pragmatics to refer to meanings that are suggested in an utterance but not necessarily expressed in the words. There is a general assumption that conversations typically proceed in an orderly manner with interlocutors understanding and sharing a focus on what is salient, and therefore relevant, in the interaction. However, it is also the case that speakers cannot assume that listeners interpret their message in the manner it was intended, an important issue in the case of communication disorders. To summarize, relevance theory suggests two principles: (a) the *cognitive principle* that states human cognition is oriented towards maximizing relevance of inputs, and (b) the *communicative principle* where "every act of ostensive communication communicates a presumption of its own optimal relevance" (Padilla Cruz 2012, 114). In addition, hearers typically follow the interpretative path that requires less cognitive effort "when testing their different interpretations of a particular utterance and stop when their expectations of relevance are satisfied" (Padilla Cruz 2012, 114). That is, relevance is satisfied when there is a great enough *positive effect* to offset the *cognitive processing effort.*

Inputs, Relevance and Dementia

In PWD the notable deficits in cognitive resources such as attention, inhibition and working memory mean that satisfying requirements of relevance can be a stressful process. Successful interactions rely on interlocutors sharing a focus on what is salient to the current conversation, while inhibiting other possible interpretations of what they hear and see. As noted above, in the context of *any* conversation there are multiple contextual inputs (external and internal) that interlocutors must attend to, and monitor, in order to adhere to the cooperative principle. External inputs may include the physical location and the purpose of the interaction, while internal inputs include such things as prior knowledge, attention, memory, and inhibition. All these factors may create added stress and increase the cognitive effort that PWD must expend in order to interpret both the propositional as well as the inferential meaning of a speaker's utterance. Hence, attempting to make an optimally relevant interpretation of a verbal utterance may require maximum effort for PWD. Furthermore, cognitive deficits may act as barriers to the PWD's processing pathways and interrupt the process before arriving at the optimally relevant interpretation (i.e. being unable to inhibit semantic competitors).

In conversations involving neuro-typical interlocutors, perceptual mechanisms assess the inputs and eventually focus the listener's attention on particular inputs or interpretations. Even though other potential exemplars may be activated (Cowan 2011) they are usually inhibited while the listener focuses on the input relevant to the context. Different inputs have different effects, and the processing effort allocated to a specific input is based on how relevant it is to the current situation. RT posits a language processing system underpinned by the notion of an economy where interlocutors balance and manage competing resources to arrive at the optimal interpretation with the least amount of processing effort. Thus, listeners are continually processing information to account for incoming stimuli, and certain stimuli, like background noise in a busy workplace, are typically given factors within an interaction that do not require the allocation of focused attention. For example, in any interaction most neuro-typical people know the following four pieces of information:

1. Where they are
2. Why they are where they are
3. Whom they are talking to
4. Why they are talking to whom they are talking

Typically, therefore, it is not necessary to expend a great deal of cognitive effort in processing such background inputs. They are factors that are either given or quickly established as new parameters in a conversation. For example, an interlocutor only has to allocate minimal cognitive resources to engaging in an interaction with people they habitually encounter (e.g. relatives or co-workers). Even in interactions with strangers, once an interactional frame is established, the factors of who one is talking to requires little processing effort, that is, the interlocutor knows he/she is interacting with a stranger and is aware of how such interactions should proceed.

Maximizing Relevance: Effort and Effect

According to RT, an utterance does not become relevant to the speaker just because it adheres to a co-operative principle or maxims of quantity, quality, relevance and manner; rather, the search for relevance is a basic feature of human communication (Wilson and Sperber 2002). RT further suggests that an input will yield positive cognitive effects when it interacts with background information in a manner that matters to the individual (i.e., the interpretation of the utterance or gesture has a meaningful effect on the listener). Wilson and Sperber believe that the 'automatic tendency to maximize relevance' (2002 , 254) is due to the manner in which our cognitive systems have evolved in response to selection pressure for efficiency. This is an important point in considering whether (a) RT can be informative in the context of dementia, and (b) whether interactions with PWD might help to extend, or support the claims of RT. If inferential mechanisms are a spontaneous reaction to an input or stimuli, and as Wilson and Sperber suggest, based on non-representational mechanisms, then it is likely that such mechanisms require optimal function in all the cognitive systems to produce inferences. This is clearly not the case for PWD: their cognitive systems are compromised. However, if seeking relevance is a hardwired cognitive behavior then it is likely to be operating even in the presence of dementia. That is, PWD will attempt to make inferences based on the most meaningful interpretation they can make given the limitations of their constrained cognitive systems and the social inputs they receive.

Thus, one (or all) of the four following cognitive processes may occur in a PWD's language system attempting to establish relevance,

(1) The PWD is unable to focus attention on only the potential relevant inputs and therefore only receives partial information about the stimuli
(2) The information relating to the stimuli may not reach the necessary locations in the PWD's brain due to cortical and/or sub-cortical damage or tissue loss. That is, the incoming information cannot

interact with, or connect to, other "bits" of information represented (stored) in other parts (neurons) of the brain that help form a connected semantic network, a processing action that may be required for full comprehension of a proposition, concept, or word (Quaid Quiroga 2012)

(3) PWD cannot inhibit other associated words or concepts activated by the speaker's utterance, in the listener's memory. This is the result of a process of spreading activation in the semantic network of the listener (Cowan 2011; Shelley-Tremblay 2011)

(4) PWD have to focus too much of their attention (cognitive energy) on inputs that should be taken as givens (e.g. knowing the identity of their interlocutor) and this action stops (or interferes with) the automatic search for the most relevant interpretation.

Wilson and Sperber (2002) suggested that generalized implicatures are typically cancelled when a speaker says (or does) something incompatible with our expectations. A hearer trying to understand a speaker's utterance uses semantically encoded information in conjunction with what is mutually manifest. As noted above, the speaker's identity is usually clear to all communication partners or, at least, quickly established in typical conversations. As a result, in dementia, where PWD may constantly forget such details, it is possible to suggest that *incompatibility* is often a default parameter in conversations. As point four above suggests, the search for generalized implicatures is likely to be cancelled if the PWD has to continually stop processing verbal propositions to consider the question of identifying whom they are talking to and why they are talking to them. Indeed, a great deal of the PWD's cognitive resources and processing efforts may be allocated to the process of trying to answer *who, what, where* and *why* questions. If PWD have to perseverate on any of the above wh-questions, it may double the processing burden or completely stall the search for relevance.

A further issue to consider is how individuals go about the business of making their intentions evident, or what Wilson and Sperber (2002) refer to as ostensive inference. They suggest it is not enough to communicate an intention to an interlocutor; a speaker also has to indicate that he/she is deliberately communicating this intention. Wilson and Sperber offer the scenario of a woman who wishes to communicate to another they want their glass refilled. The woman has conceived of an intention and may even put her empty glass in the host's line of sight but it is not an example of inferential communication unless she indicates in some manner (e.g. touching the glass) that she is intending this message and thereby affecting her host's actions. RT has developed the notion of what is termed *ostensive-inferential* communication which includes two aspects of intention, (a) the informative intention (i.e., the intention to inform person X of something Y), and (b) the communicative intention (i.e. the intention to inform X that you are intending to inform them of Y). It is this aspect of RT that enables interlocutors 'to some extent [. . .] predict and manipulate the mental states of others' (Wilson and Sperber 2002, 255). It follows that Wilson and Sperber are positing a theory that appears to include a level of meta-inferencing. That is, RT suggests that humans have a predisposition to search for features (inputs) that indicate the speaker (or communicator) is overtly indicating (or providing evidence of) a specific intention, and that because of this process the listener will arrive at a particular interpretation (the speaker's intention) of the utterance. Speakers therefore construct utterances (or make gestures) in a manner that is intended to attract the listener's attention and draw their focus towards decoding the implied meaning of the utterance. Put more simply, an ostensive stimulus makes the listener aware that this particular input is worth his/her attention. In addition, Wilson and Sperber (2002) suggest the notion of optimal relevance, the condition where a stimulus is optimally relevant if, and only if, (a) it is relevant enough to warrant the listener's processing effort and (b) it is the most relevant interpretation compatible with an interlocutor's abilities and/or preferences.

Investigating inferential theories of pragmatics is particularly challenging in the context of dementia. If we apply the classic Gricean framework to conversations involving PWD it is often the case that the PWD would be considered as violating (unintentionally) all four maxims (i.e., quality, quantity, relevance, and manner). However, despite cognitive deficits, PWD (as is shown in many of the chapters in this book) appear to work very hard to discursively fulfill the co-operative principle and maintain conversational obligations of politeness and engagement (Guendouzi and Pate forthcoming). In addition, as will be shown below, PWD also work hard to find relevance in their interactions.

Establishing the relevance of participant identity

Before discussing the data presented below, it is useful to consider how interlocutors create mental frames in which to situate the people they encounter in their daily lives. When first encountering others we create a cognitive schema related to the interaction (Minsky 1975). That is, we create and store representations of facts or attributes associated with that particular individual. Initially, we may first know them by their name, professional title, or appearance, for example Dr. Smith the dentist, or Susie the blonde girl at Starbucks who makes my coffee every day. In addition, we then store information about the functional interactions we have with these individuals, these communicative scripts are associated with the conversations we have with these individuals. The script associated with Susie might include utterances such as, "how are you today?", "can I get you a coffee today" or "would you like whipped cream with that?" Whereas the scripts associated with Dr Smith might also include "how are you today" but in addition, would contain context specific utterances such as, "open wide", "I am just going to take a look now", or 'this won't hurt much". Formulaic phatic tokens such as greetings or partings can be used in multiple interactional contexts and thus may be represented in the lexicon (or semantic network) alongside numerous cognitive schemas associated with our daily interactions. They are utterances that are multi-functional and appropriate in both formal and casual contexts. Thus, given the frequency of their use, and the flexibility of their fit to so many contexts it is not surprising that PWD appear to overuse formulaic and phatic utterances. Schemas created for people encountered regularly (e.g. friends, family, or work colleagues are activated so frequently it is likely they are processed as low level inputs that need minimal diversion of cognitive resources.

As was shown in previous work (Guendouzi and Müller 2001; 2006) people with dementia do appear to draw on cognitive schemas when they are unable to remember someone's name or professional identity. On occasions when Ms F, a woman with dementia, could not remember the researcher's name or profession she appeared to draw on a cognitive schema of things semantically associated with the researcher's profession. For example, greetings Ms F used when addressing the researcher were terms or phrases related to items or tasks associated with educational or writing contexts (e.g. "that loses me points does it", "hello the typewriter", "I didn't do my homework", or "oh the poem"). The researcher was introduced to Ms F as a professor who taught in a university. It appeared that Ms F's cognitive search for R's name or profession activated related exemplars in her working memory that she was unable to inhibit. A neuro-typical person's language processing system would disregard these competing exemplars and continue the search for relevance until arriving at the specific target word or phrase (e.g., the researcher's actual name or title). The care assistants in Ms F's nursing home at the time of data collection thought it bizarre that Ms F addressed the researcher by saying "hello (.) the typewriter" and suggested she was "totally out of it". However, this behavior reflects an automatic compensatory strategy based on a less than optimal language processing system and perhaps "the typewriter" was in fact a very good descriptor of an academic's life.

Compensatory Strategies: Cognitive or Interactional Mechanisms?

Compensatory strategies can be thought of as two separate phenomena. First, there are compensatory strategies that are deliberate interactional moves used to support an individual's communication in the face of cognitive deficits such as aphasia (e.g., circumlocution or phonological cueing). Second, there are automatic behaviors that arise because of a stressed cognitive system attempting to compensate for a deficit, for example, producing non-specific but semantically associated exemplars (e.g. 'homework' or 'poem') that are not the target word. In the data below (extract 2) Ms F's greetings to the researcher appear to reflect the second form of compensatory strategy, that is, they were cognitively rather than socially driven verbal behaviors. Unusual communicative behaviors such as Ms F's descriptors when addressing the researcher may result from a PWD's search for relevance, and as such are the product of cognitive deficits. However, despite producing a non-specific target F did show that she still comprehended that the rules of interaction dictated greeting the person who entered her room. Furthermore, the researcher's physical presence cued F's language processing system to search for a relevant identity and while not attaining the correct target, F's semantic system was in the "right ball park" and retrieved items that did reflect she understood the researcher's identity and profession. Ms F's facial expressions and accompanying smile suggested that she was pleased to be able to create a relevant context and verbally express her recognition of R. Thus acknowledging or creating an identity for a conversational partner appears for some PWD, to be default parameter of relevance that is necessary for interactions to continue. Indeed, in the interactions below it becomes a parameter of relevance that three PWD appear to need to satisfy on multiple occasions.

Formal Contexts: Clinical Interviews

The setting and type of speech event in progress also affects the listener's search for relevant inferences. A clinical or ethnographic interview that involves only a PWD and a healthcare professional is likely to be less stressful for a PWD than a social setting with multiple participants. In a healthcare interaction, there are typically less environmental distractions and the discursive interaction is more formulaic. Diagnostic history interviews follow a structured format that may allow the PWD to answer with yes/no tokens or partially repeat the interlocutor's utterances. In such contexts, the PWD does not have to contend with utterances from multiple interlocutors nor negotiate overlapping or incomplete utterances that are common in casual conversations. In addition, there is no need to try to identify the identities of the participants because the clinician is likely to be dressed in a manner that signifies his or her professional role, thus there are multiple deictic cues in such settings. This can be seen in the extract below that is taken from a structured clinical interview between a clinician (C) and a man with dementia Mr E. The corpus of data involving Mr E has been discussed elsewhere (Guendouzi and Mueller 2006) and is used with the publisher's permission (Psychology Press, *formally Lawrence Erlbaum*).

Extract 1

1. C: what did you do?
2. Mr E: I was (.4) man. I gotta think now (1.0) Uh, I guess I was responsible for (.) for getting out (.) I was in industry
3. C: oh.
4. Mr E: in (name of city) (.) I was responsible for all the production they put out
5. C: oh, geez.
6. Mr E: and (.02)
7. C: like in the administration or were **you out on the floor?**
8. Mr E: I was **out on the floor** and man, that was the last time I worked.
9. C: how **long ago** was that, then?
10. Mr E: (5.0) it's been (3.0) **how long** have we been in (name of town)?
11. M: now that I don't know I thought she (Mr E's wife) said something like **a couple of years**
12. Mr E: **Three** (.) Maybe?
13. C: Is that what it is?
14. Mr E: yeah (.) I I guess it's been **about three years.**

The above data sample was collected in a university speech-language pathology clinic. The student clinician had been instructed to ask E, a man with dementia, about his current health and life status. The environment was a clinic room containing a desk and two chairs, and the only other participant (C) wore a clinic uniform and an official name badge with the

University logo across the top. In addition, the interaction, for the most part, followed a structured question-answer format. The physical setting (i.e., a clinic room) and structured conversation were distinctly iconic inputs and this may have helped E orient to the interaction, particularly as over the past two years he had taken part in numerous healthcare interactions (e.g. health check-ups, diagnostic tests etc.). Therefore, E was not required to expend a great deal of cognitive effort to establish relevance for the interaction; that is, it was easier to draw inferences about the identity of the interlocutor because she was wearing a uniform, asking familiar questions and giving him prompts. Although Mr E's recent cognitive screener suggested he was in the moderate to severe stage of dementia he appeared to cope well in structured formal contexts.

The researcher introduced him to C and explained C was an intern clinician who was going to ask him some questions. It was noticeable that, after the initial introduction Mr E at no point in the three interviews he attended, asked questions or made comments to suggest he needed to establish C's identity. Although E experiences moments when he found it difficult to recall facts or words, overall his contributions to the interview appear to stay on topic. This is due in part, to the fact, that at times he uses partial repetitions of phrases or clauses that C had just produced. For example, in turn seven C asks if E was 'out on the floor' and he replies 'I was out on the floor', a fact which was not true because he had been an office administrator when working. This pattern of responses emerged in all three of the interviews conducted with E. Although possibly an artifact of working memory deficits and an inability to inhibit the words his interlocutor had just uttered, it helped him continue with the conversation in a seemingly coherent manner. Although caused by a cognitive deficit, E's use of partial repetitions probably functioned as a compensatory strategy and allowed the interview to continue in a relatively coherent manner. Healthcare interviews and speech-pathology assessments are interactional contexts that can generate "test anxiety" because they often involve questions or assessments that require the PWD to respond with accurate propositional content. However, the structured, and at times, formulaic nature of this type of interaction, in addition, to the dyadic interview appears to be easier for the PWD to discursively negotiate. It is notable that in many qualitative studies involving a researcher and a PWD "chatting" in a dyadic situation, PWD are able to use interactional compensatory strategies (e.g. politeness tokens, phatic tokens, formulaic items, extenders or partial repetitions) to engage and socially connect with their interlocutor (Davis 2005; Guendouzi and Muller 2006; Maclagan, Davis and Lunsford, 2008). In more structured contexts (e.g., healthcare interviews or directed research interviews) there are less cognitive stressors (e.g., multiple interlocutors, overlapping utterances) to tax the PWD's language system and the PWD is not forced to continually search for relevance in relation to interlocutor identity or interactional goals. As will be shown below, in the case of casual contexts with multiple interlocutors this is not always the case.

Social Contexts: Observations from the Day Center

The data below was collected at a day center for PWD in the early to moderate stages of dementia. The researcher visited the center as a volunteer once a week for a period of year and a half to collect ethnographic data. Her visits took place in the mornings and lasted for approximately three hours (9.00 am to 12.00 am) on each occasion. The interactions occurred in an open public access area, and the conversations might (at any time) include participants who had not given prior consent for recording therefore IRB restrictions did not allow audio-video recording to be carried out. The researcher decided that taking extensive field notes during the interactions would appear too intrusive, distract from her observations, and potentially impede the flow of conversation therefore, although some field notes were collected when the interactions occurred, most were compiled later in the day when the researcher had returned to her place of work.

The participants of these two conversations included the researcher (R) and four PWD. Ms Ann (A) was a former nun and missionary who married later in life. She had been involved in education and teaching for most of her life. Ms Betty (B) was a homemaker and mother of (she claimed) six children. Ms Caroline (C) was a former teacher of African American descent and the mother of four children, and Mr Xavier (X) was a former university professor and researcher who spoke six languages fluently (his first language was Spanish). All participants were wearing nametags. The exchanges discussed below took place while the participants were drinking coffee and eating a snack comprised of cookies. This was a daily routine while the staff arranged and set up daily activities in the lounge area. There was one care assistant present in the kitchen and she was responsible for providing the coffee and cookies but she remained at the rear of the kitchen and did not participate in the conversations.

Ms A and the first parameter of RT

The exchange in extract one below occurred just after R had sat down at the table. Greetings had taken place when R first entered the room five minutes earlier. The group was not engaged in conversation when R arrived, so R pointed to a travel magazine that was lying in the middle of the table and commented on some pictures of hotels in Italy. A conversation developed between R, Ms A, and Ms B regarding the pictures of Italy but after approximately two minutes Ms A and Ms B lost interest in the magazine. Ms C appeared to be falling asleep but she did occasionally look up and laugh. Mr X did not contribute to this segment of the conversation and was occupying himself by attempting to break up his cookie.

Extract One
Ms A: and what's your name again?
R: ge
[
Ms A: no let me read it (*leans over and peers at R's name-tag)* and how do you say that jendooza /dʒɛnduzə/ ?
R: guendouzi /gɛːnduːzi□/
Ms A: so where are you from? You're not from around here are you?
R: no I am from England.
Ms A: England mhm I thought you weren't from round here (.) so tell me again what's your name (.) and where are you from?
Ms B: they don't let us, do they? (*looking towards the care assistant and her cup)*
R: do you want some more coffee (*looking at Ms B)* or cookies?
Ms B: (*looking intently at author)* I know you oh you?
R: yes, I came last week remember?
Ms C: that's a nice one (*looking at picture)*
R: that's Italy (.) I think.
Ms A: now (*looks at author)* don't tell me you are from (0.5)
R: England
Ms A: oh England no I haven't been there and so: what is your name again?

A version of the interactional routine that occurred above was repeated on each occasion the researcher visited the center. As conversational topics developed Ms A would periodically interject a request for the author's name or nationality. This discursive pattern also continued during the activities that took place after the coffee session (e.g. making decorative cards or playing word games etc). Ms A used discourse markers (e.g., 'so' and 'now'), conjunctions (e.g.,'and'), and pre-requests (e.g., 'so tell me again) to introduce her questions into the conversation. She also frequently adds the adjunct 'again', a verbal construction that suggests she is aware of the fact that she is repeating her question. The effect of using these discursive devices helps to make her repetitions seem less out of place, and marks an awareness of appropriate politeness strategies (Brown and Levinson1987) regarding face issues. At no point, for instance, does Ms A use a bald-on-record strategy and directly ask the researcher "who are you?"

Ms A did not (in the researcher's presence) ever use this verbal habit when interacting with either the staff or her peers, nor did she manifest any noticeable signs of being distressed by the fact she could not remember R's name. However, her persistent need to ask R's name and place of origin suggests that contextualizing R's identity was an important interactional parameter for Ms A when talking to R. As noted above typically, the identity of an interlocutor is a quickly established or given piece of information in a conversation that might dictate the appropriate degree of intimacy between the participants. Indeed, interlocutors need this information to frame their conversations and choose the appropriate communicative behaviors for the context. Ms A appears to follow the path RT would predict: that is, she first establishes a relevant context for the input (i.e., the researcher). Thus Ms A's questions are an automatic cognitive strategy (albeit it one that is enacted in an appropriate interactional style), that occurs because Ms A is hardwired to continually search for relevance in the interaction. Thus, the first default parameter of RT appears to be that interlocutors must satisfy the condition of identifying their conversational partner, and if, as in the case of Ms A, that information is lost due to working memory deficits the search for relevance will continually recommence.

Ms B and the Second Parameter of RT

Ms B's interactional behaviors suggest that, in addition to knowing the identity of a conversational partner, it is important to contextualize the degree of intimacy in interlocutor relationships. The following exchange took place as the researcher was in the process of sitting down at the dining table to join the group for coffee.

Extract 2

1. R: hi how are you today?
2. Ms A: oh:: we are all very well (*looks toward R's name-tag*) so tell me (.) what's your name?
3. R: Jackie.
4. Ms B: (*stares at the researcher, appears anxious*) it's you (.) isn't it?
5. R: (*laughing*) yes (.) it's me.
6. Ms B: we are like that aren't we? *(tilts her head slightly to one side and nudges the researcher on the arm with her elbow)*
7. R: yes (.) we are *(laughs)*
8. Ms B: oh you (*laugh)* you I should (*shakes her fist while smiling)*
9. Ms A: so now tell us (.) where are you from?
10. Ms B: do you want some coffee? I should get you some coffee *(begins to get up)*

Ms B did not directly request information relating to the researcher's name or place of origin rather her comments appeared to be an attempt to establish evidence of a prior, and perhaps close, relationship with the researcher. Ms B uses the inclusive pronoun 'we' and states that they (Ms B and the researcher) are 'like that'. Her non-verbal behaviors and the manner in which she tilts her head, rolls her eyes, and then nudges the researcher add evidence to the interpretation that Ms B is suggesting that the researcher and she are old friends or, at least, close acquaintances who share an intimate relationship that can include "knowing looks" and friendly nudges. The researcher's response reflects the fact she inferred Ms B was trying to establish this joint understanding and she confirms Ms B is a close acquaintance. Ms B then gives R a friendly warning accompanied by a smile and fist shake that reinforces the notion Ms B views R as someone she knows well enough to scold. Her verbal behavior after this point suggested that, having established a close relationship with the researcher, she feels socially obligated to act as a "hostess" to her "friend" because she then enquires whether the researcher would like a cup of coffee. Establishing the nature of her relationship with the researcher did appear to reduce the anxiety that Ms B often exhibited in her non-verbal behaviors when the researcher first arrived at the center.

Mr X: Establishing common ground

Extract 3

1. Ms A: /ʒɑːkliːn/ and so where are you from?
2. Mr X: /ʒɑːkliːn/ *(smiling)* that's a nice name, parlez vous francais?
3. R: no (.) not really well I understand it (.) a bit
4. Mr X: I speak six languages (.) parlez vous Français?
5. R: une petite peu
6. Mr X: je parlez Français and Italian (.) hablo espagnol?

During her visits to the day center the researcher did not observe Mr X engage in extended conversation with either his peers or the staff. Most of his contributions to the conversations that occurred during the coffee sessions involved requests for ice for his water, statements to inform people he was going to go to the bathroom, and requests to ask if it was time to go home. He did however join in the interactions when he had the opportunity to demonstrate his linguistic abilities. Ms A was in the habit of pronouncing the researcher's name (Jacqueline) in the French manner /ʒɑːkliːn/ and Mr X, cued by this pronunciation would frequently ask if the researcher spoke French. On these occasions, the researcher would offer a reply explaining that she did not speak French fluently. Mr X would then repeat the question a few minutes later even though the researcher had provided the answer in a prior turn, or in a conversation the previous week. The use of the formal pronoun 'vous' suggests he assumed he did not know the researcher well and was attributing social distance between himself and the researcher. The researcher had been a regular visitor to the center for a year and regularly shared coffee with Mr X, yet, based on his face expressions Mr X did show any signs of recognizing the researcher when she arrived, and therefore his use of this pronoun form would be the correct social choice when talking with a new acquaintance.

Although different to the previous two examples Mr X's repeated production of this question reflects a third parameter of relevance based on the premise, *when I don't know my interlocutor and am in conversation with them I should try to establish common ground or shared interests*. Thus, three conversational behaviors associated with relevance that were observed in the researcher's interactions with this particular group of PWD were,

1. that Ms A would establish an identity for the researcher

2. that Ms B would assess the degree of social intimacy in her relationship with the researcher
3. that Mr X would attempt to establish some shared common ground with the researcher based on her name.

In a speech event that involves a casual setting such as having "a chat with friends over coffee" the interactional parameters listed above are usually given information. Therefore, typically, this interactional routine does not require a great deal of cognitive processing effort. Based on their facial expressions, it appeared that at some level Ms A and Ms B recognized the researcher but they could not recall her specific identity, nor remember how well or in what context they knew her. It appeared that Mr X perceived R as a new acquaintance, therefore when Ms A reads out R's name with a French pronunciation Mr X draws the inference from this input that R is French (or at least French speaking). This form of question is a familiar interactional strategy that interlocutors use to establish some common ground with an unfamiliar person. However, unlike a neuro-typical person, Mr X did not retain this information so, like Ms A, he continually asks the same question on multiple occasions within, and across his interactions with the researcher. It is perhaps ironic that Ms A's search for relevance also cues Mr X's repetitive behavior in establishing an interactional relationship with the researcher.

Despite their uncertainty about the researcher's identity and her status within the group, all three PWD discursively worked hard (and arguably collaborated) to create a relevant context for engaging in a conversation with the researcher during the coffee break. They did not remain silent, ignore the researcher, or fabricate an identity for her (e.g. mistake her for someone else). Although a speculative assumption, it would seem that these examples reflect a default starting parameter for RT, that is, an interlocutor should first recognize or establish the identity of other participants in an interaction before proceeding with decoding inferences from any ensuing verbal comments. This also allows participants to assess the degree of social distance between themselves and others and thus enables them to adjust or accommodate their speech style (Giles and Coupland 1991) in an appropriate manner. Thus, in the initial moments of an interaction several inputs that help to frame the relevance of any further interaction need to be cognitively processed by the PWD (i.e. others' identity.). For neuro-typical speakers, these contextual inputs are usually processed instantaneously and require only minimal diversion of an individual's cognitive resources, that is there is only one cognitive search for relevance of the inputs and once satisfied this becomes given information. In the case of the PWD discussed above, there is a repeated search for the relevance of one or more normally "low-level" inputs and this verbal behavior may disrupt the conversation or annoy their interlocutors. Thus, as table one below suggests, social activities with multiple participants are contexts that present a greater cognitive challenge to PWD than structured formal contexts such as healthcare interactions.

Table 1 Participant relevance and processing effort in two contexts

Context	*Person with dementia*	*Neurotypical person*
Social setting multiple participants	**1st parameter** → *high processing load* **re-occurring cognitive search -** context implies intimate relationship but interlocutor unknown so mismatch between input and context **2nd parameter** → *high processing load* **re-occurring search for relevance** – context implies intimate relationship therefore seeking reassurance of degree of social intimacy	**1st parameter** → *low processing load* **Search stops at initial stage of interaction -** identity of interlocutor known or quickly established **2nd parameter**→ *low processing load* **Search not necessary** - once identity established degree of social intimacy known
Healthcare setting dyad	**1st parameter** → *low processing load* **no re-occurring search for relevance** –given information contextual cues establish professional identity **2nd parameter** → *low processing load* **no re-occurring search for relevance** given information professional relationship	**1st parameter** → *low processing load* **no re-occurring search for relevance** given information **2nd parameter** → *low processing load* **no re-occurring search for relevance** given information professional relationship

Key:
Relevance theory = interlocutors hardwired to search for relevance
1st parameter to satisfy relevance principle = establish participant identity
2nd parameter to satisfy relevance principle = establish degree of intimacy in relationship to interlocutor

Conclusions

What can RT tell us about communication in dementia? In addition, what do the verbal behaviors of the PWD discussed above tell us about the claims of RT? Van der Herst and Sperber suggest that inputs are relevant to an interlocutor when processing the input within the context of available (and past) information yields a positive cognitive effect (2004). Thus, creating relevance is a top-down process that involves a listener monitoring incoming inputs to assimilate the information with previously stored cognitive schemas in their memory. Initially, for an interaction to proceed in a manner that allows speakers to create implicatures and listeners to draw inferences there are default parameters that need to be satisfied. The data above suggests that for this group of PWD two default parameters essential for interactions to continue are (1) establishing the identity of a conversational partner who behaves as if she were a close acquaintance, and (2) establishing the degree of interpersonal intimacy in their relationship with this person. If I assume I know you well I can jokingly shake my fist and scold you as Ms B did to the researcher but if I am not sure who you are then I might need to be more formal, as Mr X's behavior demonstrated when he used the pronoun 'vous' to address the researcher.

If, as RT suggests, humans are hardwired to search for relevance and this process relies on prior knowledge, then it will be a problematic process for PWD. The cognitive deficits in dementia often result in either a loss of previously known information, or fragmented memories that are incomplete representations. If searching for relevance was a volitional behavior then, given the cognitive effort would be greater than the positive cognitive effects, a PWD might abandon the search completely. However if, as Wilson and Sperber (2002) argue, the search for relevance is an innate cognitive mechanism in humans then it should be an automatic behavior that, even in the face of dementia is difficult to inhibit. Ms A's pattern of repetitive verbal behaviors when she encounters the researcher do appear to suggest that the search for this parameter of relevance is a reflexive default action of cognitive processing that she cannot inhibit. Indeed, all three PWD at the day center repeatedly asked questions that appeared related to establishing an interactional frame in which to situate a person who was acting as a friend and sharing coffee with them. In the data collected in the dyadic clinical interactions, Mr E did not appear at anytime to need to establish the clinician's identity, or to assess whether they had a prior relationship. This was also the case in similar clinical interviews collected from three other PWD; the visible cues in the clinical environment appeared to satisfy the initial parameters of relevance.

Analyzing the data from an RT perspective suggests tentative support for this cognitively based pragmatic theory. More importantly, considering the data in relation to RT's notion of cognitive processing *effort* versus positive cognitive *effects* suggests that PWD will expend a great deal of effort to satisfy conditions of relevance. Furthermore, it is not simply decoding propositional content that acts as a stressor for PWD, it is also the number of inputs they are required to process. It might be expected that a casual chat in a social setting with peers or familiar acquaintances would be a less stressful task than a clinical interview involving questions (and assessments) requiring specific propositional responses. However, the lack of structure, contextual cues, and need to situate multiple conversational partners in the social setting often results in a situation that causes greater anxiety (e.g. Ms B) or distracting repetitive behaviors (e.g. Ms A and Mr X).

It is important to understand both the nature of verbal behaviors and their interaction with cognitive processing mechanisms. If RT is a hardwired cognitive mechanism then Ms A's repetitive behavior (which her family reported as annoying) was something that she could not inhibit. It is also important to note that, even if Ms A's behavior is the result of a reflexive cognitive mechanism she did still make an effort to use the appropriate interactional devices and politeness tokens (e.g. discourse markers, pre-requests etc.) to insert her requests for information about the researcher's identity; she was, despite her memory deficits, a very considerate conversational partner. Furthermore, it appears that rehabilitation activities set up to resemble social events are more stressful than formal structured situations because PWD appear to be aware that such events typically involve people they *should* know and this mismatch of inputs and context can result in distress or anxiety.

The above observations are simply one researcher's perception of the interaction between cognitive mechanisms and interactional resources in the context of dementia. The conclusions do not claim to be a definitive interpretation of what occurred in these interactions or, for that matter, in the minds of the PWD. However, the analyses do suggest that RT has a great deal to offer researchers when they examine conversational data involving PWD. An important aspect of creating robust theories is to apply them to conversational data and assess whether the emerging pattern of verbal behaviors reflects the claims or mechanisms suggest in the theories. Using RT as a framework to analyze data collected from interactions involving PWD helps to build a clearer understanding of how cognitive mechanisms and conversational resources interact to produce verbal behaviors that are characteristic of the communication of people with dementia. Ultimately this should lead to the development of better methods to train healthcare professionals and advise family caregivers on how to manage conversations with PWD.

References

Brown, Penny and Levinson, Steven. 1987. *Politeness: Some universals in language usage*, Cambridge: Cambridge University Press.

Baron Cohen, Simon, Leslie, Alan and Frith, Uta. 1985. Does the Autistic child have a Theory of Mind? *Cognition,* 21, 37–46.

Bayles, Kathryn, Tomoeda, Cheryl and Michael W. Trosset. 1992. "Naming and categorical knowledge in Alzheimer's disease: The process of semantic memory deterioration." *Brain and Language*

Bourgeois, Michelle. 2002. "Where is my wife and when am I going home? The challenge of communicating with persons with dementia." *Alzheimer's Care Quarterly* 3, 132-144.

Cowan, Nelson. 2011. "Working memory and attention in language use." In *The Handbook of Pyscholinguistics and cognitive processing: Perspectives in communication disorders,* 75-98, edited by Jackie Guendouzi, Filip Loncke, and Mandy. J. Williams. NY: Psychology Press.

Cummings, Louise. 2009. *Clinical pragmatics*. Cambridge, UK: Cambridge University Press.

Davis, Boyd. ed. 2005. *Alzheimer talk, text and context*. NY: Palgrave-Macmillan.

Giles, Howard and Nikolas Coupland. 1991. *Language: contexts and consequences,*Buckingham: Open University Press.

Grice, Herbert P. 1975. "Logic and Conversation." In *Syntax and Semantics, 3: Speech Acts,* 41-58 edited by Peter Cole and Jerry Morgan. New York: Academic Press.

—. 1989. *Studies in the way of words.* Cambridge, Ma: Harvard University Press.

Guendouzi, Jacqueline. and Nicole Müller. 2006. *Approaches to Discourse in Dementia*. Mahwah, NJ: Lawrence Erlbaum Associates.

Guendouzi, Jacqueline and Nicole. 2002." Defining trouble sources in dementia: repair strategies and conversational satisfaction in interactions with an Alzheimer's patient." In *Investigations in Clinical Phonetics and Linguistics,*15-30, edited by Fay Windsor, M.L. Kelly &

Nigel Hewlett. Mahwah, New Jersey/ London: Lawrence Erlbaum Associates.

Guendouzi, Jacqueline and Nicole Müller. 2001. "Intelligibility and rehearsed sequences conversations with a DAT patient." *Clinical Linguistics and Phonetics,* 2: 91-95.

Guendouzi, Jacqueline and Anna Pate. (forthcoming). "Interactional resources in the presentation of self in the context of dementia: A perspective from Politeness Theory". In *Dialogue and Dementia: Cognitive and Communicative Resources for Engagement* edited by Robert Schrauf and Nicole Müller. London: Blackwell.

Hornberger, Michael and Oliver Piguet. 2012, "Episodic memory in frontotemporal dementia: A critical review", *Brain,* 135, 678 - 692

Maclagan, Margaret, Davis, Boyd, & R. Lunsford. 2008. "Fixed expressions, extenders and metonymy in the speech of people with Alzheimer's disease." In *Phraseology: An interdisciplinary perspective,* 175-190, edited by Sylviane Granger and Fanny Meunier. Philadelphia: John Benjamins.

Minsky, Marvin. 1975. "A Framework for representing knowledge." In *The Psychology of Computer Vision,* 211-277, edited by Patrick H. Winston. NY: McGraw-Hill.

Padilla Cruz, Manuel. 2007. "Phatic utterances and the communication of social information." In *Studies in intercultural,cognitive and social Pragmatics*, 112-129, edited by Pilar Garcés-Conejos Blitvich, Manuel Padilla Cruz, Reyes Gómez Morón and Lucia Fernández Amaya. New Castle-upon-Tyne: Cambridge Scholars Publishing.

Quaid Quiroga, Roderigo. 2012. *Borges and Memory*. Cambridge, MA: MIT Press.

Ripich, Danielle. 1994. "Functional communication with AD patients: A Caregiver training program." *Alzheimer's Disease and Associated Disorders* 8, 105-109.

Santo Pietro, Mary Jo and Elizabeth Ostuni. 1997. *Successful communication with Alzheimer's disease patients: An in service training manual.* Boston: Butterworth-Heinemann

Van der Henst, Jan Baptiste and Sperber, Dan. 2004. "Testing cognitive and communicative principles of relevance." In *Experimental Pragmatics* edited by Ira A Noveck and Dan Sperber. NY: Palgrave

Shelley-Tremblay, John. 2011. "The breakdown of semantics in aphasia and dementia: A role for attention. In *The Handbook of Pyscholinguistics and Cognitive processing: Perspectives in*

Communication Disorders, 625-645, edited by Jackie Guendouzi, Filip Loncke, and Mandy. J. Williams. NY: Psychology Press

Sperber, Dan & Wilson, Deirdre. 1986. *Relevance: Communication and cognition*. Blackwell: Oxford.

Sperber, Dan and Wilson, Deirdre. 2002. 'Pragmatics, modularity and mind-reading'. *Mind and Language* 17, 3-23.

Wilson, Deirdre and Sperber, Dan. 2002. "Relevance theory." *UCL Working Papers in Linguistics* 14: 249-287.

CHAPTER THREE

POSITIONING AND MEMBERSHIP CATEGORIZATION IN MONORACIAL AND INTERRACIAL INTERACTIONS OF PERSONS WITH DEMENTIA

CHARLENE POPE
MEDICAL UNIVERSITY OF SOUTH CAROLINA

From a pragmatics perspective, the use of language positions both speakers and their conversational partners in identities past, present and projected, as they perceive and categorize their social identities and group memberships in the immediate shared world and the worlds they have known. For persons with Alzheimer's disease, memories and ways of knowing may fade, but social and cultural identification and conditioning continue to appear in the talk of social interaction. Using Levinson's overview of links between pragmatics and discourse analysis, acts of positioning associated with social identity will be compared in a series of Black and White persons with Alzheimer's disease speaking in interactions with non-cognitively impaired, same-race and differing-race conversational partners. This analysis will compare particular utterances associated with membership categorizing with evidence in conversation of recognition, relevance or interpretation. Findings show the multiplicity of social identities that present beyond variations that appear in intergenerational same-race and differing race pairs, suggesting how people with Alzheimer's disease mobilize speaking resources. Particular language use practices specific to monoracial and interracial interactions suggest how intercultural pragmatics might identify markers of sociocultural contexts, power, and distance in discourse, beyond issues of sequencing and turn-taking of conversation analysis, with consequences for communicating with persons with dementia (PWD).

1. Introduction

Racial identity formation, membership categorization and the pragmatics of intercultural discourse

The comparisons of variation analysis or language use between African American and White older speakers in the United States (US) tend to focus on vernacular usage (Thomas 2007), the ability to distinguish voices (Thomas and Reaser 2004) or phonetic or phonological differences (Xue et al. 2001). Other disciplinary approaches have examined differing perceptions of or participation in health care (Joo, Wittink and Dahlber 2011) or more general language variation in the community (Wolfram 2003), rather than comparisons of social interactions potentially influenced by race, gender, and age. More general reviews of communication and aging (Harwood 2007) tend to exclude older adults who are persons with dementia (PWD) or examine ethnic differences in the experience of the disease (Manley and Mayeux 2004), rather than how people speak with one another. Some of the few studies of older adults who are PWD that examine racial differences in communication (Ripich, Fritsch and Ziol 2002) tend to look at structured tasks, rather than at the pragmatics of natural conversation in community-based circumstances.

At the societal level in the United States, racial identity formation (Omi and Winant 1994) from the desegregation of the 1960's to the current time after 2010 shifted significantly for older adults who lived through the era, suggesting that socialized communication practices and cultural habitus may affect intergenerational communication with young speech partners. In reflecting on social practice, the anthropologist Bourdieu proposes that past experiences can work actively in our present beyond our consciousness on how we perceive and act with people we identify as members of groups other than our own (Bourdieu 1990). Most relevant to the concerns of this chapter is that past experiences can work on and produce habituated communication practices shaped by bias, prejudice or lack of contact. For example, a Black speaker of middle age writes of growing up in inner city Baltimore in the 1980's and rarely speaking with White people (Blake 2013):

> *I hardly ever saw any white people in my neighborhood, and there was only one white student in my high school of 2,000.*

This observation was probably common among Blacks and Whites who lived at a similar time in history, slowly emerging first from legal and later economic segregation, with potentially conditioned expectations and speaking practices as cultural *habitus*. Bourdieu saw the concept of *habitus* as a set of predispositions or habituated practices shaped by our history and situated cultural positioning (Bourdieu 1977, 72-73), with potential effects on communication practices that would appear during social interaction between members of different social classes. Extending Bourdieu's observation, racial segregation may produce a tendency for behaviors beyond our conscious intention or the memory of their formation (Bonilla-Silva Goar and Embrick 2006), which may include tendencies for speech acts in interactions with same race and differing race conversational partners. In a study of racial identity formation in schools, Lewis (2003) introduces examples of how structural racial formation shapes the micro level social interactions when people of differing races speak with one another. The lack of such examples across generations, and particularly when one speech partner has dementia, prompts a need for comparisons, when the same PWD speaks with speech partners of both same and differing race and genders. One of the few approaches to the discourse analysis of race in a group of interviews as communication in New Zealand (van den Berg, Wetherell and Houtkoop-Steenstra 2003) did not examine older age as a factor in interaction. The analysis of the role of race in communication among older persons has tended to look at members of minority groups (Jackson and Ensley 1995), rather than racial variations within and between members of racial groups. One of the few examples of use of language use by or with older interracial dyads in social interaction concerns occasional racial slurs received by certified nursing assistants in nursing homes (Dodson and Zincavage 2007).

Aging, intergenerational interaction, and differences in social practice

This paper examines language use as a repertoire of learned and conditioned social practices that persist beyond the fading of cognitive memories, as has been described in previous qualitative analysis of discourse examples (Pope and Ripich 2005). Based on the approach of sociopragmatics to examine the potential influence of social identities (Kecskes 2012), discourse analysis provides a means to compare older speakers who are PWD with differing speech partners. In this selected sample, each PWD speaks with both a Black and White student conversational partner from a local university, visiting their assisted living residential facility. This study examined 14 paired conversational interactions, seven with an African American student and seven with a White student. Each pair interacted with a common conversational partner who was a much older person with early Alzheimer's disease. Each PWD was over 85 years of age, a category considered the oldest old and seldom found in similar qualitative studies. In contrast with more structured approaches that use standardized instruments, these comparisons use open-ended conversational interviews by a sample of university students visiting PWD, as natural conversations for this data set. Conversations were recorded and transcribed word for word. The data will be archived as part of the *Carolinas Conversations Collection,* a Web-based archive of recordings and transcriptions kept for research purposes at the Medical University of South Carolina Library in Charleston, South Carolina (Pope and Davis 2011). Though the sample is limited, the comparative examples of membership categorization for PWD in interaction can generate hypotheses and suggest best practices to promote engagement and more sensitive communication with PWD.

Most comparative analysis of interracial and same-race interactions has tended to focus on attitudes, affect, non-verbal behaviors, and particular performance outcomes (Toosi et al. 2012), rather than on discourse, with little focus on the effects of differing ages or generations. Commonly, the focus on intergenerational communication with older people examines attitudes about identity, patronizing, stereotypes about aging, and types of over- or under-accommodation (Harwood 2007). By contrast, the majority of research on communication with persons who have mild to moderate dementia tends to look primarily at communication with caregivers and providers (Smith et al. 2011; Vasse et al 2010). Yet multiple approaches similar in focus to that of sociopragmatics (conversation analysis from an ethnographic perspective, relational pragmatics, interpersonal pragmatics, and interactional sociolinguistics, as grouped by Anderson and Aijmer 2012)) offer the opportunity to look at language use in natural conversations with PWD and their conversational partners in ways that can identify variations related to social identity and sociocultural contexts (Hamilton 2008). The discursive practices that appear in talk capture indications of the cognitive process embodied in speaker participation, as Heritage describes in a broader review of cognitive processes in talk (Heritage 2005). In reflecting on cognition in discourse for example, Heritage (2005, 194) shows how words as simple as "*Oh?*" can signal a participant's shift in attention, belief, acceptance or understanding of a statement, a particular concern with adults challenged by memory. Other tokens, as simple as "*Mm-mhm*" or "*Oh really*?" used in particular contexts or in response to specific cues in talk concerning race can signal affiliation or detachment between speakers (Koole 2003).

2. Systematic Comparisons

The Potential Role of Membership Categorization in Talk with Persons with Dementia: Monoracial and Interracial Intergenerational Comparisons

This analysis begins with the premise that the identities of people are by definition social identities co-constructed in social interaction, as features of talk together displayed, attributed, inferred, and ascribed by both participants in a conversation (Edwards 1998). From the methods of conversation analysis, Sacks originally proposed that people in their use of language established membership categories in these features of talk, either explicitly in reference or implicitly in inference (Silverman 1998). The following examples present instances of membership categorization between PWD and their same race and differing race partners in which language use reflects a speaker's stance or positioning by membership category. Positioning theory suggests that speakers in conversation present themselves in relation to others with a variety of membership categorization devices in talk, such as use of pronouns, how narratives are constructed or received, words that index social or cultural contexts, and other devices (Harré and van Langenhove 1999). To select these examples, similar topics in each dyad were identified and then examined for particular discourse features. These examples illustrate only the practices of the individuals involved in each pair and do not suggest patterns by race, since the social identities involved are multiple, affected by age, gender, region of origin, years of education, socioeconomic status, past experience or interests, and other possible identities.

In the following example, Ms. W is a Black Female PWD speaking first with a White Interviewer (W-Int) and then with a Black Interviewer (B-Int), recalling her earlier life first as a teacher, and then after she changed professions to become a social worker. The transcript Extracts are presented sequentially to allow an opportunity for comparison when Ms. W recalled a past memory of herself in the larger world:

Extract -1 - Black Female PWD – Black Female Interviewer
51: Ms. W: But I like Philadelphia.
52: B-Int: You went to school there?
53: Ms. W: Let me see, undergrad in M (*school name*) graduated [?], Masters in Social Work.
54: I tried those children [?] (…) my puppy, my little puppy.
55: B-Int: (Laughter):
56: Ms. W: [?] Eating candy and writing notes. Thank you\.

57: No they didn't pay me no attention [-] so I had to give that up, teaching. [--]
58: B- Int: And you work in school? With the social work?
59: Ms. W: I enjoyed working as a social worker because I was able to [-]
60: to touch all kinds of problems [-].
Every time you saw a child was misbehaving in school
61: it wasn't because the child was a bad child. [-]
For many many reasons [-] (…)
62: B-Int: uh huh
63: Ms. W: And sometimes the kid didn't come to school because they felt [?]
64: to some of the other children. [-]
65: B-Int: Yeah.
[Narrative of the topic continues.]

In Extract 1, Ms. W, a Black PWD speaks with a Black interviewer, recalling when she attended school and changed professions from teacher to social worker. In the opening of the topic in Line 51, Ms. W offers her memory of a place. The Black interviewer builds on the story with an invitation query to continue based on Ms. W's past experience, using the referent place as a cue. This discourse move captures a feature similar to quilting in narrative (Moore and Davis 2002) and scaffolds the PWD's active engagement and participation in communication with an active response to the speaker's cue, acknowledging a shared knowledge of a city and affirming the PWD's identity and positioning as a traveler. Though pauses for recall appear in Line 53, Ms. W's joke about the children in her elementary school classroom is met by the Interviewer's laughter in the next turn, a successful sequence. In Line 56-57, Ms. W takes the opportunity to expand with examples of the difficulty she had controlling a classroom as the children ate candy and wrote notes. Within that turn, the expressive "*Thank you*" that signals an end to the children's antics and the double negation or multiple negatives of "*.**No** they didn't pay me **no** attention*" are features of African American Vernacular English (AAVE) (Bailey et al. 1998) that do not appear in the subsequent interchange with the White Interviewer. This feature may be prompted more by attention and engagement, acceptance and belief, rather than race. Yet the Black Interviewer's move in Line 58 picks up Ms. W's thread of her change of career to social work introduced in Line 53, an expression of interest and belief as well as the quilted link in turn-taking. As a result, after Ms. W has the opportunity to expand without interruption in Lines 59-61, the Black Interviewer's "*uh-hm*" is interpreted as agreement and encouragement to continue, rather than as disbelief seen in the next Extract 2. The speech act "*Yeah*" in Line 60 is interpreted as encouragement and the narrative continues.

In the next excerpt in a separate conversation, Ms. W speaks with a White Interviewer (W-Int.) who presents a different approach to positioning based on her responses in the following sequences. Ms. W presents her membership categorizations: as a professional who has retired, as a married person and as a traveler, but to considerably different responses.

Extract 2 - Black Female PWD – White Female Interviewer
111: Ms. W: I retired; I did a lot of traveling in Georgia.
112: W-Int: um hm
113: Ms. W: We traveled all the time.
114: W-Int: Oh really?
115: Ms. W: Oh yes. [-] I remember when the queen of England took the oath.
116: The person who was [?] the next one in the family..
117: W-Int: um hm
118: Ms. W: uh ... moved up. We was there when that happened.
119: W-Int: Oh really?
120: Ms. W: um hm
121: W-Int: [-] I wonder what year that was?
122: Ms. W: I don't remember what year that was; I can get my calendars at home.
123: W-Int: um hm - oh you wrote all that stuff down?
124: Ms. W: Yea I jotted that down. I have a lot of calendars in my library.
125: I have a lot of materials…
126: W-Int: Okay.
[Change of subject by Interviewer]

In Extract 2, Ms. W begins to tell her story of a memory of retirement. Her opening positions her as a person who has retired and travelled independently. In Line 112, the interviewer's *um-hm*, can be taken as either agreement or an non-committal response to maintain engagement. Ms. W echoes her premise of traveling, changing from the first person pronoun "*I*" to "*we*" referencing her husband, adding both weight to the premise and an additional identity as a married traveler. In Line 114, her interlocutor's response "*Oh, really?*" may suggest disbelief but makes no move to accept or take up the identity cue, since it prompts the assertion "*Oh, Yes*!" from Ms. W As a set of speech acts, the Interviewer's response may compromise the principle of cooperation, described in pragmatics when participants accept or do not accept the purpose of offered talk (Levinson 1983/2011), prompting the defense.

In the next turn in Line 115, Ms. W expands her experience and identity as a traveler beyond her state of Georgia to recall a trip to England when the young Queen Elizabeth took her oath, struggling only with a prosodic question of memory regarding who Elizabeth replaced in a move up, repaired in the next turn. Once again, the Interviewer's response in Line 117 is non-committal to the story, prompting Ms. W to assert "*We was there when it happened*" in Line 118. The repeated response of "*Oh, really*? in Line 119 constitutes at best conditional belief and in past analysis has been associated with disaffiliation (Koole 2003). Its repeated use in an adjacency pair after a declarative of Ms. W and in chains of "*um-hm*" without direct response to offered cues provides only marginal participation from the interviewer. When Ms. W uses tacit agreement in Line 120 instead of more detail, the White interviewer prompts a query many without Alzheimer's disease would find difficult, interrogating the year of the Queen's coronation in Line 121. Ms. W acknowledges she does not remember the year, but asserts she has calendars recording the event at home. In Line 123, the Interviewer's questioning that Ms. W has written down such information constitutes the first direct participation in this segment of conversation, but only echoes disbelief rather than positive engagement or mutual exchange of information. In this chain of conversation on the digital recording, the flat affect that characterizes the White interviewer's tone follows only superficial exchange until a double direct interrogation of Ms. W's claim in Line 121 and Line 123. The three short statements in Line 124-125 offer multiple assertions of the same premise, consistent with the use of quantity for illocutionary force when one person speaks from a contest to which their addressee does not seem committed (Levinson 1983/2011, 277). Yet in the last turn, the interviewer uses "Okay", well-documented as a discourse marker that signals an end of topic to change the subject (Schiffrin 1988), effectively rejecting Ms. W's portrayal of identity as an informed person, a world traveler and a witness of history. Based in conversation analysis, Schegloff (2007) suggests the parts of conversation considered membership categorization devices (MCD) include categories and the type of rules in talk that make the MCDs relevant. Ms. W's themes offer the membership categorization devices of *traveller*, as a wife and witness to history, yet the sequential organization of this exchange positions Ms. W differently than the portrait she offers of herself. The White interviewer's superficial participation holds a place on the conversational floor, while exchanging little information and repeatedly interrogating claims made by Ms. W in a way that positions her as a less than engaging or accepting partner. The positioning of Ms. W with each of her previous partners differs in recognition of the relevance of themes, engagement, and participation.

In the next excerpts, the same PWD, Ms. W, speaks with two different interviewers, prompted to reflect on two mealtimes.

Extract 3: Black Female PWD – Black Female Interviewer

12: B-Int:	--- Ms. W, did you eat breakfast today?
13: Ms. W:	- yes I did, but I don't usually eat breakfast,
14:	but I got- I eat breakfast this morning.
15: B-Int:	they had some good stuff today didn't they?
16: Ms. W:	yea, they did. I must say I ate three meals today.
17: B-Int:	did you?
18: Ms. W:	mmm hmm.
19: B-Int:	- now that's unusual because you said that you usually don't like to eat breakfast.
20: Ms. W:	I don't. - I don't but they woke up for some reason
21	and I just say that's why I get on up and cooperate – cause they'll um yap, yap, yap.
22:	- I say that's all right I'll just get on up and cooperate.

[*Conversation continues about Ms. W's dining companions*]

In Line 12, though the interviewer opens with a yes-no question, the cue is accepted with subsequent detail, as Ms. W positions herself as a not-usual breakfast eater who has acted out of character. In Line 14, the use of the present tense for past action in the statement, "*I eat breakfast this morning*," follows a cut off past tense and repaired statement 'I got…" The sequence positions a past action as a current observation, a use of tense observed previously in African American Vernacular English (Wolfram 2004). The Black Interviewer affirms the observation in Line 15, with "*They had some good stuff today, didn't they*?" This pair of statements as an adjacency pair positions Ms. W as an appreciative consumer with her dining service at the facility and the Black interviewer as a person who has either eaten or observed at breakfast, a move Ms. W reinforces in Line 16, with enthusiastic agreement. This choice as a listener and speaker provides the Black interviewer membership of shared experience and interest in the life of her facility. In the declarative statement in Line 16 that begins with "*I must say…I ate three meals today!" "I must say…"* functions as a retrodictive or reflective declaration in pragmatics (Levinson 1983, 240), to mark a different practice than Ms. W's usual. In successive Lines 17 and 19, the Black Interviewer first interrogates the eating as noteworthy and then in Line 19 marks how unusual Ms. W's breakfast eating was as a practice, confirming her understanding of the Line 16 "*I must say…*" as a declarative utterance marking the unusual membership category of Ms W as an enthusiastic breakfast eater. This type of adjacency pair marks attention and response to the context of an utterance and the significance to a speaker of what might be taken as a minor remark by one less attentive as a listener or conversational partner. Though the differences in engagement and enthusiasm between the previous White Interviewer and this Black interviewer cannot be attributed to race, the comparison establishes an interesting contrast and suggests possible hypotheses that could be explored with larger samples of same-race and interracial intergenerational dyads to consider the possibility of patterns.

Reflecting on the social interaction in this dyad, an observer might consider theories and evidence from social psychology addressing social identities and how people categorize themselves and one another (Crisp and Hewstone 2006), interracial communication (Orbe and Harris 2008) and intercultural communication (Scollon, Scollon and Jones 2012). Using social psychology to consider interactions between members of minority and majority groups, McGarty (2006) summarizes how people categorize social identity in hierarchies where self-perception and perception of the person with whom they interact may lead them to infer accessibility and cooperation when similar or salient and merit resistance or mobilize other identities when less so. When people interact, stereotypes may not only function as attributions, but may act subliminally in communicating to set boundaries for what speakers or listeners consider normative roles or expectations for people (Gandy 1998, 84) and how they position themselves and others in conversation. For example, Extracts 1 and 3 when compared with Extract 2 present attention to and a readiness to pick up Ms. W's cues and build narrative that positions her as a competent speaker with more detail to offer, a concern in promoting interaction for a PWD. Given the history of race in US society, when communication is perceived as interracial or race is salient for one of the participants, usual expectations of communication as mutual transaction, message exchange, and disclosure may vary (Orbe and Harris 2008). Past and current racial segregation may produce less comfort with contact and interaction, as well as the pressure on minorities who balance the "double vision" of continual awareness of commonalities and their marginal position as power outsiders (Orbe and Harris 2008, 13). In considering the potential of interactions as intercultural, language use provides endless potential for observing inferences drawn quickly and talk as ambiguous, until positioned by a number of context cues, whether in message form, reaction, sequence, vernacular, or politeness strategies signaled by involvement or dropped or rejected cues (Scollon, Scollon and Jones 2012).

By contrast, in the next excerpt, Ms. W discusses the possibilities for dinner to a different sort of response with a White Interviewer. From the first inquiry, the White interviewer controls the conversation with interrogation, positioning Ms. W's identity as a member of an 'other' group with "*y'all,*" yet not taking up cues for participation when offered.

Extract 4: Black Female PWD – White Female Interviewer

187: W-Int: What time ya'll usually eat?
188: Ms. W: [?] about 4 o'clock.
189: W-Int: [?] (Talking low, though muffled, a query by prosody)
190: Ms. W: [?] Because we been on a bus ride today.
191: W-Int: (um hm)
192: Ms. W: I wonder if it's worth going over there eating.
193: W-Int: [-] I don't know.
194: Ms. W: [?] eat them black eyed peas, [-] collard greens. I ate that salad [?]
195: they have that old stuff over there.
196: W-Int: [?huh] (Laughter)
197: Ms. W: I'm tired of that. We used to get tired of chicken [?]...[interruption].
198: W-Int: What is in the paper today? [-] Ain't hitting on nothing. [*referring to the newspaper*]

[*Change of subject*]

In Line 187, the White Interviewer asks when Ms. W and perhaps others at the facility eat their dinner, with "*What time ya'll usually eat*?" In referencing identity, in this case without a verb ("*ya'll*" functions as a form denoting assumed *do*), the inferred term *You all* is considered a common standard for Southerners of all races as well as a feature of particular AAVE (Davies 2007, 78). This use positions the White Interviewer as either referencing a common Southern bond or employing what she considers Black vernacular as a performance perhaps for accommodation but as an inauthentic self, while positioning Ms. W as a member of people living in the facility. In some circumstances the White use of what the performer considers Black dialect can be considered inauthentic and a way of signaling inappropriate access to a culture not one's own (Johnson 2003). Ms. W explains the change in dinnertime answering a muffled query in Line 189. In Line 190, she explains that a bus trip had changed the meal time. As a cue, the bus trip is not taken up in the next turn, so Ms. W returns to the potential for dinner as a theme.

Ms. W's expressive utterance in Line 192 shows her wondering whether it is worth going to the dining room thus positioning herself as an experienced member of the facility, raising the inference that the meal offering might not be worth the effort. The White Interviewer's response that she doesn't know in the next line prompts Ms. W to list in Line 194 foods common in the South and especially staples in the Black Southern diet (black-eye peas and collards) followed by an "*I ate that salad,*" a comment that marks context for Ms. W as having eaten even something not common to the style of the first two foods. The representative utterance in Line 195 summarizes an opinion about the food offerings in this Southern facility, in which the food they offer is typical of the "old stuff" people in a particular context eat. In Line 196, the White Interviewer does not pick up the context cue about common foods but laughs, though the laughter is not heard as shared. Ms. W attempts to speak of chicken as another offering that has grown tiresome, but the White interviewer interrupts to introduce a new topic in Line 198, first inquiring *"What is in the paper today?"* without dialect or vernacular and then following with an informal comment *"Ain't hitting on nothing."* The use of "*ain't*", a non-standard grammar form of the negative of "*is not*" in this case, is followed by informal slang.

The use of nonstandard English and slang by a White speaker in an interracial interaction as supposed dialect has been considered "*styling,*" and inauthentic in the presentation of an identity when performed by Whites (Strausbaugh 2006). More significantly for the PWD, the dropping of the invitation to speak about the topic of their choosing, food and eating choices, in preference to an empty attempt at styling, leads to exclusion and a change of topic. This apparent dropping of cues and attention by the White Interviewer with a Black conversation partner evokes the description of attention as a non-material commodity for exchange in conversation by the sociologist Derber (2000, 59), a negotiation in interaction influenced by perceived social status. The contrast between the engaged, attentive and more interactive prompting by the Black interviewer raises the possibility that the White interviewer may be influenced by race, given the inauthentic speaking practices that mark racial contexts. Though others may interpret such interactions with young White interviewers who drop cues and control the conversation as more related to the perceived frailty or dementia of the PWD with whom they are interacting, the contrast with same race dyads suggest patterns worth pursuing in future observations.

The following two excerpts were produced by a Black Male older speaker in conversation with first a Black Female interviewer and then with a White Male interviewer on a different day. In each case, the Black PWD reflects on an event of discrimination, with differing discursive practices by their speech partner and differing reactions in consequence.

Extract 5: Black Male PWD with Black Female Interviewer

130: Mr. T:	And, um, my Daddy, he had a restaurant up the street there on Beatty's Ford Road.
131:	And, he say, "X_____, why don't you go to [College Name]?
132:	And, that way, you can come and be with me and help me in the restaurant."
133:	I say, "Daddy, I'm leaving here."
134:	And, he didn't say another word, cause he knew I was going.
135: Int:	Yeah.
136: Mr. T:	I couldn't stand it. Going to the back of the bus. And, oh, it was really bad.
137: Int:	Yeah. Yeah. It, I couldn't imagine.
138: Mr. T:	It was bad.
139: Int:	I could not imagine.
140: Mr. T:	I could tell you some things that, it was bad.
141: Int:	Well, I'm glad you got out of that.
142: Mr. T:	Yeah. I got away from it.
143:	It, it really, um, surprised me the way the place has changed, you know.
144:	We got some good people every place you go, but, uh, Charlotte is a nice place.
145: Int:	Yeah, now, yeah, it does seem like (overlap)
146: Mr. T:	It's a nice place.
147: Int:	It'd be a lot better now.
148: Mr. T:	Oh, yeah. Oh, yeah.
149: Int:	Okay. (Pause.) What were your parents like?

[*Change of subject*]

In Line 130, Mr. T, the Black male PWD introduces a new topic to a Black female interviewer, with the tentative "*And, um...*", a repair described as a speech practice that can preface a delay to hold the conversational floor while the speaker retrieves an important topic or sufficient details (Clark and Fox Tree 2002). As a constructed delay signaling a context, this type of filled pause can signal a relevance to the speaker that will be filled in later. The story's introduction, "*...My Daddy, he had a restaurant up the street there on Beattie's Ford Road....*" uses a pronoun as a double referent to the speaker's father. Although repetition of a pronoun at the start of a spoken narrative is quite common, speakers with mild Alzheimer's disease have been observed to use more frequent pronouns when compared with non-cognitively impaired speakers of similar age (Amor et al. 1999). Lines 131-134 build a narrative with situated contexts: a father in a particular place, who cared for him and hoped he would pursue his education nearby, who offered the possibility of working together in a family business.

This type of example of direct reported speech allows a narrator to set the stage for a narrative, framed by what will be most significant for him in selection within the event and interpretation, rather than the reported facts of an account (Holt 1996). With "*And, he say…*" in Line 131, Mr. T selects an AAVE form of a quotative verb used by African Americans born before 1955, according to a study of the transition of the verb form over time to other forms used by younger Black speakers such as '*he goes*' or '*he be like*' (Cukor-Avila 2002). The use of AAVE to another Black speaker stands as a potential offer of common indexical ground, to be recognized or not recognized.

In Line 133, Mr. T shifts the narrative from a father's invitation to stay in the South to a declarative statement, where the narrator takes agency for a decision that places him in his memory in a role of dramatic conflict, "*I say, "Daddy, I'm leaving here."* The summary statement in line 134, "*he didn't say another word, cause he knew I was going*" holds the echoes of the unsaid. The lack of reported discussion offers the interlocutor opportunity to request details, since the reported silence effectively ends the narrative and presages subsequent events where the speaker enters a new context, place, and life. The Black Female interviewer offers only a "*Yeah*" that holds her place on the conversational floor without reaction or request for the details of this life-changing event.

Mr. T.'s response in Line 136 provides his feelings for the historical context he has evoked with three short, successive sentences. The listing provides his frustration and rejection, the primary theme of discrimination, and the summary of the historical period for Southern Blacks: "*I couldn't stand it. Going to the back of the bus. And, oh, it was really bad.*" The Black Female interviewer acknowledges her speech partner's experience with two affirmatives and a personal reflection in Line 137: "*Yeah. Yeah. It, I couldn't imagine.*" In the next Lines 137-140, Mr. T and the interviewer echo one another, as he affirms her observation that "*it,*" the troubling time in his history and their shared history, "*was bad.*" His repetition of this evaluation in Lines 136, 138 and 140 in successive turns takes a particular stance as a speaker with the type of generalization that suggests to a listener that this is a claim that needs to be unpacked (Scheibman 2007). Listeners in conversation faced with this type of repetition as a discourse move are expected to understand that this reference captures a speaker's intention to discuss the details behind the expression (Brown 1995). The decision of the Black Female interviewer in Line 141, "*Well, I'm glad you got out of that,*" effectively closes the door on continuing a narrative of the past with an affirmative evaluation that turns them away from the experience of discrimination. The use of the pronoun "*you*" positions racial discrimination as a category of experience owned by Mr. T and an event of an unshared past. There is no token of self-disclosure from the younger Black Female, nor are there any pronouns of "*we*" in subsequent turns where place referents and neutral interrogation of parents follow.

In Lines 142-144, Mr. T chooses to follow his speech partner's positivity, first echoing that he had got away from the unnamed "*it*", and then in mirroring affirmations that there are now "*good people*" around and that their shared town in the present is a "*nice place*". This turn exemplifies a politeness strategy, to follow the interviewer's turn of topic and goal and not cause trouble, representing a choice that acknowledges a differing goal in conversational turn-taking (Coulmas 2005, 84-89). It is not possible to speculate on the motive for the Black Female interviewer's choice to not categorize herself as part of this experience or to drop the cue of discrimination. Mr. T demonstrates willingness to explore this topic in exchange with a subsequent interviewer, suggesting that racial discrimination has had significant influence on retained memories. Findings that racial socialization is associated with positive adjustment and internalized Afrocentric identities to negative adjustment to life in predominantly White Universities for Black students (Anglin and Wade 2007) may suggest a possible reluctance to accept discrimination as a common theme in the discussion.

Mr. T's choice to not insist on retrieving his version of this memory of the past may be tied to his positioning of his perceptions of the gender or younger age of his listener, or perhaps to positioning himself as a willing speech partner not wanting to invoke conflict. In Line 147, the Black Female interviewer sets the final course for control of the discussion with the observation of preference, "*It'd be a lot better now,*" a choice that positions them away from a particular disadvantaged past. Her choice to change topic in Line 149 and ask about "*What were your parents like?*" represents a particular challenge to Mr. T. as a PWD; she asks him to choose a neutral biographical topic of a past with less turmoil and asks him for difficult retrieval that will challenge his memory far more than the recall of a history over which he had triumphed. Limited somewhat by a dependency on laboratory exercises rather than community-based observations, theorists of positioning in the social identity theory of intergroup relations point out that there has been a lack of attention to dynamics in interaction, how histories affect people in practice, and differences in power relations (Tan and Moghaddam 1999). Though Extract 5 is a same-race pair, their participation as an intergenerational dyad does not position them as sharing a common history yet a story of discrimination receives a different reception, a contradiction that may or may not be influenced by differing politeness norms by gender.

In the next selection, Mr. T. speaks of another episode of discrimination with a young White Male Interviewer in a slightly longer segment that reflects somewhat differing speaking practices that resulted in a longer narrative and more discussion of discrimination. The presentation demonstrates yet again that social identities are multiple and that variations in talk cannot be reduced to race alone.

Extract 6: Black Male PWD with White Male Interviewer

357: Mr. T: When he say “sleet, you in trouble, now.”
358: I say, "My name is not Sleet, my name is Sergeant X____ .”
359: And, put me in the back and told me,
360: "You go in the back and stay, until it start raining.”
361: I went back there, had my gun right there.
362: W-Int: Uh huh.
363: Mr. T: I start thinking… I better get out of here.
364: W-Int: Yeah. Yeah.
365: Mr. T: And, I took off and got through that mountain
366: and looked around trying to find a place to turn around and come back.
367: W-Int: Uh huh.
368: Mr. T: I couldn't.
369: W-Int: Uh huh.
370: Mr. T: And, a big eighteen wheeler passed by me and parked,
371: come out and he told me, say, "Sarge, you in trouble, huh?"
372: I say, "Yes, I am." He say, "Follow me and my lights."
373: And, we got to a place putting it in park,
and he say, uh, "You want a drink?"
374: I say, "Yeah." I gave him the money, he went in there and got a drink.
375: I gave him money to get another drink,
376: and he say, "I see you been to Korea, and I was in Korea."
377: W-Int: Uh huh.
378: Mr. T: He say, "It's a shame that we can't go in the bar together."
379: So, that just go to show you that everybody is not bad,
because of your (overlap)
380: W-Int: Right. (overlap)
381: Mr. T: color. You know.
382: W-Int: Right. Right. Right.

383: Mr. T: Yeah.
384: W-Int: Yeah, you have your good ones.
385:Mr. T: You got your good and you got your bad.
386: W-Int: You sure do.
387: Mr. T: But, you got more bad in the White than you have good,
388: because if it wasn't, we'd be more closer,
389: but they think they can go get them drugs and stuff
390: for you to use to keep everything confused.
391: W-Int: Yep. Yep.
392: Mr. T: Because, if they didn't,
393: if we'd loved each other and do what we supposed to do,
394: we'd be the most powerful nationality in the world.
395: W-Int: Yeah.
396: Mr. T: To do everything.
397: W-Int: You're right. Yeah.
[*Discussion continues]*

Summarizing from the entire transcription, this episode opens as Mr. T recalls an episode that occurred when he had been working as a truck driver over long distance. In Line 357, he uses reported speech to recount the threat of a White police officer who has stopped him on a mountain road where traffic has been backed up by weather. He recalls being singled out and sent to the end of the traffic line to wait behind other drivers, presumably White. With the policeman's comment, "*Sleet, you in trouble, now,*" Mr. T. positions himself in the account as not only a truck driver in bad weather, but a person singled out for an accusation. In Line 358, his correction and presentation of a full name asks for respect. This stance as a Black man who feels disrespected by a White policeman alludes to a social and cultural context that infers differences in power and threat that he has no way of knowing if a young White listener will understand. The prevailing pattern by White speakers in the US has been to deny racism exists through a variety of discourse practices, described in the use of exceptions, disclaimers, excuses for mitigation, blaming the victim, and other practices used to save face (van Dijk 1992). In Lines 359-360, Mr. T when sent to the back and told to stay there in reported speech, ends this portion of the narrative with Line 361, "*I went back there, had my gun right there.*"

As a dramatic device, the juxtaposition of gun possession in an account of weather positions the telling as a conflicted stance that requires agency in the face of trouble, but in a form where the category of societal membership one assumes may be considered trouble-making. The phrase "*had my gun right there*" ends with what is considered an indexical expression or words that signal a particular context considered a hierarchy of relevance to which the listener is compelled to respond (Lepper 2000, 40). From Lines 362-369, the White Male interviewer responds with a series of affirmatives and secondary prompts that function as support for active listening, as Mr. T. builds the narrative with the interviewer's scaffolding of first "*Uh-huh*" and then "*Yeah-yeah*" in Line 364, responding with affirmation to Mr. T's conclusion that he needed to "*get out of there*," acceptance of the common indexical ground. The succeeding elements of the story unfold because the White Male interviewer participates as an active and engaged listener, with a series of practices that signal attention, interest in the story, without defense, and that taken as a whole are consistent with shared context and shared information in listener behavior (Brown 1995, 217).

In Lines 370-376, Mr. T continues the narrative with a new character, another driver who sees him stopped and offers help. Though the truck is identified in Line 370, the person has no name or racial identity in direct categorizing. The driver's rationale for the use of "*Sarge*" in reported speech greeting in 371 is not made clear, whether he was present for the traffic stop and over-heard or in memory was identified by uniform or linked to Mr. T's self-categorizing with the police officer. Later, by inference in Line 378, the inability to go into a bar together for a drink in segregated times infers White racial identity for the second driver as indirect categorization. The indirect recall of the constructed social episode of drinking together outside a White establishment in Lines 374-375, precedes the direct report of the White driver establishing a shared social context in Line 376, in which they had both served in the Korean conflict. After the White university student prompts with the "*Uh-huh*" of listening, Mr. T in Line 378 presents the White driver's reported assessment, considered a representative utterance in pragmatics that commits the speaker to a type of truth or conclusion (Levinson 1983, 240). The White driver's reported statement that "*It's a shame that we can't go in the bar together,*" offers a different type of White person that Mr. T. summarizes in Line 379, with the idiom, "*So, that just go to show you...*" to draw a lesson about racial identity and differing types of White people in his memory. The White male interviewer's interruptions in Lines 380 and 382, with repetitions of "*Right!*" represent the type of interruption considered rapport-building in their support and affirmation of a story (Goldberg 1992).

In Line 384, the White Male interviewer for the first time in this sequence positions himself as part of Mr. T's dialogue, with "*You have your good ones...*", a sequence that Mr. T echoes and expands. The mirrored use of their shared pronoun "*you*" for two turns in the co-

constructed declaration exhibits the cooperative principle in pragmatics (Levinson 1983, 101), with shared assumptions about racial experience (Line 386). The next sequence raises potential trouble when Line 387 suggests, "*But, you got more bad in the White than you have good,*" a generalization from Lines 387-390 that could have been interpreted as accusation. The lack of defense from the White Male interviewer shows that he has not categorized himself in a White group that needs defending.

Yet the PWD tendency to overuse pronouns provides a deft use of shifting positioning and membership categorizing with the White listener to mediate potential trouble. First, Mr. T infers his White conversational partner's relationship to Whites with "*you*", then attributing potential shared relationship with "*we*" in Line 388, then positioning other Whites causing troubles with drugs in the Black community as "*they*", and with that pronoun positions his White listener as not part of the group being discussed. This shifting continues in Lines 390-394, ending with a shared "*we*" vision of shared nationality as Americans. The White Male interviewer affirms these ideological assessments in Line 397, with "*You're right. Yeah,*" in a subsequent discussion that lasts almost twice as long as the Black Female interviewer who did not pick up the cues offered in Mr. T's previous storytelling of discrimination. Rather than implying patterns related to race or gender in these different interactions, particular speech practices, attending to cues, and more active listening resulted in more engagement and participation in speaking by the PWD in this dyad.

Earlier in the transcript that precedes this next example, the young White Male interviewer has prompted discussion of tractors and farming with Mr. J, a White Male who is a PWD, using a picture on Mr.'s J's wall as a prompt. He accepts the categorization that Mr. J had been a farmer and offers shared membership as drivers who wrestle with gas prices, even though in differing historical periods.

Extract 7 – White Male PWD with White Male Interviewer

135: W-Int:	Well the way gas is now-a-days, as high as it is,
136:	it (uh) almost better to get animals to do everything anyway. (*Laughter*)
137: Mr. J:	Gas high, I hear. I don't know what it is a gallon [-] (uh)
138:	my brother tells me what it was but I forget.
139: W-Int:	Well I filled up my car yesterday and it was 3.66 a gallon.
140: Mr. J:	Whew! 3.66.
141: W-Int:	(um hm)
142: Mr. J:	(gah!) [-] I'm glad I don't have a car.
143: W-Int:	How much was it when you were driving around?
144: Mr. J:	(*Laughter*) (uh) [-] I believe around a 1.40.

145: W-Int: 1.40?
146: Mr. J: I believe that's what is …was, I'm not sure.
147: W-Int: The lowest I ever seen since I started driving was [-] about 2 I want to say,
148: I'll give it about 2.50 is the lowest I ever seen it and that's since I was sixteen
149: so seven years ago since I saw it that low.
150: Mr. J: It's been lower than that.
151: W-Int: Yeah.
152: Mr. J: Yeah.
[*Extended conversation follows*]

The opening Lines 135-136 offered by the White Male interviewer to Mr. J, a White PWD begins with the discourse marker "*Well*", followed by an indirect reflection on the price of gas and finishes by tying the topic to the picture of the farm on Mr. J's wall, as indicated by the referent to animals. As a discourse marker, the word "*Well*" can introduce a new context and send the listener the message that a new subject is being framed (Jucker 1993). In this case, it frames the high price of gas, a topic that Mr. J. takes up readily for reflection, perhaps more readily than a yes/no or direct question would produce. Mr. J affirms the gas price is high, though not remembering exactly in Line 137, and invokes his brother in Line 138 with "*my brother tells me what it was but I forget.*" The link with his brother is also a link to the family farm where his brother still lives, so links the speakers to the original prompt of conversation. The White interviewer does not challenge the challenged memory, but uses self-disclosure in Line 139 to announce he had filled his tank with an amount Mr. J. is able to take up in the next turn, marveling at the cost. The recognition of the offered cue and the ability to use it for more reflection shows evidence of the strategy of quilting (Moore and Davis 2002) that accommodates the PWD in their ability to participate. This approach prompts him first to joke in commiseration in Line 142, "*I'm glad I don't have a car*" and then to respond more easily to the interviewer's direct query for price in Line 144 with an amount considerably less decades earlier.

The White Male interviewer echoes the amount which continues a reflection, that is first repaired from a present tense to a past interrogative where memory falters in Line 146: "*I believe that's what is …was, I'm not sure.*" The interviewer continues the theme of low prices instead of picking up the cue of remembering, with two specific prices he has seen in a younger driving life that allows Mr. J to re-enter as a driver who remembers still lower prices in his own time. This gentle categorizing of shared membership as drivers who have faced gas prices and choices scaffolds their exchange beyond specific recall, reinforces their ability to communicate and extends the possibilities of conversation. Additionally, the same race pair share experience as drivers with details of self-disclosure. This type of sharing corresponds with positioning theory that portrays how people build positive positioning, in which they show a capacity, willingness, and power in interaction to position themselves and others similarly. This type of common positioning has been noted previously in people with Alzheimer's disease as a strategy that can transcend cognitive impairment (Howie 1999, 53).

In the last excerpt, Mr. J, a White PWD speaks with a young Black Male interviewer who prompts Mr. J similarly to reflect on his time living on the family farm. The sociologist Goffman described the concept of footing as a person's attempt to align or take a stance that invites a conversational partner to accept or respond to an utterance (Goffman 1981, 128). In contrast with the previous interaction, the ability of the speakers to connect falters because of Mr. J's lack of recognition of cues, unwillingness to take up offered cues or group memberships even when recognized, and continued corrections or qualifications that undermines the Black Male interviewer's attempts to seek a footing or position in the conversation.

Extract 8

53: B-Int:	And growing up on the farm?
54: Mr. J:	huh?
55: B-Int:	growing up on the farm
56: Mr. J:	yeah 85 years ago
57: B-Int:	That's a long time ago
58: Mr. J:	Yeah it is
59: B-Int:	W____ [location name] right?
60: Mr. J:	huh?
61: B-Int:	W____ [location name] right?
62: Mr. J:	yeah. Out in the country
63: B-Int:	that's nice
64: Mr. J:	not in the town
65: B-Int:	kinda out to yourself, not a whole lot of neighbors or anything
66: Mr. J:	well there were people around but none real close by
67: B-Int:	Yeah [*silence*]

[*Change of topic, shorter interview*]

In Line 53, the Black Male interviewer is also querying the picture of a farm on the wall with Mr J. With the response of "*Huh*?" in Line 54, Mr J does not take up the cue, whether from issues of comprehension or relevance cannot be interpreted. The young interviewer tries again with the same cue, positioning the topic and group membership, "*growing up on the farm*" in the past. Mr J's response in Line 56 "*yeah, 85 years ago*" distances Mr J from the past and the interviewer, as he positions himself in the present. The discourse marker, "*yeah*" also can be used to raise contention or disaffiliation rather than agreement (Koole 2003), as it does in this case. The Black interviewer's attempt at agreement that it was indeed long ago does not produce engagement or reflection, but instead finds Mr J ending the topic with the "*Yeah it is*" in Line 58, a second dismissal as a discourse marker by the PWD.

In Line 59, the interviewer tries again with a referent to the name of the area or place Mr J grew up. Once again, Mr J responds with a "Huh?" in Line 60, a discourse marker in repetition that can signal a lack of attentiveness or willingness to recognize a conversational partner that a speaker/listener has positioned as the Other (Bolden 2006). In Line 62, Mr J admits to living in the referent place, but modifies it as being "*out in the country*", a modifier that suggests they do not share the same concept of the place or indexical ground. When the young Black interviewer offers an affirmation in Line 63 that the place is "*nice*," Mr J. does not take up the cue but counters with an inferred correction that they did not live in the town for which the young man has offered the affirmation. The attempt in Line 65 to prompt Mr J to reflect once more, "*kinda out to yourself, not a whole lot of neighbors or anything*" receives another modified observation and no subsequent detail from Mr J, as the interviewer ends his attempt at the topic. This episode corresponds in sociopragmatics to the concept of misunderstanding when trying to create a situational context in conversation (Tzanne 2000, 85-125), an example of miscommunication that finds participants in conversation speaking in cross-purposes.

3. Conclusion

Reviews of discourse frameworks that consider intercultural and interracial communication include the Anxiety/Uncertainty Management (AUM) theory proposed by Gudykunst (1995) and Communication Accommodation Theory (CAT) as described by Gallois and colleagues (1988). The examples selected for these comparisons capture instances that seem to exemplify both theoretical approaches. In three of the four members of same-race dyads, conversational partners in the presented dyads provide illustrations of particular linguistic devices whether as speakers or listeners that signaled approval, desire for more information exchange that drew members closer, used speech practices that inferred group membership, demonstrated attention to speaker intentions, and clarified communication with narrative building quilting, consistent with CAT (van Dijk 1997). The exception can be seen in Extracts 3 and 4, where the young White Male interviewer demonstrates more willingness to accommodate and encourage a narrative concerning the lived experience of discrimination than the young Black Female interviewer.

Members of differing race dyads seemed more likely to exhibit discourse practices more consistent with AUM, where feelings of awkwardness or discomfort in participation with a person perceived as different by race may contribute to disaffiliation linked to uncertainty, anxiety, less willingness to exchange and concern about face (van Dijk 1997, 162-163). In these interactions, participants seemed more likely to infer or express disbelief, to not recognize conversational cues as readily, or to request person-based information in forms more difficult for PWD to provide. The potential of social habitus to contribute to difficulties in social interaction beyond the awareness or identified intentions of speakers (Bonilla-Silva 2006) may play a role in the practices observed in these dyads. The potential for this selection of speaking practices to contribute to patterns of engagement and participation with PWD when race, gender and generation may play a role requires further study. The practices that promote engagement and active listening can be taught, potentially leading to more sensitive care of PWD. Sociopragmatics could provide a significant lead in this necessary area of investigation, using membership categorization analysis to show how speakers invoke, maintain, or resist the situated meanings of categories (Stokoe 2012), as a method to systematically structure monoracial and interracial comparisons.

References

Almor, Almit; Kempler ,Daniel; MacDonald, Maryellen; Andersen, Elaine; and Tyler, Lorraine. 1999. "Why Do Alzheimer's Patients have Difficulty with Pronouns? Working Memory, Semantics, And Reference in Comprehension and Production with Alzheimer's Disease." *Brain and Language*, 67: 202-227.

Anglin, Deidre and Wade, Jay. 2007, "Racial Socialization, Racial Identity, and Black Students Adjustment to College." *Cultural Diversity and Ethnic Minority Psychology*, 13: 207-215.

Bailey, Guy; Baugh, John; Mufwene, Salikoko; and Rickford, John. 1998. *African American English: Structure, History, and Use.* New York: Routledge.

Blake, John. 2013. "I Was an Affirmative Action 'Imposter'." *CNN-US Online,* July 2, 2013. Taken from the Internet (7/12/2013): http://www.cnn.com/2013/07/02/us/imposter-affirmative-action

Blommaert, Jan. 1991. "How Much Culture Is There in Intercultural Communication?" In *The Pragmatics of Intercultural and International Communication*, edited by Jan Blommaert and Jef Verschueren, 13-32. Benjamins Publishing Company.

Bonilla-Silva, Eduardo; Goar, Carla; and Embrick, David. 2006. "When Whites Flock Together: The Social Psychology of White Habitus." *Critical Sociology* 32: 229-253.

Bolden, Gina. 2006. "Little Words that Matter: Discourse Markers "So" and "Oh" and the Doing of Other-Attentiveness in Social Interaction." *Journal of Communication*, 56: 661–688.

Bourdieu, Pierre. 1977. *Outline of a Theory of Practice*. Cambridge, UK: Cambridge University Press.

—. 1990. *The Logic of Practice.* Translated by Richard Nice. Stanford, CA: Stanford University Press.

Brown, Gillian. 1995. *Speakers, Listeners, and Communication: Explorations in Discourse Analysis.* Cambridge, UK: Cambridge University Press.

Clark, Herbert and Fox Tree, Jean E. 2002. "Using *Uh* and *Um* in Spontaneous Speaking." *Cognition,* 84, 73-111.

Coulmas, Florian. 2005. *Sociolinguistics: The Study of Speakers' Choices.* Cambridge, UK: Cambridge University Press.

Crisp, Richard and Hewstone, Miles (Editors). 2006. *Multiple social Categorizations: Processes, models and applications.* NY: Psychology Press,.

Cukor-Avila, Patricia. 2002. "*She Say, She Go, She Be Like:* Verbs of quotation over time in African American Vernacular English." *American Speech,* 77: 3-31.

Davies, Catherine Evans. 2007. "Language and Identity in Discourse in the American South: Sociolinguistic Repertoire as Expressive Resource in the Presentation of Self." In *Selves and Identities in Narrative and Discourse*, edited by Michael Bamberg, Anna de Fina, and Deborah Schiffrin, 71-88. Amsterdam, NE: John Benjamins Publishing Company.

Derber, Charles. 2000. *The Pursuit of Attention: Power and Ego in Everyday Life,* 2nd ed. Oxford, UK: Oxford University Press.

Dodson, Lisa and Zincavage, Rebekah. 2007. "It's Like a Family: Caring Labor, Exploitation and Race in Nursing Homes." *Gender and Society,* 21: 905-928.

Edwards, Derek. 1998. "The Relevant Thing about Her: Social Identity Categories in Use, in *Identities in Talk,* edited by Charles Antaki and Sue Widdicombe, 15-33. London, UK: Sage Publications.

Fix, Sonya. 2010. "Representations of Blackness by White Women: Linguistic Practice in the Community versus the Media." *University of Pennsylvania Working Papers in Linguistics,*16: Article 8. Taken from the Internet (7/10/13): http://repository.upenn.edu/pwpl/vol16/iss2/8/

Gallois, Cynthia; Franklyn-Stokes, Arlene; Giles, Howard; and Coupland, Nikolas. 1988. "Communication Accommodation Theory and Intercultural Encounters." In *Theories in Intercultural Communication*, edited by Young Kun Kim and William Gudykundst, 157-185. Newbury Park, CA: Sage Publications.

Gandy, Oscar H. Jr. 1998. *Communication and Race: A Structural Perspective.* NY: Arnold/Oxford University Press.

Goffman, Erving. 1981. *Forms of Talk.* Philadelphia, PA: University of Pennsylvania Press.

Goldberg, Julia. 1990. "Interrupting the Discourse on Interruptions: An Analysis in Terms of Relationally Neutral, Power- and Rapport-Oriented Acts." *Journal of Pragmatics*, 14: 883-903.

Gudykunst, William. 1995. "Anxiety/Uncertainty Management (AUM) Theory: Current Status." In *Intercultural Communication Theory,* edited by Richard Wiseman, 8-58. Thousand Oaks, CA: Sage Publications.

Hamilton, Heidi. 2008. "Language and Dementia: Sociolinguistic Aspects." *Annual Review of Linguistics,* 28: 91-110.

Harré, Rom and van Langenhove, Luk (Eds.). 1999. *Positioning Theory.* Oxford, UK: Blackwell Publishers.

Harwood, Jake. 2007. *Understanding Communication and Aging.* Thousand Oaks, CA: Sage Publications.

Hazen, Kirk. 2002. "Identity and Language Variation in a Rural Community." *Language,* 78: 240-257.

Heritage, John. 2005. "Cognition in Discourse." In *Conversation and Cognition*, edited by Hedwig te Molder and Jonathan Potter, 184-202. Cambridge, UK: Cambridge University Press.

Holt, Elizabeth. 1996. "Reporting on Talk: The Use of Direct Report in Conversation." *Research on Language and Social Interaction*, 29: 219-245.

Howie, D. 1999. "Preparing for Positive Positioning." In *Positioning Theory,* edited by Rom Harré and Luk Van Langenhove, 53-59. Oxford, UK: Blackwell Publishers.

Jackson, Jacquelyne Johnson and Ensley, Donald. 1995. "Minority Elders Really Aren't All Alike." In *Communication in Older Life,* edited by Ruth Huntley and Karen Helfer, 127-156. Boston, MA: Butterworth-Heinemann.

Johnson, E. Patrick. 2003. *Appropriating Blackness: Performance and the Politics of Authenticity.* Durham, NC: Duke University Press.

Joo, Jin Hui; Wittink, Marsha; and Dahlberg, Britt. 2011. Shared Conceptualizations and Divergent Experiences of Counseling Among African American and White Older Adults. *Qualitative Health Research,* 21: 1065-74. doi: 10.1177/104973231140424

Jucker, Andreas. 1993. "The Discourse Marker *Well:* A Relevance-Theoretical Account." *Journal of Pragmatics*, 19: 435-452.

Kecskes, Istvan. "2012. Sociopragmatics and Cross-Cultural and Intercultural Studies." In The Cambridge Handbook of Pragmatics, edited by Keith Allen and Kasia Jasczholt, 599-616. Cambridge, UK: Cambridge University Press.

Koole, Tom. 2003. "Affiliation and Detachment in Interviewer Answer Receipts." In *Analyzing Race Talk: Multidisciplinary Approaches to the Interview,* edited by Harry van den Berg; Margaret Wetherell; and Hanneke Houtkoop-Steenstra, 178-199.. Cambridge: Cambridge University Press.

Levinson, Steven. *Pragmatics.* Cambridge, UK: Cambridge University Press, 1983/2011.

Lewis, Amanda. 2003. "Everyday Race-Making: Navigating Racial Boundaries In Schools." *American Behavioral Scientist,* 47: 283-305.

Manly, Jennifer and Mayeux, Richard. 2004 . "Ethnic Differences in Dementia And Alzheimer's Disease." In *Critical Perspectives On Racial Differences In Health In Late Life,* edited by Norman Anderson; Rodolfo Bulatao; and Barney Cohen, 95-138. National Research Council (US) Panel on Race, Ethnicity, and Health in Later Life. Washington, DC: National Academies Press,.

McGarty, Craig. 2006. "Hierarchies and Minority Groups: The Roles of Saliences, Overlap, and Background Knowledge in Selecting Meaningful Categorizations from Multiple Alternatives." In *Multiple Social Categorizations: Processes, models and applications* edited by Richard Crisp and Miles Hewstone, 25-49. NY: Psychology Press,.

Moore, Linda and Davis, Boyd. 2002. "Quilting Narrative: Using Repetition Techniques to Help Elderly Communicators." *Geriatric Nursing,* 23: 262-266.

Orbe, Mark and Harris, Tina. 2008. *Interracial Communication: Theory into Practice.* Thousand Oaks, CA: Sage Publications.

Omi, Michael and Winant, Howard. 1994. *Racial Formation in The United States: From the 1960's to the 1990's*. 2nd ed. NY: Routledge.

Pope, Charlene and Davis, Boyd. 2011. "Finding A Balance: The Carolinas Conversations Collection." *Corps Linguistics and Linguistic Theory,* 7: 143–161.

Pope, Charlene and Ripich, Danielle. 2005. "Speak to Me, Listen to Me: Ethnic and Gender Variations in Talk and Potential Consequences in Interactions for People with Alzheimer's Disease." In *Alzheimer Talk, Text, and Context: Enhancing Communication,* edited by Boyd Davis, 37-59. NY: Palgrave Macmillan.

Ripich, Danielle; Fritsch, Thomas; and Ziol, Elaine. 2002. Everyday Problem Solving in African Americans and European Americans with Alzheimer's Disease. *International Psychogeriatrics,* 14: 83-95.

Schegloff, Emanuel. 2007. "A Tutorial on Membership Categorization." *Journal of Pragmatics,* 39:462-482.

Scheibman, Joanne. 2007. "Subjective and Intersubjective Uses of Generalizations In English Conversations." In *Stancetaking in Discourse,* edited by Robert Englebretson, 111-138. Amsterdam/ Philadelphia: John Benjamins Publishing Company.

Schiffrin, Deborah. 1988. *Discourse Markers.* Cambridge, UK: Cambridge University Press.

Scollon, Ron; Scollon, Suzanne Wong; and, Jones, Rodney. 2012. *Intercultural Communication: A Discourse Approach*, 3rd edition. Malden, MA: Wiley-Blackwell.

Silverman, David. 1998. *Harvey Sacks: Social Science and Conversation Analysis.* New York: Oxford University Press.

Smith, Erin; Broughton, Megan; Baker, Rosemary; Pachana, Nancy; Angwin, Anthony; Humphreys, Michael; Mitchell, Leander; Byrne, Gerald; Copland, David; Gallois; Cindy, Hegney, Desley; and Cherey, Helen. 2011. "Memory and Communication Support in Dementia: Research Strategies for Caregivers." *International Psychogeriatrics,* 23: 256-263.

Stokoe, Elizabeth. 2012. "Moving Forward with Membership Categorization Analysis: Methods for Systematic Analysis." *Discourse Studies,* 14: 2-77-303.

Strausbaugh, John. 2006. *Black Like You: Blackface, Whiteface, Insult and Imitation in American Popular Culture.* NY: Penguin Books.

Thomas, Erik. 2007. "Phonological and Phonetic Characteristics Of African American Vernacular English." *Language and Linguistics Compass,* 1: 450–475. doi:10.1111/j.1749-818x.2007.00029.x

Thomas., Erik and Reaser, Jeffrey. 2004. "Delimiting Perceptual Cues Used for the Ethnic Labeling of African American and European American Voices." *Journal of Sociolinguistics,* 8: 54-87. doi:10.1111/j.1467-9841.2004.00251.x

Toosi, Negin; Ambady, Nalini; Babbitt, Laura; and Sommers, Samuel. 2012. "Dyadic Interracial Interactions: A Meta-Analysis." *Psychological Bulletin*: 138, 1-27.

Tzanne, Angeliki. 2000. *Talking at Cross-Purposes*: *The Dynamics of Miscommunication.* Amsterdam/Philadelphia: John Benjamins Publishing Company.

van den Berg, Harry; Wetherell, Margaret; and Houtkoop-Steenstra, Hanneke (Eds.). 2003. *Analyzing Race Talk: Multidisciplinary Approaches to the Interview.* Cambridge: Cambridge University Press.

van Dijk, Teun. 1992. "Discourse and the Denial of Racism." *Discourse and Society* 3:87-118.

Vasse, Emmelyne; Vernooij-Dassen, Myrra; Spijker, Anouk; Olde Rikkert, Marcel; and Koopmans, Raymond. 2010. "A Systematic Review of Communication Strategies for People with Dementia in Residential And Nursing Homes." *International Psychogeriatrics,* 22: 189-200.

Wolfram, Walt. 2004. "The Grammar of Urban African American Vernacular English." In *Handbook of Varieties of English* edited by Bernd Kormann and Edgar Schneider, 111-132. Berlin: Mouton de Gruyter.

Wolfram, Walt. 2003. "Language Variation in the American South." *American Speech,* 78: 123-129

Xue, Steve An; Neeley, Richard; Hagstrom, Fran; and Hao, Jianping. 2001. "Speaking F_0 Characteristics of Elderly Euro-American and African-American Speakers: Building a Clinical Comparative Platform." *Clinical Linguistics and Phonetics,* 15: 245-252. doi:10.1080/026992001300054856

CHAPTER FOUR

'AW, SO, HOW'S YOUR DAY GOING?': WAYS THAT PERSONS WITH DEMENTIA KEEP THEIR CONVERSATIONAL PARTNER INVOLVED

BOYD DAVIS
UNC CHARLOTTE
MARGARET MACLAGAN
U CANTERBURY
AND JULIE COOK
UNC CHARLOTTE

Abstract

Interpersonal pragmatics deals with the role of language in relational work, specifically how "social actors use language to form relationships in situ" (Locher & Graham 2010, 1), making it a good framework for the examination of key features in discourse between persons with dementia (PWD) and their unimpaired interlocutors. The progression of dementia curtails verbal communication in several ways: the ability to access words and story components diminishes, as does the ability to process conversation and respond to others. However, over much of the course of the disease, the PWD wants to communicate, and to be seen as responsive, even competent. With some speakers, repetition of stories and story fragments becomes a shorthand way of signaling memory and emotion (Davis 2011; Schiff. 2005); with others, extenders and pauses allow a PWD to involve the conversation partner in completing a sentence or a story (Fox Tree and Schrock 2002; Davis & Maclagan 2009; Maclagan, Davis and Lunsford 2008). Many PWD draw on a repertoire that includes extenders, pauses and formulaic utterances: here, we look at their association with head nods and gestures in video-recordings of "Maureen

Littlejohn." By adding the analysis of head nods (Aoki 2011; Stivers 2008), we better identify what embodied interpersonal skills the speaker retains as her impairment increases.

Introduction

Taking a multimodal perspective on the pragmatics of interpersonal or intercultural relationships allows us to better understand the dynamics of interaction between two conversationalists, especially when one of them is cognitively impaired. By a multimodal perspective, we mean that we consider gestures, facial expressions, body posture, and eventually prosody as well as initiation and maintenance techniques such as turn taking and topic shading, and speech content. All of these are part of conversation with someone with dementia.

In this discussion, we examine a set of video-recorded interactions and analyze head nods, hand gestures, speech content and style, looking particularly closely at how "Maureen Littlejohn" (pseudonym) a person with dementia (PWD) works to keep her unimpaired interlocutors interested in reminiscences about the importance of apples in her childhood. Her primary techniques, which we hear also in the fifteen audio-only conversations with her, include telling her stories as well as possible, with few repairs, enthusiastic intonation, and self-commentary, so that she sounds competent; introducing her own topics which will let her perform a story; and avoiding anything with which she cannot associate a ready, handy rehearsed narrative or narrative fragment. When she can no longer add another fragment to her narrative, she falls back on asking the listener "Aw, so, how's your day going?" This phatic utterance, a form of "small talk", (Boxer 2002) does not expect voluminous self-disclosure or awkward questions in response from her conversational partners, and she can then try to find a way to include another of her stories in the discussion.

According to her family, Ms Littlejohn has always been known as someone who tells interesting stories. As long as she can find a way to hook one of her practiced stories into the conversation, she does not seem to need to work at keeping her conversation partner involved. Her stories are repeated across conversation partners, and more recently within the one conversation. She often uses phrases like "as I've just said" which sound like an apology for this repetition. Analysis of linguistic features such as repetition of key words, use of extenders, phrasal verbs and filled pauses, allows us to see the formulaic nature of her stories. Multimodal analysis of her gestures allows us to distinguish which features of her conversations are directed at her conversational partners, and which sections, no matter how other oriented they may sound, are actually directed at herself.

Ms Littlejohn has lived in a secure memory care unit in a retirement village for several years and has just moved to a new village. Staff in such units usually expect people with dementia to have highly impaired communication skills and do not therefore expect to be able to engage them in meaningful conversation (Davis and Pope 2010). Ms Littlejohn was more communicatively fluent than the other people in the first unit she lived in, a fact that was often commented on by the staff. She is more communicatively fluent than her room-mate in her new village. For someone like Ms Littlejohn, low staff expectations mean that she receives little communicative stimulation in her daily interactions, and she chooses to stay in her room most of the time, rather than mix with the other residents.

In the terms developed by Gubrium for his masterful study of Murray Manor (Gubrium 1975), Ms Littlejohn has chosen to be socially isolated from most of the "network of social ties and avoidances" (107) inside both of her residences. She is not part of an "alertness clique" that gathers to chat after breakfast, or read a section of the morning paper, though she is slightly annoyed by the low level of alertness of her roommate at the new residence. She does not join groups of residents in complaining about the aides or in discussing toileting aches and pains to pass the time (see Chapter 5), and has not shown any inclination to develop friendships or to offer support to another resident. In her previous residence, staff told us that they had learned to leave her alone, that she wanted to read and listen to music and, while friendly enough at mealtimes with staff and residents, and willing to take walks with staff, she did not consider herself to be like the others and did not want to be with them. Many people in retirement communities distance themselves from people who appear to have memory problems (Williams and Guendouzi 2000) and Ms Littlejohn is not unusual in her desire to remain aloof, even after having been moved to a memory care unit.

It is too soon to tell if she feels as different from the others in her new residence: she was far more verbal and more fluent than the residents in her previous residence but that situation may change if her own abilities decrease. Given the continued emphasis on task-focused care as opposed to patient-centered care as reported in the ethnographic study by McLean (2006) over twenty years later than Gubrium's work, staff may actually be comfortable with leaving her in relative isolation. She has weekly visits from family, does not like television, and her relatives assert that she makes no trouble for staff, something that is corroborated by the staff.

In this chapter, we first provide background on the language of people with cognitive impairment. We then use stories about apples from conversations with Ms Littlejohn to illustrate the repetitive, formulaic nature of apparently fluent speech from a PWD who is still able to keep the casual listener interested in her stories. Finally we examine her apple stories and illustrate her combination of speech and gestures for one such story.

Interpersonal/intercultural Pragmatics and Cognitive Impairment

The study of Alzheimer's discourse involves both social and cognitive aspects of interpersonal pragmatics (Davis 2010), for which study the researcher can draw on the clinical and discourse literatures as well as what Ainsworth-Vaughn (1998) calls the praxis literature, which together examine specific patient outcomes in response to various communications interventions. As researchers expand their analyses of the range of pragmatic abilities retained by persons with dementia across the course of the condition, they can develop interventions designed to further facilitate their conversation and their co-construction of narrative-in-interaction. Studies that examine PWD's retained abilities may be particularly suitable for planning interventions because they indicate the conversational levels achieved by many PWD. Woods et al. (2012) reviewed interventions that present some form of cognitive stimulation (which can include conversation and memory stimulation, usually in small groups) and showed that they do, indeed, provide some benefits. In addition, studies that emphasize what is retained and manipulated by PWD may contribute to studies of listener expectations about speaker competencies, as well as to acquisition and loss of particular language features. This is particularly important in that the very institutions in which PWD live often impose lowered expectations on residents. The residents are cared for, but not expected to be fluent or coherent conversationalists (Davis and Pope 2010).

We follow Locher and Langlotz (2008) in assuming that pragmatics allows the examination of relational, affective, and emotional signaling in addition to informational content. Relational work is itself placed "at the intersection of cognition, interaction and emotion" (Locher and Langlotz 2008, 165) in that "the display of emotional states allows the interactants to signal their evaluation of both the transactional state of the shared practice as well as the ongoing linguistic negotiation of their social relationship" (176). Such a definition accords with the recent explanation of sociopragmatics as an approach, which Aijmer and Andersen (2010, 2-3) explain as incorporating interactional sociolinguistics, linguistic anthropology, variational pragmatics, as well as conversation analysis from an "ethnomethodological perspective" (p. 3), corpus linguistics, sociophonetics and critical discourse analysis. The examination of interaction with PWD allows us to identify which features of practice are retained and thereby infer their stability.

Relational aspects of language use are conveyed by lexicon, syntax and phonology (Locher and Graham 2010, 3); we add that gestures are part of the way people signal their identity or negotiate relationships in interaction. With a multimodal lens, we can begin to grapple anew with issues of whether and how PWD might construct the relational: can they, for example, initiate and manage rapport, which is how Spencer-Oatey (2011) begins her discussion of relational work. She sees rapport, a term she prefers to relational work, as being "subjective perceptions of disharmony, smoothness-turbulence and warmth-antagonism in interpersonal relations" (Spencer-Oatey 2011, 3567). Davis and Maclagan (2013 in press) discuss how alignment between speakers can give rise to the establishment of such rapport. Aspects of speaker alignment are often described in terms of language accommodation or as the result of grounding in which "interlocutors provide evidence of their understanding e.g., attentiveness, eye contact and seek this type of evidence from their conversation partner" (Riordan et al. 2011, 2411). Often, this alignment and its rapport are accomplished through small talk, which is also referred to as phatic communication. Coupland (2003, 4) comments that "in small talk, relational issues are paramount." Its emphasis on safe topics and ritual exchanges allows speakers to establish shared alignments. Padilla Cruz (2007, 118) comments that phatic utterances have social importance and convey information "about the politeness system in which interlocutors carry out social interaction." They account for the power and social distance displayed via solidarity, deference and hierarchical variables, as discussed by Scollon et al. (2012). With phatic communication, speakers can signal and also infer social communication needs, as explained by Davidson et al. (2008) for aphasic speakers. Video recordings of conversation partners, one of whom had aphasia, showed the pleasure of initiating social interaction and extending relational goals, finding connectedness and the reaffirmation of social bonds.

As they are frequently conceived to be unable to take the perspective of the other conversant and furnish needed information, an extended analysis through the lens of interpersonal pragmatics may give us real-world examples of what the PWD can or cannot do. Bara (2011, 452), for example, in a discussion of intentionality in pragmatics, comments that "the impairment in understanding others' intentions exhibited by paranoid patients and autistic patients can be considered as the two extremes of a continuum." Our analysis of Ms Littlejohn indicates that she is at neither end of this continuum. While she can no longer fully understand others' intentions, her interaction, and especially her gestures, indicate that she is still well aware of her interactants and the pragmatic requirements of conversations, such as turn-taking and some degree of topic maintenance.

Characteristics of Dementia-compromised Speech and Interaction

Almost any discussion of communication with PWD will include the following challenges over time as their condition advances, listed in a recent Alzheimer's Association brochure:

> Difficulty finding the right words. Using familiar words repeatedly. Inventing new words to describe familiar things. Easily losing train of thought. Difficulty organizing words logically. Reverting to speaking in a native language. Using curse words. Speaking less often. *Relying on gestures more than speaking.*
>
> (Alzheimer's Association, 2012, our italics).

We have used this reference because of its emphasis to a lay readership on using gesture to compensate for the lessened ability to produce coherent speech, an emphasis which we think warrants further study, as discussed below.

As the disease progresses, working memory is reduced; domains in which people enjoy talking are similarly reduced, as well as the ability to handle referentiality. The following are affected: memory, language, perceptual skills, attention, orientation, problem solving, and functional abilities of daily living. Singh et al. (2001, 1) note the presence of "difficulties with word-finding, decreased verbal fluency, increased paraphasic errors, circumlocutory speech due to anomia, and general impairments of discourse, all of which worsen over the course of the disease." In addition, as short-term memory becomes increasingly compromised, many PWD become increasingly uncomfortable talking about recent events that they cannot have rehearsed as often, and prefer to return to earlier memories that are still available for access.

Over the last two decades, a number of researchers have moved from a clinical, largely deficit perspective to incorporating sociolinguistic features in their analyses (Hamilton 1994, Ramanathan 1997, Davis 2005). This has led to a number of studies by linguists, clinical linguists, communications specialists, and clinicians (Davis 2010) expanding and in some cases challenging earlier clinical findings and assumptions. For example, the increase in "empty speech" noted as a characteristic of moderate and severe Alzheimer's is now seen as referring only to semantic content. It is now acknowledged that PWD can still interact even when their speech is apparently "empty." As Schiffrin (2001, 65) noted with respect to filled pauses,

> even vocalizations that are themselves semantically empty can provide an option within a set of paradigmatic choices that includes semantically meaningful markers…. Thus, vocalizations that have no inherent meaning at all, and that occur elsewhere for very different reasons … can also provide markers through which to structure discourse (for a parallel argument about gestures, see Kendon 1995).

Extenders "and stuff like that", pauses, and filled pauses are similarly semantically empty, but play multiple functions in Alzheimer talk. In its earlier stages, PWD use extenders like unimpaired speakers, usually as part of a list of objects or actions, and can retrieve or refer to other components in the list (Jefferson 1990). As the disease progresses, however, while PWD continue to use extenders, they typically produce only the first item of the list followed by the extender and depend on their unimpaired conversation partner to finish the list. The use of the extender stimulates a regular flow of expression, and keeps the unimpaired speaker "involved with the larger effort of co-constructing meaning and understanding" (Maclagan et al. 2008, 185).

We have found changes in the functions for pauses as the condition progresses. In mild dementia pauses signal difficulty in finding words as they do for non-impaired persons. As dementia progresses, PWD tend to lose the gist of their stories, and pauses signal problems in finding key components in the thread of the story (Davis and Maclagan 2009). In addition to buying time for location of key elements, PWD also use pauses for social interaction as part of a repertoire of compensatory language behaviors (Davis and Maclagan 2010).

The ability to initiate and maintain topics diminishes as the disease continues: Mentis, Briggs-Whittaker and Graminga (1995) find that PWD grow less able to maintain topics or to contribute new propositions to a topic. Garcia and Joanette (1997) note that problems with coherence and relevance interfere with ample topic development and topic shift. That is, given increasing problems with memory and pragmatics, "they would have problems holding propositional information in memory and searching for information which may make a shift in conversational topic relevant" (Garcia and Joanette 1997, 96). However, a number of researchers have identified preserved features of topic and of retained self-identity, well into the disease (Orange and Purves 1996), with PWD using a number of compensatory techniques that can support collaboration in conversation and in narrative. In particular, some PWD rely "on a schema, an already familiar path that provides the speaker with a sort of recipe for the ideas to be verbalized and the order in which to verbalize them" (Chafe 2008, 28-9). Such schema often crystallize around familiar stories that PWD have shared with family members and others. PWD can become adept at working these story/schema into interactions, often adjusting them slightly so they fit into the current context (Davis 2011). When PWD find it difficult to answer questions, they can often segue into one of their story schema and so continue as a partner in the conversation.

Maureen Littlejohn's Speech Characteristics

In this analysis we focus on interactions with "Maureen Littlejohn" who was born in 1929 and was close to 80 when the conversations analyzed here started. She lives in a secure memory care unit of an assisted living residence. Between October 2008 and November 2012, we have twenty-five recordings of her conversations either with student volunteers or with the researchers. Approval for the recordings was granted by the IRB at the University of North Carolina-Charlotte. Formal permission for both audio and video recording was obtained from Ms Littlejohn's niece and from Ms Littlejohn herself. The recordings average approximately 20 minutes each for a total of roughly 455 minutes. At the start of our interactions with her, Ms Littlejohn was in the mild stage of dementia and able to hold a relatively normal conversation with students. By the end of 2012, she was moving into the moderate stage of dementia, and her conversational ability was more compromised. In particular, she found it difficult to introduce a new topic into the conversation. By preference, she would resume a story she had told earlier in the session often with variations from the earlier telling, segue into a new story or ask a question of her conversation partner in order to keep their interest. Even though both the volunteer students and the researchers visited Ms Littlejohn multiple times in any given academic semester, it was not on a daily basis. We cannot therefore presume that she necessarily remembered any of the interactants. In essence, everyone had to reform a social relationship at each visit and renegotiate interpersonal stances toward each other.

Ms Littlejohn is highly fluent in certain domains that are of interest to her, as long as she is directing the conversation by asking questions of the unimpaired partner, or telling stories as she associates them with some feature of a previous topic. She gracefully dismisses or evades topics about which she does not have some sort of ready-to-go story-chunk or schema reflecting an incident from her past. In fact, Ms Littlejohn is so well versed at incorporating such schema that it would be difficult, were it not for the context of the physical setting, to mark her as being impaired if one were to only have a single, short interaction with her. It is not until one analyzes details of her language production or interacts with her on a regular basis that one sees how much of her discourse is comprised of her stories which are made up of formulaic utterances: colloquialisms, idioms, phrasal verbs, and idiosyncratic phrases she repeats, as shown in Fig. 4-1 on page 94. In addition, within the one conversation, she has begun to repeat narratives she enjoys telling, given her smiles and nods when she presents them, and small stories (Georgakopoulou, 2006a; b) that may well be parts of earlier rehearsed narratives.

If Ms Littlejohn feels that her interactant is not really engaged in the conversation or is not listening closely, signaling such by gaze, head nods or backchannels (see Stivers 2008), she is more likely to ask questions and less likely to try to introduce a new story fragment. Overall, in her earlier conversations, Ms Littlejohn tends to say less and produce less complex language with volunteers who do not expect her to be a particularly good partner (Davis and Maclagan 2013 in press) and her standard phatic question "Aw, so, how's your day going?" appears more often in such interviews. As dementia progresses, we expect to see more of such questions. For the present analysis, we focus on stories Ms Littlejohn produced about apples.

The apple stories discussed here are only one set of Ms Littlejohn's repeated stories. Across all 20 conversations, she repeats several stories and accounts: accounts of how she and her sister made mountain crafts; how she had worked in health services as a radiologist; accounts of feeding dogs and birds and finding flowers; observations – but no details - about the book, *Cold Mountain*, since the mountain was near her home; small stories about her parents: her mother's education and her father's reading; and reminiscences about giving one of her handmade baskets to a visiting Archbishop.

These repeated stories, accounts, and small stories have several features in common. Most importantly, they are not totally identical repetitions: they may be rehearsed narratives or fragments of such that have become incorporated into schema, but they are not parrot-like. As with another repetitive narrator we have studied, Lucinda Greystone (Davis 2011), details may be added or subtracted, as the repeated story illustrates different aspects of the identity Ms Littlejohn is co-creating with her audience. She positions herself as a person who knows what she is talking about, as an Appalachian narrator presenting rehearsed narrative retaining some Appalachian habits. She is a woman who is using some of her lifetime acculturation from Western North Carolina and is very proud of it; she also happens to be a person with dementia. She is not adopting a persona, she is privileging a style that she has grown up in, and she may be exaggerating certain parts as she shifts in and out of her register as part of her interpersonal pragmatics. Her preferred conversation style consists of narrating, rather than responding to the conversation partner, and she is constructing herself on the spot (van de Mieroop 2009), positioning herself by her monophthongized [a:] as a Western North Carolina native (we note, for example, the way she says "spices") who is a fine teller of tales. Her rehearsed stories are ones that she has told to herself or to family members. She is sprinkling her stories with Appalachian pronunciations but presents no syntactic or lexical signals of that dialect. She has been gone a long time and has adapted to other speech regions (Hazen et al. 2010). As long as she can control the airspace, she appears happy to continue talking. This is easier for her to do when she is interacting with BD than with some of the student volunteers, since BD uses associative prompts as opposed to typical interview questions and thus facilitates Ms Littlejohn's preferred interaction style.

In the conversations, Ms Littlejohn initiated a small number of repeated topics about her family and the mountains where she lived. The topic of apples came up by accident, originating as a detail in her comments about the kinds of foods mountain people canned or stored during the depression:

> But no, it was just then, the women of the, and the men too, of the mountains during the depression years and so on; like I just got through saying. They didn't sit and woe on me type, they got busy, and canned. Well, it was just, there were just so innovative and now you go to the grocery store for it, IF you can find it. That's the problem, you can't find it. <*No, and my pickles are still better than what you can buy*>. Well I'm not gonna; I'll make that a basket you can buy … I wouldn't buy pickles, I don't think. But no, we were never hungry. And apples! My grandparents had an apple orchid and I LOVE apples. I would always have at least two apples to go to school with. (October 2011).

Maureen Littlejohn and Multimodal Analysis

As well as introducing the topic of apples, this short extract emphasizes the importance of the multimodal approach we take. In it, we see one of Ms Littlejohn's frequent idiosyncratic formulaic phrases, an apologia for repetitions, "like I just got through saying." However, the phrase is not a way to monitor her listeners or to give them a chance to comment: no pauses surround it, although Lin (2012) notes that formulaic language is often associated with prosodic features including alignment with pauses, intonation units and fast speech rhythms. In addition, no head nods or chin movements accompany the phrase any time it is used across all three samples analyzed in detail or across the total recordings. Rather than inviting the listener to take part, Ms Littlejohn is punctuating her own conversational contribution, and allowing herself to continue with her narrative. Had we not taken a multimodal approach, but just analyzed the words of the text, we would have thought that Ms Littlejohn was carefully checking with her conversational partner. It is the analysis of pauses and gesture that allows us to see that her apologetic comment is most probably self-directed rather than being an indication of good pragmatic interaction. As is the case with a number of her other apologetic comments, it is more likely to be part of her dementia.

Repetition and Formulaicity in Ms Littlejohn's Stories

The extract in Fig. 4-1 shows Ms Littlejohn using repetition of topic and theme within a 41 second exchange. The themes of eating apples instead of candy and of having most of her teeth because of eating apples surface in other conversations during a three months period in which apples played a primary role. In those conversations she often adds a corollary theme, that her family did not have much money, but shared generously with others and never went hungry, as they had apples to spare, and also inserts comments about her mother.

Additional clips from adjacent conversations suggest the extent of her repetition. On 10 October 2011, see *a*, Ms Littlejohn focused her conversation on her mother, who was a school teacher and who made good use of everything their small farm provided. She canned produce i, made sure there was plenty of firewood ii, fed her husband and four children well iii. In iv, Ms Littlejohn concludes all her small stories, three of which include a repetition of the small story *never hungry*. In the first clip, *never hungry* is expanded by the canned goods; in the second, *never hungry* is replaced by a parallel story familiar from oral histories of rural speakers,

{laughter} Oh I never went s~ Oh - I ate **apples** until they *just*
- I guess that's why I still have most of my teeth now because I ate **apples** instead of candy cos we didn't have money to buy candy so we
- we just always ate **apples**
- Had my - grandparents house
- they got this
- had an orchard
- And we had this lean to built
- and it in the fall - it ah, at the back of the house
- they'd go up to the **apple** orchard and *just* pick bushels and bushels and bushels of **apples** and come

Put a lot of straw in the bottom around it <Mmm hmm>

And they would *just* load these **apples** in there and instead of eating candy
- cos didn't have money for candy but we could sure eat the **apples** –

Figure 4-1: Formulaic speech in an extract from an interview with Maureen Littlejohn recorded on November 10, 2011.
Legend used here or in other extracts: boldface = repeated topic keyword, italics= repeated discourse particle, - = pause between 0.5 and 1.0 seconds, - - = pause between 1.0 and 2.0 seconds. < > = brief feedback utterance by conversational partner. All caps=strong emphasis.

that they *made do* with what they had. In the third clip, *never hungry* is because they had plenty to eat, and in the last clip, *never hungry* leads into the announcement of the family's orchard.

a *10 October 2011*

i.

We all were, we never were hungry.
- Didn't have much money
- but she always can had a basement or canned closet somewhere that was full of pickled beets and beans and

ii.
well see I grew up in the country, and we had plenty of firewood, and plenty of trees to cut down. You didn't uh, you didn't have plenty of money to go out and buy a bunch of stuff you just made do with what you ha –had

iii.
Yeah, but we always just had a - plenty to eat
- Didn't have much money but, we were never hungry.

iv.
I wouldn't buy pickles I don't think.
- But no, we were never hungry.
- And apples! My grandparents had an apple orchard and I LOVE apples
- I would always have at least two **apples** to go to school with.

A month later in November, Ms Littlejohn had begun to conflate her good teeth with the continued themes of eating apples as opposed to candy, which was largely unavailable. She was happy to share short reminiscences and opinions, repeating topics and themes within a single conversation and often within seconds of each other. For example, sections b i and ii are within 6 seconds of each other, and ii is 7 seconds from iii, though thematically, they are separate; sections iv – vi are within a 12 second burst of talk, and not quite a minute later, sections vii and viii are within 7 seconds of each other.

b 10 November 2011 [Clips in addition to the clip in Fig. 4-1]

i.
Oh, - I ate apples until they just
- I guess that's why I still have most of my teeth now because I ate **apples** instead of candy cos
- we didn't have money to buy candy so we,
- we just always ate **apples**. -

ii.
And they would just load these apples in there and instead of eating candy
- cos didn't have money for candy but we could sure eat the **apples** –

iii.
I went back and one of the persons there had known me before they says "you know what I remember most about you?" and I thought,
- oh yeah it's gonna be something great.
- And I said "well what?"
- "You always had an **apple**" –

iv.
And we grew up on, we didn't eat candy.
- Didn't have candy
- we ate **apples**. We had a just a little lean to and it
- piled in with straw and just fill it full of **apples** and we had **apples** all winter long. -

v.
that's what's kept me and made me as healthy as I am today is just
- eating **apples**, cos we, - you got Chris~ candy at Christmas time
- But that was the only time.

vi.
Yeah oh yeah
- You got your stick candy,
- ah, - but we
- well literally really we just ah we could sit and eat a bucket of **apples** a night.

vii.
- Well, ah, and as I say in ah, we just ah
- we grew up, I've forgotten how my grandfather got this ord~ orchard it was on some kind of bad debt
- But, we ah, - I've still got all my teeth, *{laugh}* at least part of it. *{laugh}*

viii.
The way we grew up it kids would be so
- underpr~ underprivileged and
- just if they had
- go back and
- didn't couldn't go to the grocery store and get a bag full of candy for
- five cents almost! *{laugh}*
- - But ah, - we n~, we n~ were never hungry.

- That's for sure. -

Thematically, the first two segments emphasize the family's lack of money; the third segment represents her later awareness of how she was perceived; segments four – six conflate eating Christmas candy with daily apples, and the last two segments highlight her good health and her family's never going hungry, with the inference that having bushels and bushels of apples kept them full and healthy.

Three weeks later, Ms Littlejohn was still offering comments about apples and candy, but now they were set inside an elegiac threnody lamenting the changes that had come to the mountains of western North Carolina, spread throughout a collection of reminiscences of growing up in the mountains.

c *29 November 2011*

i.
we've just become so accustomed to being able to go to the store and buy
- ah store bought bakery cake and
- <u>all the candy</u> that we've forgotten the little things that really
- mean more. -

ii.
she would get up early enough to bake at least six plus
- there were no less than six.
{unclear speech BD} and then then you would just put one cookie dough down then you would have this mixture
- **apple** sauce, and spices and what have you
- and you would keep stacking 'em up until you had a stack of cookie dough cake
- or well it was a cake about that high and we just they were just called stack pies. - -

iii.
and ah we just ah
- - we just never worried you just never worried that ah that there was always enough
- I loved **apples**
- I still do

iv.
[Sheepnose] that is an old old **apple**
- and i~ it was it was
- about this big around at the top and it d~ did graduate down until it
- it had a n~ it wasn't a nose it's just that they were b~

v.
well
- there was no ah nothing like just
- crunching down on a good old **apple**
- but ah and they were so plentiful back then
- but not anymore.

Unlike the clustering of discourse chunks in conversation *b*, the excerpts from conversation *c* are scattered throughout, and are not as thematically cohesive: section i laments the changing values brought by growing materialism, section ii remembers her mother's stack pies which were filled with a spicy apple mixture. Section iii is near section ii, and may be thematically connected to the long-ago apples. In section iv, Ms Littlejohn talks about a heritage apple, the Sheepnose; in section v, Ms Littlejohn remembers the crunch of a crisp apple, plentiful in her childhood, but no longer available.

These three sessions in 2011 are the only times she has talked about apples. She did not discuss apples in two conversations in 2012 in which we attempted to reintroduce the topic. However, in a conversation with the researcher and a young male student in May, 2013, given the cue by the researcher that she "has told me stories about living in the mountains," Ms Littlejohn commented that her family had "a storage area" into which they put "bushels and bushels" of apples for the winter.

Multimodal Analysis: The Apple-story Clips

Methodology and Background

We now turn to a detailed analysis of Ms Littlejohn's gestures in her stories involving apples. All these stories occurred in three video-recorded conversations, which were collected by the researchers on October 10, November 10 and November 29, 2011. The first author had been visiting Ms Littlejohn for three years, and Ms Littlejohn appeared to be completely comfortable conversing with her. Ms Littlejohn had given permission for the filming, and again appeared completely relaxed in these video-recorded sessions. The first author conversed while the third author used a Kodak flip-cam to record the interaction. The videos were converted to QuickTime video and AVI formats. Transcription was done in Transcriber http://trans.sourceforge.net/en/presentation.php, which supports acoustic analysis in Praat (Boersma and Weenink 2010) and pause analysis. For this discussion, three samples were taken, one from each video, in which Ms Littlejohn is talking about apples and some topics she associates with them, such as her mother. The samples chosen for analysis were typical of her usual speech; the one requirement was that they should include gestures. The sample clips about apples were made using QuickTimePro and iMovie, and the clips themselves were reviewed and annotated first in Elan and then in QuickTimePro. Figs 4-2a and 4-2b display the initial stages of annotation in each. The first and third authors made the initial analysis. The second author carried out an independent analysis. Where there was disagreement, we re-checked our analyses until we came to a consensus.

All of the videotaped conversations were face-to-face. Mendoza-Denton and Jannedy (2011, 266) contend that face-to-face interaction incorporates "semiotic layers" of parallels between gesture and speech on three planes, structure, content and meaning, where gesture aids in the structuring of the other two planes and in cuing speaker stance p. 291. Their analysis shows the convergence of discourse semiotics with the grammar of intonation. Depperman (2013) reviews the fairly extensive use since the mid-1970s and particularly since the early 1990s of the analysis of multimodal interaction within the perspective of Conversation Analysis and its utility when combined with ethnographic analysis. As Depperman comments,

> Video data can enhance our understanding of participants' understandings, because the analyst can draw on the participants' bodily displays of how they interpret others and how their own actions are coordinated with and oriented to other events, objects and participants (2013, 4).

In the next sentence, however, he cautions that such an interpretation needs embedding in ethnographic analysis, because "bodily displays are implicit and therefore often very ambiguous" (*Ibid.*) and the term "multimodality" is by now quite "fuzzy" (2013, 3).

Our specific interest in viewing and reviewing the clips about apples in these three videos of Ms Littlejohn has been to see which types of gestures she retains, the appropriacy of her gestures to topic, situation and conversation partner, and how she may be using them to keep her partner interested in continuing to converse, which would argue a certain degree

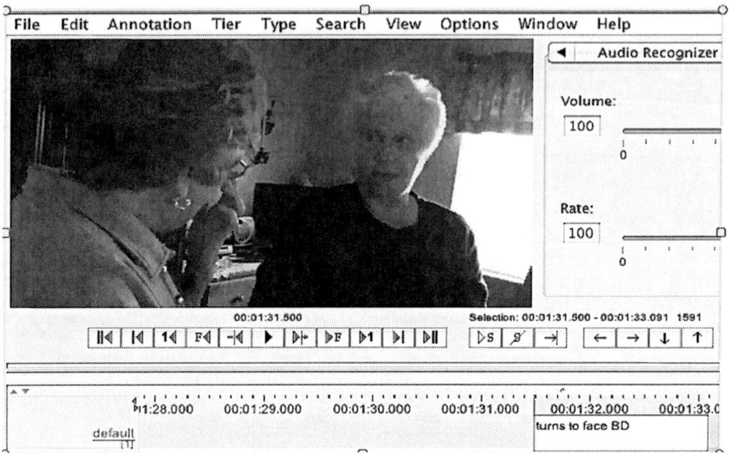

Figure 4-2a: Initial annotation using Elan.

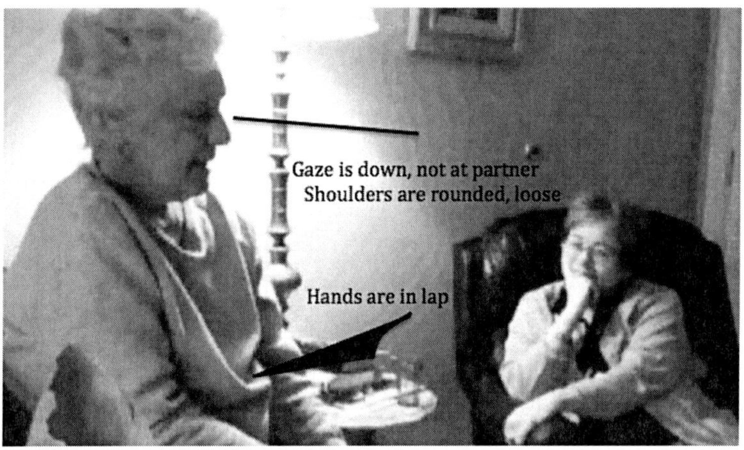

Figure 4-2b: Initial annotation using QuickTime Pro ® with Photoshop.

of awareness and intentionality, a layering assumed and argued in the study by Mendoza-Denton and Jannedy (2011). Since much of our discussion of apples over two months stems from BD's gift of an actual apple to Ms Littlejohn, who touches and turns it in her hands throughout one video-recorded conversation, we turn to Streeck for appropriacy, (2013, 72):

> Although speakers utilize a variety of methods to depict objects, including drawing their shapes or performing schematic acts of making them, the most common method for depicting things by gestures is to perform some schematic act of handling them: lifting them, putting them down, or performing a characteristic motion that identifies the object more specifically (Streeck 2008).

Maureen Littlejohn's Gestures and Head Nods

Older PWD often use nonverbal behavior "in meaningful ways for others to interpret, and as a way of self-communication" (Hubbard et al. 2002, 155). Aoki (2011, 11) cites Kendon (1967) who found "that speakers tend to look away in the beginning of or prior to an utterance to forestall responses from recipients" and at the end, look back at recipients. Ms Littlejohn seldom leaves a beat open for the recipients to say anything, but her gestures and head nods appear to have specific functions: they help her to hold the floor for her stories, and they support her reacting to her hearers and perhaps taking the part of her hearers in terms of how much information she provides about packing the apples into the lean-to (compare Table 1b and Table 2). In Fig. 4-3, Ms Littlejohn is in her usual story-telling posture, and here, she is holding and turning the apple BD gave her. During the interactions, Ms Littlejohn faces towards her conversation partner, BD, most of the time, but at key moments in her narratives, she regularly turns to face JC who is doing the filming. The relative positions of the interactants are suggested in Figure 4-4.

In our short clips, we have repeated stories about Mother and apples. Mother went off to school on her brother's tuition and is an excellent and generous cook. Apples are stored in a lean-to, eaten instead of candy, and have helped her keep all her teeth. At the end or at the tellable high point of each of these stories, Ms Littlejohn turns her face to JC, and presents a larger-than-usual for her smile, turning almost immediately back to BD. The head turn and the smile signal the completion of her story and show emphasis, show her awareness that JC is there filming her, identify boundaries of discourse chunks that may or may not include routines and small stories, and keep the floor, although they can also show that she is getting ready to shift perspective (Maury-Rouan 2011) or start a new, frequently related story.

There are other examples of Ms Littlejohn using gesture to react to her hearers. One occurs when BD asks "Is there anything better than fried green apples?" Ms Littlejohn responds "Well I don't remember that too

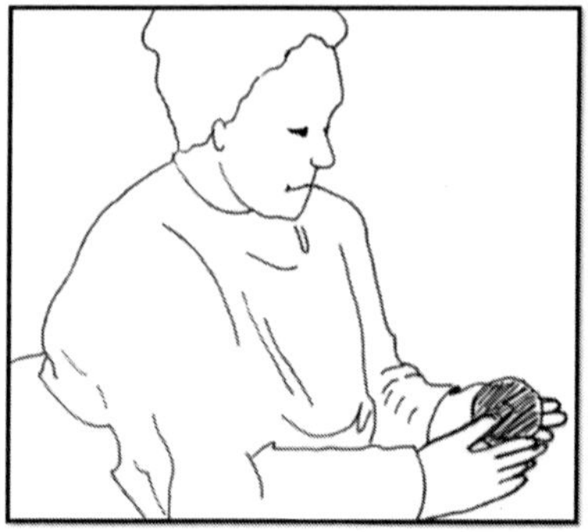

Figure 4-3. Ms Littlejohn's typical posture when telling stories.

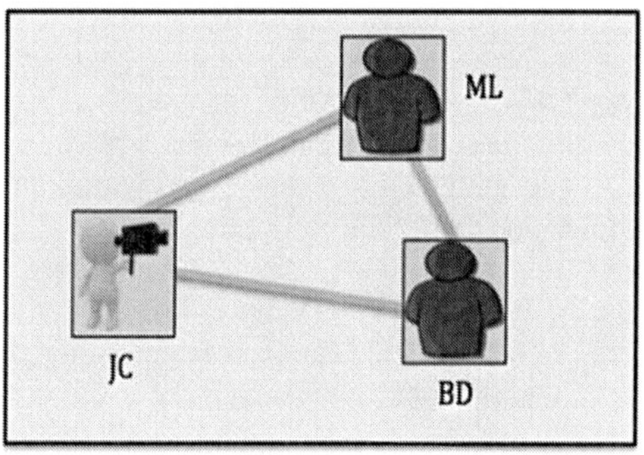

Figure 4-4: Ms Littlejohn's placement relative to BD and JC.

much" hesitates and finally says "it's, nothing's relevant anymore" with a wide back and forth gesture with her left hand, palm held horizontally facing down. The gesture clearly underlies how irrelevant what her hearer has said is. She then segues back into one of her story schemas that are related to her mother.

However, many of her gestures do not seem to be other-directed. Because Ms Littlejohn likes to keep the conversational floor, her discourse chunks are large; routines and repetitions occur within them. The repetitions of short collocational phrases "as I said before" buy her a beat or two with which to resume the gist of her story; they are like kennings in oral-formulaic poetry. She does not pause before or after them, nor does she look to see how her listeners respond: accordingly, our interpretation is that these phrases are not directed to her listeners but rather to herself.

Nor, as far as we can tell, are her head nods and shakes directed to her listeners: again, that is because she does not look at either BD or JC when she moves her head.

Although speaker head nods are typically used to prompt or to proffer backchannel feedback (Aoki 2011; McClave 2000; McNeill 1992), they are also used for "emphasizing words and phrases uttered" like batons; "self-affirmation … repeated head nods are used after statements as an expression of self-reflection, acceptance and reinforcement of what the speaker him/herself has said"; and "citation and imitation" to mark a switch from direct to indirect discourse (Boholm and Allwood 2010). Ms Littlejohn offers head nods and head shakes, but they are intended to reinforce what she is saying, and appear to be directed as self-affirmation to herself rather than to her listeners. The nods and shakes typically mark the initiation of a topic, or the introduction of a new proposition, as seen in Table 1.

In what follows, we intersperse sketches of head nods and hand movements with an outline of a single story schema from the interview recorded on November 10, 2011. Throughout the excerpt, Ms Littlejohn is involved with the apple, beginning by holding it in both hands. She continues to hold it in her right hand throughout most of the extract; most of the gestures are with her left hand and are described using conventional terms for gestures (McNeill 1992; Kendon 1967). (See Table 1a.)

The story continues with very little pause; the intonation contour marks the close of the preceding utterance and, with it, the first story-chunk. In the upcoming story-chunk, she is at pains to have listeners understand that the orchard and the lean-to are important. (See Table 1b.)

In the two stories in Table 1, Ms Littlejohn's hand movements are usually iconic and support her narrative, as with the gesture describing the lean-to. However, at "bushels and bushels and bushels," when she pats the air three times, this seems to be a baton-like gesture emphasizing what she is saying rather than an iconic gesture. The head nods/shakes and the head turns are what signal the high points and boundaries within the discourse and appear to be self-reinforcing rather than directed to the listener. The tellable high points of both the stories in Table 1 are marked, as usual, by her turning from BD to JC and then back to BD. If Ms Littlejohn is talking about childhood, and her mother is associated with anything she is telling, she almost *has* to fill in with a small story about her mother because she has clusters of small stories and little short rehearsed narratives tangled in an associative web.

Table 1a Head nods and hand moves in a story schema

Story component	Transcript of spoken story	GESTURES/NODS TYPICALLY BARELY PRECEDE SPEECH
    Start of story	Oh I never went s~. Oh, - [pause] - I ate apples until they just. -	AT SECOND "OH," DROPS HANDS HOLDING APPLE, CLASPS THEM IN LAP, AT "ATE." DROPS HEAD, AT "JUST," SHAKES HEAD HORIZONTALLY
Tellable high point of story	- I guess that's why I still have most of my teeth now because I ate apples instead of candy	AT "THAT'S," NODS HEAD VERTICALLY, VERY SLIGHTLY AT "CANDY," LOOKS AT JC, LAUGHS, SMILE 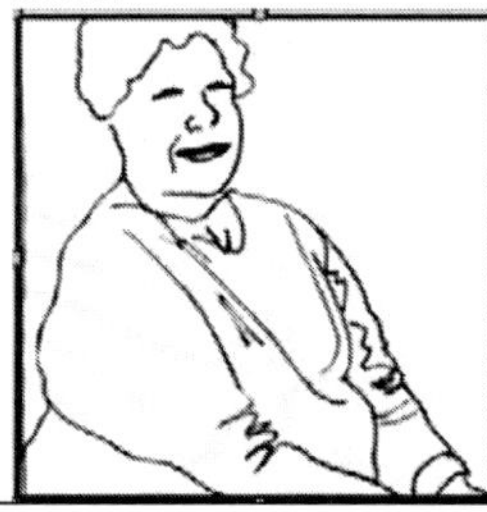
	cos we didn't have money	AT "WE" TURNS APPLE WITH RIGHT HAND AT "DIDN'T," LOOKS BACK AT BD
	to buy candy so we [pause]	HEAD NOD AT "CANDY" 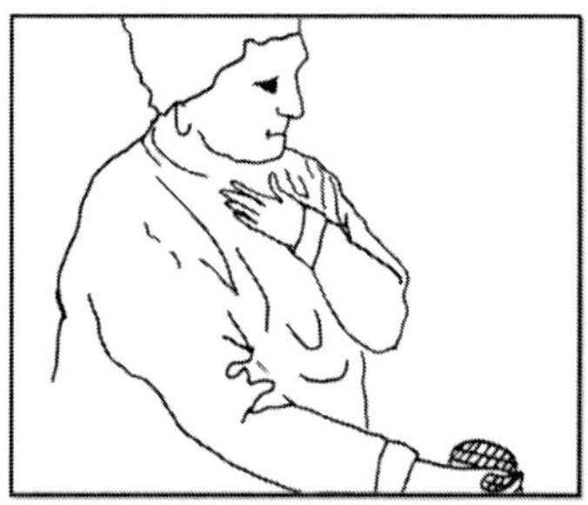 AT "WE" BOSOM CLUTCH WITH LEFT HAND, LOOKS DOWN TO RIGHT, STILL HOLDING AND TURNING APPLE
End of story	we just always ate apples.	AT "WE," RAISES HAND HOLDING APPLE, LOOKS DOWN AT IT, AT "ALWAYS," BEGINS TURNING APPLE OVER IN BOTH HANDS

Table 1b: Hand movements and head nods in a story schema

Story orientation	Had my, grandparents’ house - they got this - had an orchard.	Continues turning apple over in hands.
Start of story	- And we had - this lean-to built 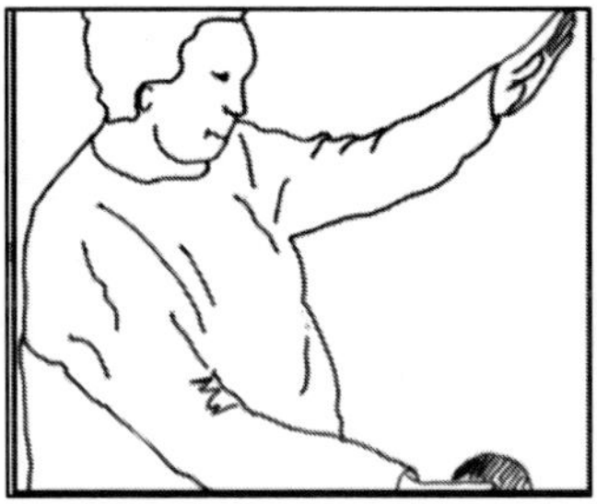	At “this,” raises left hand to mark a height. At “lean-to,” sharply brings hand back to lap at a slant, suggests shape, size 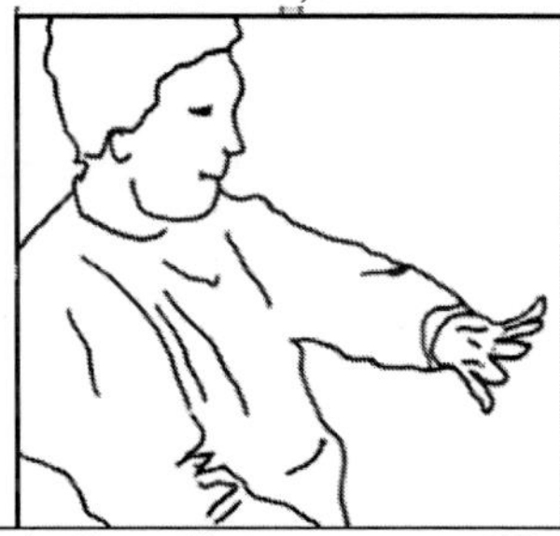
	and it in the fall - it ah at the	At “fall,” turns to face BD, looks directly at her
High point of story	back of the house they’d go up	At “back,” draws circle in air with left hand, palm down. Hand remains slightly raised. At “they’d,” turns to look at JC 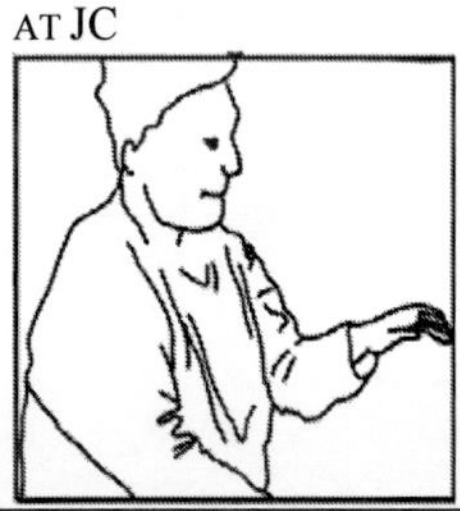
	to the apple orchard and just pick bushels and bushels and bushels	At “apple,” turns back to face BD. Hand flat and still raised, palm down, fingers slightly spread, half way to shoulder, pats air three times in time with “bushels and bushels and bushels”

		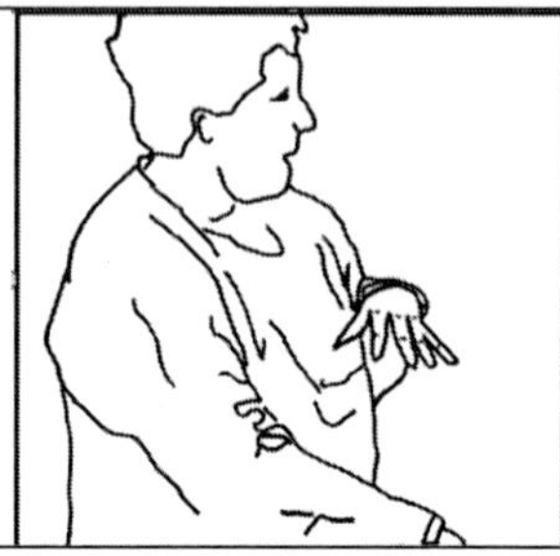
	- of apples and come - - Put a lot of straw in the bottom around it 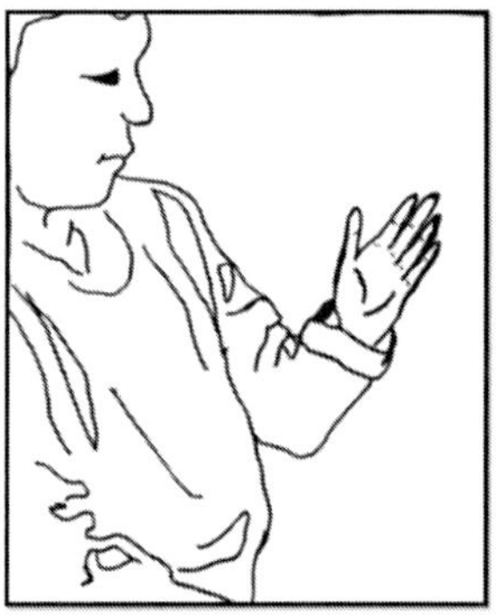	AT "AND" RAISES SLIGHTLY CUPPED LEFT HAND TO SHOULDER HEIGHT. FROM "COME" TO END OF PHRASE, SCOOPS AIR IN SMALL CIRCLE AND THEN LARGER CIRCULAR SWEEP PUTTING STRAW AROUND 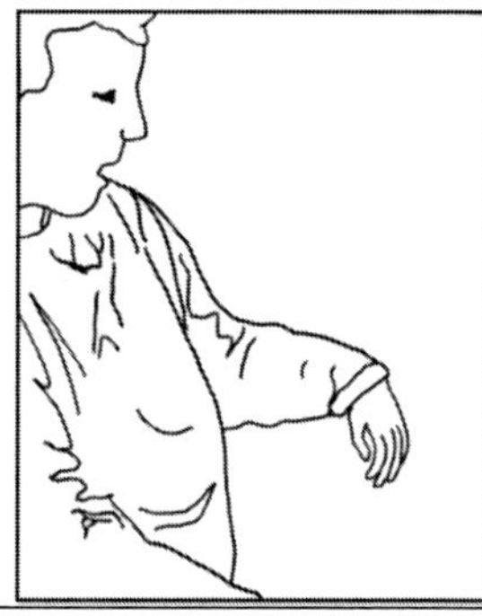
Starts final section	And they would just load these apples in there and instead of eating candy	AT "AND," DROPS HAND TO LAP. AT "INSTEAD," SLIGHT HORIZONTAL SHAKE OF HEAD
End of story	- cos didn't have money or candy but - we could sure eat the apples	AT "SURE," NODS HEAD VERTICALLY AT "APPLES," PAUSES, CHIN DOWN, MOUTH CLOSED, UNDERSCORES STATEMENT

However, the rehearsed narratives are definitely not all identical, nor are they merely ideational perseveration: their "sameness" is connected to her embodied and performed identities. Her "rehearsed, routinized retellings become something more than ideational perseveration or her stepping into a rehearsed self" (Davis 2010, 97). Later in the same conversation as that in Table 1, the interaction shown in Table 2 occurred.

Ms Littlejohn is using the same story schema as in Table 1, but this time the iconic gestures are absent, there are no details about the "apple house" the *lean-to* in the earlier extract, and long silent pauses begin to stack up. Ms Littlejohn appears to lose track of her narrative, so that BD provides the information about the straw, and this time Ms Littlejohn provides new information and describes how the apples were built up against each other.

Table 2: Second, later extract from November 10, 2011 conversation

ML: And we, we as you just got through saying, you know that's one thing they always did is,
- had this old **apple** house and, we would have **apples** all winter long. - And, - I do - -

BD: Well the straw kept them from freezing.

ML: Yeah. Right and you could build 'em up against another b~ so that they were not ah, - oh.
- - Gone, - gone are the days that you just ah -

Implications

Although persons with mild to moderate DAT will often reply to questions or other requests with gestures either to supplement or substitute for the gist of a story or the word they cannot find, we are not sure that PWD increase their meaningful and intended gestures over the course of the disease as suggested by the pamphlet produced by the Alzheimer's Association and quoted on page 88 above. Nor, in our analyses, do gestures seem to substitute for speech. The analysis of gesture in DAT is complicated by the increased apraxia that often accompanies moderate and late dementia: indeed, the combination of apraxia, aphasia and agnosia is often claimed to be a major characteristic of the disease http://www.alzheimer-europe.org/. Giannakopoulos et al. (1998) note that apraxia typically occurs in late dementia. Rousseaux et al. (2012) find apraxia in moderate as well as late dementia. Studies reporting gesture have worked with DAT populations who have early or mild to early moderate dementia, which is the case in the present study. Glosser et al. (1998) evaluated arm and hand gestures in persons with aphasia and persons with probable DAT, anticipating impairments in gesture as speech became impaired, but assuming that the two cohorts would have different patterns of problems.

Their study found differing patterns, with PWD having "semantically ambiguous gestures when compared to content-bearing gestures" (1998, 6). Carlomagno (2005) finds that the nature of the cognitive impairment underlying poor information content and lack of reference in DAT discourse constrains the production of conversational gestures by patients with this disease. Accordingly, we would anticipate that Ms Littlejohn's gestures will diminish in some as yet undetermined way as her stories become either fragmentary or less frequent, or both. We have not yet found that certain gestures continually accompany formulaic language or repeated chunks of tales, which is part of our ongoing study of her language production over time.

Mittelberg (2010) points out that gestures provide multimodal evidence for conceptual and spatial metaphor: we see this in the gestures connected with the lean-to, in Table 1. In Ms Littlejohn's stories, those are iconic gestures, which depict physical properties of referents such as the lean-to or wrapping the apples in straw over winter, giving information that complements co-occurring speech. As with Ms Littlejohn's rehearsed narratives, her co-occurring gestures are not identical. However, this observation does not necessarily suggest that her gestures and non-verbal modes of communication, as seen through head nods and headshakes, are "empty". On the contrary, thus far Ms Littlejohn's gestures and head movements are pragmatic. Moreover, gesture catchments can be either partial or complete (McNeill 2000). As McNeill et al. note, "gesture and speech arise from the same semantic source but are non-redundant; each modality expresses its own part of the shared constellation" (2000, 2). We have already seen how a multimodal examination of Ms Littlejohn's stories showed that her "apologies" were for her benefit, not for her listener. As Ms Littlejohn moves farther into the moderate stage of dementia, a multimodal approach will be even more important as we explore how much she is still able to interact with other people, how she will continue to produce formulaic expressions and performed narrative, and under what conditions she will continue to gesture with her hands and with head nods and where she may direct her gaze.

The extracts presented in Tables 1 and 2 show how Ms Littlejohn's repeated stories are not repeated word for word. The story fragment in Table 2, which occurred later in the interaction, is not as detailed as the earlier story in Table 1. It is possible that Ms Littlejohn was getting tired, but it is also possible that she retained some sense that she had already given information about this, "And we, we as you just got through saying" with an unusual use of *you* where she means *I*. As with the speaker analyzed in Davis (2011), Ms Littlejohn's interaction demonstrates that more is going on than simple repetition of often repeated tales. Her story schema allow her to remain a part of the conversation and are slightly different with each telling, being slotted into the on-going discourse with greater or less finesse.

From the perspective of multimodal analysis, there is much to investigate around the semiotic impact or function played by her speech and her gestures. Understanding the interpretation drawn from multimodal analysis involves us with both social semiotics and pragmatics, and thus with looking more closely at aspects of indexicality. That is, we need to examine what repeated stories and fragments of stories index in the performed conversational narratives of a person who, because she has dementia, has already been positioned as a semiotic object in and of herself (Sabat 2005). Mertz (2007, 343) comments that "Performance and audience are both issues that require us to examine indexical connections between speech and social context." Certain repeated motifs in Ms Littlejohn's stories could be said to index aspects, areas or times in her life that she wishes to emphasize. These motifs are basically memorized strings: though they are remembered for their own sake, some perform an additional function of "signalling identity in some culturally significant way" (Wray 2002, 72). For example, frequent mentions of the book, *Cold Mountain* surface when she is identifying herself to listeners as being from Western North Carolina. When she learns that the region is somewhat familiar to two of her twenty-five conversation partners, she increases her references to regional scenery and events, and slips in and out of monophthonging /aɪ/ so that a word like "fire" sounds more like "far." Interestingly, she does not produce other features of the Appalachian dialect she grew up using, such as a-prefixing *I'm a-goin'* or deleting *–ly* from adverbs *She's awful tired.* We are continuing to monitor pronunciation and lexicon in her repeated stories: bilinguals often revert to their first or mother tongue as their dementia increases (Nold 2005), and it will be interesting to learn if, as a bidialectal speaker, she reverts to earlier speaking habits, even in situations where she is story-sharing with strangers. Here, we follow Johnstone and Kiesling (2008, 6), who note for Pittsburgh that certain dialect features, such as /aw/, are stylistically variable: "Such variation arises because indexical meaning is created and reinforced in local practices in which different people participate in different ways, if at all." Ms Littlejohn may or may not have a semiotic association between Appalachian features and her chosen presentation style, and she may or may not be directing her occasional, and we think stylized (Coupland 2001), use of the /aɪ/ to persons she perceives as being familiar with the region.

Conclusion

Our analysis of Ms Littlejohn indicates that she is still well aware of her interactants and can still adapt her retained conversation skills to meet their pragmatic needs. She uses stories to keep her conversational partner involved, falling back on questions like "Aw, so how's your day going?" only when she can no longer hook another story fragment onto the current story. Such questions are phatic on her part: they serve to maintain the rapport between the interactants by inviting her conversational partner to make a contribution on a "safe" topic, a topic where there is no expectation either of great self-disclosure or of something specific she will have to retrieve and produce. When both researchers are with her, she focuses mainly on BD who serves as a primary partner, but turns to include JC by smiling at what she must assume are the tellable high points of her repeated stories. The repeated stories to visiting conversation partners show Ms Littlejohn tailoring a story's theme and motifs to fit some kind of situation, suggesting that she retains some sense of what can keep her audience aligned with her viewpoint or affiliated with her as a speaker. Her caregivers speak with admiration of her fluency: at least one norm for residents in her setting is the expectation of low competence. There are other expectations lurking in the social context for PWD, few of them positive: institutional caregivers are reputed to talk over their clients, in effect, "ghosting" their embodiment as thinking conversationalists (Davis and Pope 2010).

In this analysis, we have explored interpersonal aspects of how Ms Littlejohn, as a social actor, uses "language to shape and form relationships" (Locher and Graham 2010, 1) through real-world examples of what she as a PWD may or may not do in forming brief relationships with a constant stream of strangers through her story practices. Even though both the volunteer students and the researchers have visited Ms Littlejohn multiple times, it has not been on a daily basis and we may not presume that she necessarily remembers any of us, either generally or particularly. In essence, we reform a social relationship at each visit and must renegotiate our interpersonal stances toward each other. Multimodal analysis has allowed us to differentiate when gestures that would usually be considered interpersonal, like head nods, were actually self-reinforcing and when gestures, such as those related to the apple stories, were instead appropriately directed to her listeners. It is often assumed that PWD are no longer able to take the perspective of another person in conversation. However, a closer look at Ms Littlejohn's apple stories shows her using gesture to clarify for her listeners just how a lean-to was built to store apples in winter, and verbally introducing different information into a story that was repeated within the one interaction. This is one way she can retain personal agency in an institutional setting that typically assumes its residents have very little such agency. Retaining agency by her story-telling allows her to establish what degree of closeness or distance she feels appropriate to the situation and to the conversation partner: for example, in one conversation with a student volunteer, she used exquisite tact to suggest that her partner talk to somebody else Davis, Maclagan and Shenk, (2013 in press). By setting her own boundaries, she can still retain some control over the choice of conversation partner; by speaking rapidly and injecting rehearsed stories that have elicited warm response in previous interactions, she can maintain agency as a competent conversationalist and experienced raconteur. She is almost obligated to pull from a readymade store of stories. Her stories do not rise out of the conversation in the usual sense *well that reminds me... you know, I always...* in that they are not used to explain a point or to share a recent experience with a friend *you'll never believe who I saw today* because she has very little "today" to talk about: no TV, books, movies, friends, or encounters with others. The only "today" things she mentions are routine comments about living in the facility, and these are performed comments, such as saying she no longer needs to do dishes or her bed is made for her. She is beginning to use her performed stories and small stories as substitutes for ordinary small talk, in social situations. Sabat and Gladstone (2010) note that cognitive function in social situations is a far different phenomenon from that as measured by standardized tests, and problems in social interaction may often, at least during mild dementia, arise from PWD having been malignantly positioned. Ms Littlejohn's interpersonal interactions position her as a person with a social self who happens to have a progressive and debilitating condition, not as a disease that has a person.

References

Aijmer, Karin and Gisle Andersen. 2012. Introduction. In Andersen, G., Aijmer, K., eds. *Pragmatics of Society,* 1-27. Berlin: Walter de Gruyter.

Ainsworth-Vaughn, Nancy. 1998. *Claiming power in doctor-patient talk.* Oxford: Oxford University Press.

Alzheimer's Association 2012. *Communication.* http://www.alz.org/national/documents/brochure_communication.pdf

Aoki, Hiromi. 2011. Some functions of speaker head nods. In *Embodied interaction: Language and body in the material world,* edited by Juergen Streeck, Charles Goodwin, and Curtis LeBaron. Cambridge: Cambridge University Press pp. 93-105.

Bara, Bruno. 2011. Cognitive pragmatics: The mental processes of communication. *Journal of Intercultural Pragmatics* 8, 443-485.

Boersma, Paul and Davis Weenink. 2010. Praat: Doing phonetics by computer. Last downloaded 4 October 2012. http://www.fon.hum.uva.nl/praat/.

Boholm, Max and Jens Allwood. 2010. Repeated head movements: their function and relation to speech. In *LREC 2010: Proceedings.* Mediterranean Conference Centre, Malta: LREC Workshop on Multimodal Corpora, 2010

Boxer, Diana. 2002. *Applying Sociolinguistics: Domains and face-to-face interaction*. Philadelphia, PA: John Benjamins.

Carlomagno, Sergio, Maria Pandolfi, Andrea Marinia, Gabriella Di Iasi, and Carlos Cristilli. 2005 . Coverbal gestures in Alzheimer's type dementia. *Cortex* 41, 535-46.

Chafe, Wallace. 2008. Aspects of discourse analysis. *Brno Studies in English* 34: 23-37.

Coupland, Nikolas. 2001. Dialect stylization in radio talk. *Language in Society* 30, 345-375.

Coupland, Justine. 2003. Small talk: Social functions. *Research on Language and Social Interaction* 361, 1–6.

Davidson, Bronwyn, Linda Worrall, and Louise Hickson. 2008 . Exploring the interactional dimension of social communication: A collective case study of older people with aphasia. *Aphasiaology* 22, 235-57.

Davis, B. ed. 2005. *Alzheimer talk, text and context*. NY: Palgrave.

Davis, Boyd. 2010. Intentional stance, selfhood, and Lucinda Greystone: Twice-told tales from a digital corpus of Alzheimer talk. In *Language, body, health,* edited by Paul McPherron and Vai Ramanathan, 75-104. NY and The Hague: Mouton de Gruyter.

—. 2011. Interpersonal issues in health discourse: Caregiver-resident interaction in Alzheimer talk. In Locher, M. & Graham, S., eds., *Interpersonal Pragmatics* pp. 381-404. Vol. 6 of *Handbooks of Pragmatics* Series. NY and The Hague: Mouton de Gruyter

Davis, Boyd, and Margaret Maclagan. 2009 Examining pauses in Alzheimer's discourse. *American Journal of Alzheimer's Disease & Other Dementias,* 24, 141-54.

Davis, Boyd, and Margaret Maclagan. 2010. Formulaicity, pauses and fillers in Alzheimer's discourse: gluing relationships as impairment increases. In *Fillers and placeholders in discourse and grammar*, edited by Nino Amiridze, Boyd Davis, and Margaret Maclagan. 189-215. Amsterdam/Philadelphia: John Benjamins.

Davis, Boyd, and Margaret Maclagan. 2013 in press. Talking with Maureen: Extenders and formulaic language in small stories and canonical narrative. In *Dialogue and Dementia: Cognitive and Communicative Resources for Engagement*, edited by Robert Schrauf and Nicole Mueller. NY: Psychology Press.

Davis, Boyd, Margaret Maclagan, and Dena Shenk. 2013 in press. Exploring communicative interactions between visitors and assisted-living residents with dementia. In *Routledge Handbook of health discourse*, edited by Heidi Hamilton and Wen-ying Sylvia Chou.

Davis, Boyd, and Charlene Pope. 2010. Institutionalized ghosting: policy contexts and language use in erasing the person with Alzheimer's. *Language Policy* 9, 29-44.

Depperman, Arnulf. 2013. Introduction: Multimodal interaction from a conversation analytic perspective. *Journal of Pragmatics* 46, 1-7

Fox Tree, Jean and Josef Schrock. 2002. Basic meanings of *you know* and *I mean*. *Journal of Pragmatics* 34, 727-747.

Garcia, Linda and Yves Joanette. 1997. Analysis of conversational topic shifts: A multiple case study. *Brain and Language* 58, 92-114.

Georgakopoulou, Alexandra. 2006a. Thinking big with small stories in narrative and identity analysis. *Narrative Inquiry* 16, 129-37.

—. 2006b. The other side of the story: Towards a narrative analysis of narratives-in-interaction. *Discourse Studies* 8, 235-257.

Giannakopoulos, Panteleimon, Myriam Duc, Gabriel Gold, Patrick Hof, Jean-Pierre Michel, and Constatin Bouras. 1998. Pathologic correlates of apraxia in Alzheimer disease. *Archives of Neurology* 55, 689-95.

Glosser, Guila, Mary Wiley, and Edward Barnoski.1998. Gestural communication in Alzheimer's disease. *Journal of Clinical and Experimental Neuropsychology* 20, 1-13.

Gubrium, Jay. 1975. *Living and dying at Murray Manor*. NY: St. Martins.

Hamilton, Heidi. 1994. *Conversations with an Alzheimer's patient.* Oxford: Oxford University Press.

Hazen, Kirk, Paige Butcher, and Ashley King. 2010. Unvernacular Appalachia: An empirical perspective on West Virginia dialect variation. *English Today* 26, 13-22.

Hubbard, Gill, Ailsa Cook, Susan Tester, and Murna Downs. 2002. Beyond words: Older people with dementia using and interpreting nonverbal behaviour. *Journal of Aging Studies* 16: 155-167

Jefferson, Gail. 1990. List-construction as a task and resource. In *Studies in ethnomethodology and conversational analysis,* edited by George Psathas. Maryland: the University Press of America.

Johnstone, Barbara and Scott Kiesling. 2008. Indexicality and experience: Exploring the meanings of monophthongization in Pittsburgh. *Journal of Sociolinguistics* 12, 5-33.

Kendon, Adam. 1967. Some functions of gaze direction in social interaction. *Acta Psychologica*, 26: 22-63.

—. 1995. Gestures as illocutionary and discourse structure markers in Southern Italian conversation. *Journal of Pragmatics* 23, 247-279.

Lin, Phoebe. 2012. Sound evidence: The missing piece of the jigsaw in formulaic language research. *Applied Linguistics* 33 3, 342-347.

Locher, Miriam and Sage Graham, eds. 2010. *Interpersonal Pragmatics*. Mouton, 2010.

Locher, Miriam, and Andreas Langlotz. 2008 Work at the intersection of cognition, interaction and emotion. *Bulletin vals-asla, bulletin suisse de la linguistique appliquée*, 88, 165-191.

Maclagan, M., Davis, B., & Lunsford, R. 2008. Fixed expressions, extenders and metonymy in the speech of people with Alzheimer's disease. In Granger S. and Meunier F. eds *Phraseology: An interdisciplinary perspective.* Philadelphia: John Benjamins.

Maury-Rouan, Claire. 2011 Do listener's facial expressions influence speaker's discourse? http://www.gesturestudies.com/Contributions/Maury-Rouan/Maury-Rouan.html

McClave, Evelyn. 2000. Linguistics functions of head movements in the context of speech. *Journal of Pragmatics*, 32, 855-878.

McLean, Agatha. 2006. *The person in dementia: A study of nursing home care in the US.* Toronto: University of Toronto Press.

McNeill, David. 1992. *Hand and mind.* Chicago: University of Chicago Press.

McNeill, D. ed. 2000. *Language and gesture*. Cambridge: Cambridge University Press.

Mendoza-Denton, Norma, Jannedy, S. 2011. Semiotic layering through gesture and intonation: A case study of complementary and supplementary multimodality in political speech. *Journal of English Linguistics* 38, 265-299.

Mentis, Michelle, Jan Briggs-Whittaker and GD Graminga. 1995. Discourse topic management in senile dementia of the Alzheimer's type. *Journal of Speech and Hearing Research* 5, 1054-1066.

Mertz, Elizabeth 2007. Semiotic anthropology. *Annual Review of Anthropology* 36, 337-53.

Mittelberg, Irene. 2010. Geometric and image-schematic patterns in gesture space. In *Language, Cognition and Space: The State of the Art and New Directions* edited by Vyvyan Evans, Paul Chilton Eds,. London: Equinox. 351-385.

Nold, Guenter. 2005. Alzheimer's speakers and two languages. In *Alzheimer talk, text and context*, 102-127, edited by Boyd Davis. NY: Palgrave.

Orange, JB and Barbara Purves. 1996. Conversational discourse and cognitive impairment: Implications for Alzheimer's disease. *Journal of Speech-Language Pathology and Audiology* 20, 139-150.

Padilla Cruz , Manuel. 2007. Phatic utterances and the communication of social information: A Relevance-Theoretic approach. In *Studies in intercultural, cognitive and social pragmatics*, edited by Pilar Blitvich, Manuel Padilla Cruz, Reyes Gómez Morón, and Lucia Amaya, 112-129. Newcastle, UK: Cambridge Scholars Publishing

Ramanathan, Vaidehi. 1997. *Alzheimer discourse: Some sociolinguistic dimensions*. Mahwah, NJ: Lawrence Erlbaum.

Riordan, Monica, Rick Dale, Roger Kreuz, and Andrew Olney. 2011. Evidence for alignment in a computer-mediated text-only environment. *Proceedings of the 33rd annual meeting of the Cognitive Science Society*, pp. 2411-2416. Austin, TX: Cognitive Science Society.

Rousseaux, Marc, J. Rénier, L. Anicet, Florence Pasquier, and Marie Mackowiak-Cordoliani. 2012. Gesture comprehension, knowledge and production in Alzheimer's disease. *European Journal of Neurology* 19, 1037-44.

Sabat, Steven. 2005. Capacity for decision-making in Alzheimer's disease: Selfhood, positioning and semiotic people. *Australian and New Zealand Journal of Psychiatry* 39, 1030-1035.

Sabat, Steven, and Caroline Gladstone. 2010. What intact social cognition and social behavior reveal about cognition in the moderate stage of Alzheimer's disease. *Dementia* 9, 61-78.

Schiff, Brian. 2005. Telling it in time: Interpreting consistency and change in the life stories of Holocaust survivors. *International Journal of Aging and Human Development* 60, 189-212.

Schiffrin, Deborah. 2001. Discourse markers. *The Handbook of discourse analysis*, edited by Deborah Schiffrin, Heidi Hamilton, and Deborah Tannen, 54-75. Malden, MA: Blackwell.

Scollon, Ron, Suzie Scollon, and Ronald Jones. 2012. *Intercultural communication: A discourse approach*. NY: Wiley-Blackwell.

Singh, Sameer, Romola Bucks, and Joanne Cuerden. 2001. Evaluation of an objective technique for analyzing the variables in DAT spontaneous speech. *Aphasiology* 15, 571-583.

Spencer-Oatey, Helen. 2011. Conceptualising 'the Relational' in pragmatics: Insights from metapragmatic emotion and impoliteness comments. *Journal of Pragmatics* 43, 3565-78.

Stivers, Tanya. 2008. Stance, alignment, and affiliation during storytelling: When nodding is a token of affiliation. *Research on language and social interaction* 41, 31–57.

Streeck, Juergen. 2008. Depicting by gestures. *Gesture* 8, 285-301.

—. 2013. Interaction and the living body. *Journal of Pragmatics* 46, 69-90.

Williams, Amanda and Jacqueline Guendouzi. 2000. Adjusting to the home: Dialectical dilemmas and personal relationships in a Retirement Community. *Journal of Communication* 50, 65-82.

Woods, Bob, Elisa Aguirre, Aimee Spector, and Martin Orrell. 2012. Cognitive stimulation to improve cognitive functioning in people with dementia. *Cochrane Database of Systematic Reviews* 2012, 2. Art. No.: CD005562. DOI: 10.1002/14651858.CD005562.pub2.

Wray, Alison. 2002. *Formulaic language and the lexicon*. Cambridge: Cambridge University Press.

CHAPTER FIVE

MISLAYING COMPASSION: LINGUISTIC TRIGGERS FOR INADEQUATE CARE-GIVING IN ALZHEIMER'S DISEASE CARE

ALISON WRAY
CARDIFF UNIVERSITY

This paper explores the possibility that formulaic language might be part of the explanation for the high incidence of stress and mental health problems in those caring for people with dementia, and also for the much—publicised problems in health care regarding lack of compassion on the part of caregivers. Specifically, it is proposed that the increased levels of use of formulaic language that are typical in people with Alzheimer's Disease have a powerful impact on the pragmatics of communication. As the symptoms of Alzheimer's increase, the incidence of formulaic language is bound to rise, because it is a means of accommodating reduced cognitive capacity and anchoring important information (Wray 2002, 2011). However, caregivers will find it difficult to set aside their standard sensitivities to the significance of an overuse of formulaic language, and as a result, a conflict in relation to the pragmatics of interaction will emerge. A 'perilous' communicative environment will ensue, that makes it difficult for carers to sustain compassionate behaviour. Carers are at risk of experiencing stress unless they can find an alternative approach to the interaction. Techniques of mindfulness and meditation may be one such approach, offering carers a means of acknowledging and managing their own needs more independently of those of the person they are caring for.

Section 1: Communication, compassion and mental health in caregivers

In 2011, a report by the UK ombudsman into the care of older people highlighted within the health service "an attitude—both personal and institutional—which fails to recognise the humanity and individuality of the people concerned and to respond to them with sensitivity, compassion and professionalism" (Abraham 2011, 7). A year later, the NHS Confederation offered ten recommendations for improvement, including:

> Hospitals should recruit staff to work with older people who have the compassionate values needed to provide dignified care as well as the clinical and technical skills. Hospitals should evaluate compassion as well as technical skills in their appraisals of staff performance. (NHS Confederation 2012)

Generally, the root cause of the endemic problems is viewed as being the commodification of healthcare in a competitive market-driven environment (Goodrich and Cornwell 2011; Youngson 2011; Zigmond 2011). However, in this paper it will be proposed that language can also play a role in creating conditions in which care ceases to be compassionate. The focus here will be on one sub-group of caregivers—those looking after people with Alzheimer's Disease (AD). However, some elements of the account may apply to other types of care situation too, not least because key parameters are the respective sense of agency and need for self-protection experienced by the caregiver and cared-for: factors that are not restricted only to AD care. Following Webster's dictionary, the term 'caregiver' will be used in this chapter to refer to any "person who provides direct care", irrespective of whether the person is paid (e.g. nurses, care assistants) or an unpaid family member. Merging paid and unpaid caregivers in this way is not intended to deny that there may be significant differences in how they approach their role. However, the question of how language might lead to stress, and stress to a reduced capacity for compassion, applies to both types and in the present discussion it would be misleading to differentiate between them.

It will be proposed that the linguistic environment in which caregivers operate when looking after people with AD is "perilous". That is, a double-bind is created in which caregivers are trapped into non-compassionate behaviour, because of a clash between fundamental principles governing communication. It will be shown how this trap will be extremely uncomfortable for caregivers, creating personal tensions that result in extreme stress. That caregivers do experience such stress is well-illustrated in the following posting on an Alzheimer's forum, headed "Lost it this morning and feeling incredibly guilty"

> I'm ashamed to say that after a number of phone calls from 6.30am from dad and then him ringing the doorbell at 7.45am this morning, I shouted at him and subsequently broke down in tears in front of him, he knew I was mad at him (I'm not, I'm furious at this awful disease) and exhausted from lack of sleep and his constant need for me. Have returned him home now where he's apologetic saying it's his fault reassured him it's not at all and is mine but I feel awful ....
> (http://forum.alzheimers.org.uk/showthread.php?3442)

Guilt is a significant problem amongst caregivers, and is a destructive and stressful emotion to cope with (Alzheimer's Society 2012). Brereton (2012) reports that "nearly 60% of [unpaid adult caregivers] suffer with mental health problems." Although the Chair of the Royal College of General Practitioners, calling for preventative support for the UK's 7 million caregivers, cites a more modest 40% suffering psychological problems, particularly depression (Guardian 2013), both figures are strikingly high. These statistics cover all caregiving, but the home care of people with dementia is a major component of the total. Leaving aside the personal impact of stress on the caregiver and cared-for, these high levels of mental health problem carry considerable cost to the health service. Lilly et al (2012, 103) recommend "A fundamental re-orientation towards caregivers and caregiver support … rather than resorting to costly patient care for caregivers who have reached the point of burnout." As the Chair of the UK's Royal College for General Practitioners has pointed out "If caregivers fall ill you lose two patients. You lose the person they are caring for and also the caregiver so it makes financial sense to keep caregivers well" (Guardian 2013).

In what follows, some suggestions are made about the role that language might play in the creation of stressful environments. Nevertheless, it is not to be inferred that the proposals offered in this paper constitute the only explanation for caregiver stress.

In section 2, the relevant aspects of the general nature of AD language are reviewed. In section 3, formulaic language in AD communication is discussed in the light of the roles played by formulaic language more generally. Sections 4 and 5 introduce the proposal that the excessive use of formulaic language violates fundamental pragmatic principles of communication, resulting in an almost intractable dilemma for caregivers (section 6). Section 7 concludes by exploring one possible solution.

Section 2: The nature of AD and language, with particular relevance to cognitive load and memory loss

Alzheimer's Disease involves the progressive death of brain cells due to the development of 'plaques' (amyloid deposits) and 'tangles' (accumulations of the tau protein). There is a typical progression pathway, according to which the language areas of the brain are not directly affected until the moderate stage of the disease (ADERC 2011). However, earlier changes in the entorhinal cortex and hippocampus (Hampel et al. 2008), which control the efficiency with which short term memories are converted to long term memories, already impact on language, by affecting recall and planning. Consequently, even at the mild stage, linguistic symptoms exist, including word-finding difficulties, word substitutions and neologisms, and repetitive questioning (National Institute on Aging 2009). Repetition has a number of functions in normal discourse as well (e.g. Levinson 1983; Tannen 1989), and it behoves the analyst to avoid assuming that all repetition in AD discourse is a product of the disease (Shakespeare 1998, 175ff). By the moderate stage, repetition is more common, including anecdotes and favourite words and expressions (*Ibid.*). Repetitive language may be produced with a fluency and grammatical complexity well beyond that of novel language. Hamilton (1994, 73-4), for example, observes, "it is interesting to note that one of Elsie's residual abilities is repetition—both repetition of other's talk as 'read-made' to incorporate into her utterances … as well as repetition of her own previous utterances … to continue holding on to her turn-at-talk."

There are many reasons why a person with AD might increase the frequency of their repetitions, relative to non-disordered discourse. Directly, repetition is associated with frontal lobe dysfunction (Asp et al. 2006, Cullen et al. 2005). But repetition can also have local functional causes. They include emphasis, salience, and simply having forgotten what one has previously said. For example, in Shakespeare's (1998, 178ff and 224ff) 197-line conversation between Tilly, a "confused person" and her interviewer Moyra, Tilly describes the effect of Deep Heat lotion in relieving her rheumatism, compared with the "greasy …rubbish" that the doctor prescribed as alternative, which "messed my vest and my nightdress up" after which "I threw the whole tin in the bin." She returns to her core themes several times in the conversation, making the account very repetitive, despite Moyra's attempts to develop the theme in different directions.

Tilly's repetitions contain the same information but are not lexically or grammatically identical, which indicates that this is not verbal perseveration. Conversely, while verbatim repetition can indicate verbal perseveration (Cullen et al 2005), it need not. It is also a common option for expressing a thought anew, since we have preferred ways of putting our ideas into words (Wray 2002), which will naturally lead to repetitions of form if the meaning is repeated. Reformulating an idea in slightly different ways is, in this context, simply a variation on reformulating them in the same words: in both cases, the person has an idea and then encodes it in a convenient way. For example, Lily, recorded by Brown and Clegg (2010, 135-8), has an extensive account of her day that she repeats over and over in almost identical words. For instance, one sub-routine begins "I get up … put my socks on … put my shoes on … comb my hair." It occurs six times in their transcript (Brown and Clegg use three dots to indicate the end of a phrase). Yet the coherence of her account, and its relevance to her daily life, suggest that her monologue is motivated by content, rather than being the empty repetition of a memorised narrative.

Another reason why repetition may occur is a sense of insecurity or a loss of confidence, both likely to attract repetition of the form. As explained in section 3, statements that seek to anchor a person's identity will tend to be identical each time, because they are social signatures. Repetition can also occur because of self-priming. Asp and De Villiers (2010, 182-192) discuss in detail a conversation in which the person with dementia, Cleo, offers "a monologue that is genuinely incoherent" (p.191). One feature of it is the repetition of *lucky* in different expressions (*I'll be lucky... I'll be lucky … you're not lucky*), which they interpret as a superficial echoing response to her own speech.

Overall, repetition needs to be interpreted in context, and also with reference to wider changes in discourse that result only indirectly from the cognitive deterioration itself. Triggers include uncertainty (Hamilton 1994, 72), depression, altered power relationships, the social construction of AD as an illness (Ballenger 2006), and the discourse contexts in which people with AD find themselves, such as how caregivers speak to them. Of course, people's varying tendency to adopt compensatory linguistic strategies may create individual differences in the trajectory of symptom development or the overt evidence of a problem (see Davis et al., Chapter Four, this volume; Wray 2010). That may be one part of the reason why the brain pathology of AD does not result in consistent levels of translation into discernible cognitive and linguistic impairment (Prince and Jackson 2009, 6).

Section 3: Interpreting formulaic language in AD communication

In a context in which communication is increasingly impeded by the multiple complications of reduced memory capacity, general disorientation, rapid change in social power and status, and, often, changes in the physical environment, a person's linguistic resources will be put to the test and must be mobilised as effectively as possible. It is important to recognise that people bring into their AD a sophisticated lifelong portfolio of communicative skills, interactional agendas and personal priorities, enabling them to respond resourcefully to their new difficulties.

The typical deficit perspective on AD may tend to eclipse evidence of how people display resilience in adjusting to changes by drawing on the compensatory strategies that have worked well through a lifetime of occasional lapses in concentration, embarrassing linguistic incidents and breakdowns in communication. For instance, Wray (2010) shows how "Joan", a singing teacher with noticeable AD symptoms, successfully taught master classes for an entire weekend. Joan was a former international opera singer in her mid-80s, who had for many years given master classes to amateur and professional singers. This particular weekend workshop had recruited 13 singers. They had travelled up to 250 miles, and had paid for the opportunity to perform three or more songs to the assembled group and receive feedback on how to improve them. Joan had very noticeable symptoms consistent with AD, that participants from previous years' workshops confirmed had been evident, though far less severe, in the past. Joan's husband commented, "Well she's got dementia. We're not going to do this [i.e. master class teaching] anymore. She knows but she doesn't mind. I prompt her a lot. I know all the stories and I fill it in for her". However, he was adamant that the dementia could not be AD "because if it were, she'd be talking to you one minute, turn to talk to someone else, and then turn back to you and not remember she'd been talking to you before". For more details of this study, see Wray (2010).

It has been observed in a number of studies that accomplished musicians retain their musical abilities relatively intact in AD (e.g. Beatty et al. 1999). One of the participants in the weekend master class commented by email afterwards: "I was very struck by how she could frequently remember more or less all the words of songs she had sung in the past, and was mouthing them throughout people's performances, even though much of the rest of the time she couldn't string words together in a way that made sense." She used the songs as a vehicle for expressing her ideas, often singing a phrase to demonstrate what she wanted, rather than explaining (Wray 2010). One of her strategies was to draw on the turns of phrase and formulaic responses that she had developed over many years of teaching, prior to her illness. These word strings were easily retrieved and effectively deployed because they had been frequently used for an appropriate function in the past. They were, one might say, rat-runs through the maze of communication, enabling her to anchor her intentions to "islands of reliability" (Raupach 1984) that were sufficiently apposite to deliver the information she intended.

In defining "formulaic language," researchers prioritise different characteristics of word strings, according to their primary concerns—concerns which extend from general language description, through first and second language acquisition, to models of discourse, of grammar and of processing. In these different contexts, features of interest may include non-compositionality (e.g. *face value; pull strings*), grammatical unpredictability (e.g. *come a cropper; sure as eggs is eggs)*, developmentally precocious structures (in which language learners can produce a form they have not yet mastered the grammatical components of, because it is embedded in something memorised), fossilisation (in which learners continue to use an incorrect form that they now know how to correct, because it is embedded in something they have previously memorised), frequency or infrequency in the language (associated with, for instance, collocational pairs and idioms respectively), social and discourse roles (e.g. ways of holding the turn, signalling identity, etc) and resilience to brain damage (as noted in studies of aphasia as well as AD). For overviews of the types and features of formulaic language see, for instance, the collections by Corrigan et al (2009a, 2009b) and Granger and Meunier (2008) and Meunier and Granger (2008), and the reviews and discussions of Wray (2002, 2008, 2009). What all researchers accept is that the core characteristic of formulaic language is some sort of privileged processing, whether because of holistic lexical storage and retrieval or automaticised procedures (e.g. Segalowitz 2010).

Wray (2002) proposes that the reason formulaic language is so useful and prevalent in normal communication is that there are key survival advantages in deploying fast-track linguistic production. Specifically, it is in individuals' interests to create and sustain a beneficial level of control over their environment in order to ensure they can meet their physical, emotional and psychological needs. The success of the human species is due in large measure to the capacity to offset potentially lethal physiological changes by developing social structures that reinforce collective survival. For example, bipedalism and large-brained offspring have resulted in enforced shorter gestation, complex childbirth and extremely immature neonates. Midwifery support and a long period of dedicated child-rearing have developed to offer a counterbalance to the high risk of mother and child mortality. More generally, humans are successful because they have built social structures that enable them to rely on others. However, this means that a significant amount of an individual's control over his or her environment is through the agency of others. This is most acutely seen in infancy, but in fact it extends throughout life, if we consider emotional security and shared information as contributors to survival and successful reproduction. In old age, reliance on others increases towards the levels in infancy, and this requires adjustments to the modes of interaction with others. The effect of this social interconnectedness for survival means that humans have had to develop ways of manipulating other humans, to ensure they have access to everything they need. Wray proposes that fast-track language processing helps achieve this, in several ways.

Firstly, directly manipulating the actions of others is more reliably achieved if the other person immediately recognises the formulation of a command or request, without having to engage in extensive decoding. Since the best way to deliver a message that others will easily understand is to use one you have already heard them use, speakers will naturally become highly sensitive to the forms of words used by others in their community. Secondly, as a result of this sensitivity, speech communities and sub-communities will develop, in which certain ways of expressing ideas are shared. Consequently, it will be possible to differentiate groups according to the precise ways in which they use language to sound like each other. Language will thus develop as a marker of identity, and will operate, as necessary, as a means of protecting the integrity of communities (Wray and Grace 2007).

Thirdly, shared familiarity with certain turns of phrase and their functions will create contours of given and new information within discourse, that enable speaker and hearer to coincide in their attention. For instance, discourse markers such as *On the one hand... on the other hand* are used to help the hearer share the speaker's organisation of information into a relationship of opposition. Familiar, formulaic material may be used to package up new information, being marked phonologically and/or lexically in a manner that enables the hearer to recognise its function and reduce attention to it (Kuiper 1996, Lord 2000).

Routine interactions such as customary greetings can be downplayed in terms of their intellectual content, in recognition that their role is social: it matters *that* one greets someone one knows in the street, not whether *how are you doing?* is received and responded to as a genuine request for detailed information (Austin 1962). Filler words and expressions can be used, by mutual agreement between hearer and speaker, to enable the speaker to buy time during the formulation of new ideas (Wray 2002). A hearer will not usually challenge a speaker's *you know* by saying *no, I don't,* because the expression has a recognised filler role that obviates any internal examination of its literal meaning (Aijmer 1996).

However, all of these uses of formulaic language are balanced on subtle social norms of interaction, to which we are highly sensitive. If someone uses a formulaic response when a novel one was expected, we will take it that the respondent is transgressing a social rule—normally that of giving adequate attention. If someone uses a turn of phrase that is inappropriate for the situation, we will wonder why they are marking themselves out socially as a non-group member. And, in certain circumstances, we will create an identity for a speaker that makes them different from ourselves—whether as a non-native speaker or, if the signs indicate it, as an 'abnormal' communicator (Shakespeare 1998). It is this last judgement that will be examined in what follows, in relation to the excessive use of formulaic language by people with AD.

Importantly, we should neither assume that people with AD have to be entirely 'abnormal' communicators on account of their formulaic language, nor that older people more generally who use an increased amount of formulaic language are necessarily 'abnormal' communicators. Firstly, people with AD can often operate rather successfully as communicators if the circumstances are such that they are not precipitately or uniquely labelled as incapable of normal communication (Sabat 2001). Wray (2010) found that the supportive context in which the singing teacher Joan operated during her weekend master classes enabled her to be treated more like a healthy non-native speaker with poor English skills (not uncommon in international music training contexts) than like someone with a communication disorder. This was possible because the priority for everyone was accessing her expert knowledge.

Secondly, some of the characteristics of communication that are associated with AD are also characteristics of ageing more generally. Mild Cognitive Impairment (MCI) is a condition that features short term memory loss, which can result in some repetitive linguistic behaviour. However, although MCI is a marker of early stage AD, only 5-15% of cases of MCI develop into AD (Alzheimer's Society 2010), and Milwain (2000) urges caution about conflating two different conditions: mild memory loss as a natural function of ageing, and mild memory loss as a precursor of AD. For models of communication in normal aging see, for instance, Backhaus (2011), Coupland et al. (1988) and Nussbaum and Coupland (2004).

Wray (2011, 2012) identifies four ways in which formulaic language might be increasingly deployed in AD communication, as a result of changes in cognitive function and social context:

a) Sustaining fluency, as planning and retrieval become increasingly difficult.
b) Marking routine and low-level social activity so as to anchor what is happening, as short term memory deteriorates.
c) Getting others to do, think and feel things, when personal agency decreases as a consequence of physical frailties, cognitive decline and reduced social freedoms.
d) Expressing personal and group identity, as memory problems challenge the person's capacity to be sure of who they are and who others around them are.

As outlined in section 6 below, Wray (2011) offers evidence that caregivers are themselves triggered into producing formulaic responses as a defence against "the sense of dehumanisation that arises from being treated disrespectfully or inappropriately by the [person with] AD" (p.447). In particular, in accordance with (b), caregivers use formulaic language to "create a detached, automatic approach to interaction, never expressing any new information or personal feelings" (p.447) and, in accordance with (d), to reassert their sense of worth and identity, which can be severely undermined by the repetitive behaviour of people with AD. It is these responses that will be further probed in the following sections, by considering how formulaic language affects the pragmatics of communication.

Section 4: Pragmatics and the interpretation of AD communication

According to Kitwood (1997, 20) "[t]he prime task of dementia care ... is to maintain personhood in the face of the failing of mental powers... [which requires] the sensitive meeting of [a] cluster of needs, and in a way that corresponds to the uniqueness of each individual." Such attention to the individual is radically different from what he terms the "old culture of care, with its malignant social psychology and pervasive neglect" (p.17), which Goffman (1961) also recognised as a context that removes an individual's sense of identity.

Studies of how to maximise the effectiveness of conversations with people with AD (e.g. Kitwood 1997, Orange and Purves 1996, Tappen et al. 1997) show the importance of understanding and accommodating the challenges they face. Since it is generally recognised that turn-taking behaviour is resilient until a late stage in AD (Orange and Purves 1996), and that there is likely to be an intention to communicate, focus is placed on helping the speaker release meaning from its often inappropriate or underspecified linguistic framing. For instance, Orange and Purves (1996, 145) suggest as strategies: using cueing questions, stating topics overtly, restating what has been said previously, providing a lot of context, and guessing possible meanings.

However, as Asp and De Villiers (2010, 154) note, Alzheimer's talk raises challenges for some of the assumptions that speakers and hearers bring to communication under the auspices of pragmatics. Table 1 reproduces their list of likely challenges to Gricean maxims in AD.

Table 1: Gricean maxims and Alzheimer's Disease, adapted from Asp and De Villiers (2010, 155).

Quality	Truthfulness: don't say things you know to be untrue or for which you lack evidence	- Confabulation - Paranoid suspicions
Quantity	Too little information; too much information	- Underspecified, deictic reference - Repetition, verbosity
Relevance	Be relevant (cohesive and coherent), topic sharing assumes mutual interest or at least socially conditioned behaviour norms that allow performance of mutual interests	- Tangential (can't track conversation, so incoherent) - Perseverative ideation: return to same topic despite current one
Manner	Be clear, avoid obscurity, avoid ambiguity, be orderly	- Poor planning, information-processing problems lead to fragmented incomplete, unplanned, 'disordered' discourse which may affect cohesion and/or coherence

It is central to Grice's model that, in normal communication, a speaker's intentions can extend beyond simply applying the maxims in Table 1. The maxims gain their power precisely from the frequent contexts in which they either are, or appear to be, flouted. This is why the features in the right hand column of Table 1 are not automatically regarded by the hearer as abnormal (Wray, in press). When a hearer is unable immediately to see how a speaker's utterance conforms to one or more of the maxims, the hearer is obliged, on the basis of assuming the Cooperative Principle (i.e. that the speaker intends to be relevant), to look for an interpretation that restores the statement to within the maxims' parameters. This is achieved by assuming that the locutionary element (the surface meaning) does not directly match the underlying illocutionary properties (the social intent) (Austin 1962).

However, if the speaker has AD, the hearer has the option of bringing to bear an alternative interpretation: that the utterance is erratic and cannot be interpreted on the basis of normal expectations of relevance. This choice on the part of caregivers in how they respond to what they hear is central to understanding how the situation can become stressful.

Different choices will be made in different circumstances. In particular, it may be easier to write off an utterance as uninterpretable when there is no strong need on the part of the hearer to understand it—such as with general chat or passing remarks. The stronger the belief on the part of the hearer that meaning was intended, and that this meaning is worth pursuing, the more likely it is that the utterance will be viewed as an attempt at relevance.

Thus, in the case of the singers studying with Joan, the fact that they recognised her as an expert practitioner with a lot to teach them meant that they were prepared to make considerable efforts to interpret her disordered output within the bounds of relevance. One singer commented after the weekend, "I realised when I sang my song that it was up to me to work out what she wanted to tell me because she couldn't say it herself." This singer did not appear to contemplate—and indeed had no grounds to on the basis of Joan's behaviour—that Joan's cognitive difficulties might extend to the delivery of inappropriate or inaccurate advice.

The examples that follow explore the parameters determining how Joan's turns were responded to.

(1)	Joan	I think sometimes the German
	Beryl	the vowels?
	Joan	yes, the vowels and everything like that

(2)	Joan	sometimes you're a bit dithery
	Beryl	do you mean I'm behind the beat
	Joan	oh yes I know

(3)		(Joan has been speaking in content-less formulas, while holding Emma's shoulders back)
	Joan	if you can only just you know

	Emma	stand still (laughs)
	Joan	stand still

In these examples, Beryl and Emma respectively have just performed a song, and Joan is now advising them on how to improve it. In (1), Beryl infers from Joan's comment that the German pronunciation needs work. She offers a suggestion about what precisely Joan means, probably on the basis of having been told before that her vowels are not very accurate. It is not possible to tell whether Joan does in fact mean the vowels, since she would often repeat part of the previous turn as the anchor for her response, even if she then went on to disagree. However, there were plenty of instances like (2) and (3) where there did seem to be an alignment of meaning.

Examining the data as a whole, it is noticeable, that Beryl, one of the older participants who had known Joan for some years, was particularly willing to seek clarification. In (4), the reference to 'holding it more' regards the length of the note on the German word *Tränen*.

(4)	Joan	do that thing
	Beryl	do what thing (laughs)
		(Joan demonstrates by singing)
	Joan	you've got to do that, darling
	Beryl	here? shall I hold it more
	Joan	that's right you've got to do it more (.) and *Trä::::nen* (sung) and put the n on the end

In (5), Joan's formulaic response could be interpreted as a challenge to David, the piano accompanist, who acted throughout the weekend as a major provider of input to the singers, albeit disguised as input from Joan (Wray 2010). Only her 'yes' at the start seems to contradict the rest of her statement. However, David's application of pragmatics means that he interprets it as a confirmation of his observation, rather than a comment on the singer's German, and thus suggests a repeat of the song, so that she can intervene on Chris's pronunciation.

(5)	David	(to Chris) your German needs some work
	Joan	yes that's very good it's very good really
	David	do you want to do it one more time
	Joan	oh yes I want to do it one more time darling

Yet even in this particularly supportive interactional situation, there were times when Joan's inability to express relevant meaning had to be managed. In (6), the singer is unable to extract any useful meaning from

Joan's statement (regarding an aria from Bach's *Magnificat*). But she does not follow up.

(6) Joan you know sometimes um I'm (2.0) oh well never mind (.) so you know *Bach Magnificat* if you do that

In (7), Joan's response to David does not furnish him with the information he needs for continuing with the class. He uses his experience as a singing coach to repair the situation. In (6) and (7) Joan's interlocutors set aside the standard pragmatic response, which would be to interrogate Joan for her meaning and, in David's case, pursue further an answer to his question.

(7) David what else do you want to do
Joan yes want to do it darling
(Stuart proceeds to give the singer advice)

As we see from examples (5), (6) and (7), given an incongruous answer to a question, a hearer will have to decide whether or not it is intended to be relevant and/or whether relevance should be sought; indeed, whether the fact of the speaker's responding in the right place, albeit with something apparently irrelevant, is sufficient indication of an intention to mean.

Only on one occasion in the entire weekend was there a more challenging negotiation of the communicative capacity of Joan. Muriel was a similar age to Joan and was one of those most reluctant to admit that Joan had a problem, observing during the weekend that she could see Joan had changed, but could not say in what way. In (8), Muriel is keen that Joan tell the anecdote, but Joan does not want to try. David replies to Muriel as if she were addressing him.

(8) (David asks Muriel to tell the story behind the song she is singing)
Muriel (to Joan) you tell it you know it
David no you tell it you told it to ME
Muriel (to Joan) oh you tell it please
Joan oh no I don't
Muriel oh please you tell it
Joan oh no I
(Muriel tells the story)

Section 5: The impact of excessive formulaic language on pragmatic norms

Not all situations will be as supportive as the one in which Joan found herself, not least because not all people with AD are able to command respect and authority in the way that she could in that context. Interestingly, although all but one of the singers, when interviewed, admitted that they had not got as much out of the master class as they had hoped, none expressed any deep frustration. As noted above, this may be indicative of the power of engaging in negotiated meaning, driven by a genuine need to access it. In contexts where the hearer is less committed to, or less able through context to, pursue or construe meaning, the failure to understand the speaker's intentions will mean that the communication cannot proceed, and this can be a fast track to negative feelings. A caregiver in a study by Ekman et al (1991, 168) observed, "When you cannot get into contact with the patient you feel insufficient, without hope, dissatisfied or burnt out. Care seems meaningless. You lose your commitment" (quoted in Allan and Killick 2008, 219).

Yet guidelines for effective communication typically take as their starting point the assumption that caregivers are able to overcome any personal feelings associated with the negative experience of the interaction. How can caregivers reliably get to that position of personal strength, and what exactly is it that is likely to prevent them doing so? Allan and Killick (2008) observe,

> Kitwood's concept of personhood emphasizes that one can only be truly a person if we are recognised as such by others, and ... *this applies as much to staff as it does to the person with dementia* (p.219, emphasis added).

So, what are the main threats to a caregiver's sense of being recognised? Bayles and Kaszniak (1987) list among the problems with communication by people with AD, their "being insensitive to others in the conversation, saying either too much or too little, and failing to repair misunderstandings" (p.175). To this we can add the potential impact of excessive repetition, both in questions and in statements. While such formulaicity may be an anchor-point for the person with AD, and while caregivers themselves may have been advised to deploy a measure of repetition to scaffold the conversation (Orange and Purves 1996), nevertheless there are ground-rules for repetition in normal conversation. If the caregiver continues to apply these rules in interpreting conversations with a person with AD, the inferences may be uncomfortable.

In normal interaction, if someone asks me the same question more than once, I may certainly infer, benignly, that they would not have asked me so often if they had not needed to. That is, I will apply pragmatics to interpret the repetition as relevant (Tannen 1989). On the other hand, being sensitive to the difference between flouting a maxim and a speaker's capacity to operate outside of the cooperative space entirely, I will also not be slow to wonder if the reason they need to repeat themselves is that they didn't attend to my previous answer to their question. Thus, if someone tells me the same thing more than once, I may soon come to the conclusion that they haven't really noticed that I have heard that statement before. It may well be that a person with AD is indeed signalling these things: the problems that AD brings for short term memory, attention and semantic representations (ADERC 2011; Hampel et al. 2008) may certainly explain why a person with AD might fail fully to take in the presence and roles of a person caring for them.

Nevertheless, as outlined in section 2, there may be other reasons for them to repeat statements and questions too, including gaining reassurance, and reanchoring their own sense of identity. Joan several times announced to the group of students that she had performed a famous operatic role a certain number of times at a particular opera house. This seemed not to be for the benefit of her audience but rather a device for Joan to demonstrate to them and to herself the legitimacy of her expert role.

The puzzle, then, is not so much why a person with AD might use an excess of repetitive language, nor why doing so might transgress certain pragmatic norms that, on first hearing, could make the caregiver feel ignored or undervalued. Rather the puzzle is why this negative response from caregivers would persist. After all, the problems with memory and attention associated with AD are well-known. Advice from the Alzheimer's Association (2012, 2) in relation to behaviours including repetition is that "It is important to understand that the person is not acting that way on purpose." Yet it is not easy to suppress feelings of anger and frustration, which can, indeed, be viewed as "healthy responses to challenging circumstances" (Alzheimer's Society 2012, 1). In order to understand why a caregiver cannot simply reason that this is the disease talking, and brush it off, we must examine how the roles played by language in human communication might be fanning the flames of frustration and hurt.

If you ask me a question of information, I will try to answer it. If you make a request for me to act in a way beneficial to you, I will evaluate my capacity and willingness to fulfil your request, and respond accordingly. This is a matter of co-operation in the general sense (see note on Grice's

Co-operative Principle in section 6 below), and it is a choice I make. There are many contexts in which I can choose whether or not to respond to questions and requests, such as when, on the street, someone approaches me with a survey. Whatever my response is, I will expect the survey researcher, when I walk back along the street, to remember that I already answered the questions, or that I declined to, and not approach me again. But, as this indicates, the pragmatics of tracking the context within which the next interaction will occur are complex and highly sensitive to local events. They fundamentally depend on attention and on memory—two things that a person with AD is not able to deploy all that well.

Clark (1992), examining the interface between pragmatics and memory observes:

> people's memory must be organized to enable them to get access to evidence they will need to make felicitous references. What this implies is that their memory must contain a diary of significant personal experiences cross-indexed with an encyclopedia organized both by subject matter and by the communities who possess the knowledge. It also suggests that people have selective access to information that is pertinent to each person they talk to. They have a model of what is in the other person's mind, a model they have built up from previous contact and which they continue to update as they go on talking. It is that model that enables people to make and understand references so quickly and accurately (p.57-8).

Clark's proposal explains why a person with AD might struggle to conform to the pragmatic norms of communication—the 'common ground' of knowledge that is established and shared by interactants is undermined by the cognitive deficit, leaving them unable to judge what information they will be expected to omit, as given (see also Guendouzi's chapter in this volume). However, it also gives us a clue to why the caregiver is unable easily to accommodate this problem. For the caregiver also needs to have "a model of what is in the other person's mind"—yet this model is unstable against the evidence coming from the person with AD. For instance, a caregiver might wonder if it really is the case that a straight repetition of previous information is required because the person has forgotten it. Hoadley (2008), on an advice blog, notes:

> As Alzheimer's disease progresses, people often repeat the same question over and over—as if their mind is caught in an endless loop. This behavior can be tiresome for caregivers. But it is important to know that your loved one is not trying to annoy you. Instead, your Mom or Dad may be feeling insecure or fearful. They repeat questions to feel in control – a feeling that

> is being lost slightly more and more each day. Repeating questions can drive you crazy but it provides comfort to your loved one!

In similar vein, Coste (2003) recommends “keep[ing] in mind that [the person with AD] wants to articulate some feeling behind the [repeated] question” (p.110). Thus, a caregiver might wonder if the words spoken, although formulated as a particular question, are actually an attempt to ask or express something quite different, to which they have not yet given a satisfactory response. The mind-reading that a caregiver may attempt to engage in will be stressful even before any of the other factors are added in.

This destabilising of the common ground on which pragmatically appropriate interaction is built might, even so, seem little more than a troublesome hurdle that the caregiver must overcome. Hoadley advises, “Try to remain calm and patient and answer the question. Try to understand what your Mom or Dad may be feeling. And, don’t point out that your Mom or Dad has asked the same question repeatedly” (see also Alzheimer’s Association 2012). Why, then, is this so difficult to achieve?

Section 6: The “perilous” environment of the caregiver

It will be argued here that the caregiver is not, as it might at first seem, simply located in a new kind of interaction that requires adjustment. Rather, making adjustments results in an equally troublesome alternative, leaving the caregiver stressed about which of these options to select.

Language is a window into another person’s thoughts and feelings, and connects them rather directly with our own. Although we can examine what passes along this conduit for its reliability and veracity, doing so is cognitively burdensome, and the basis on which we are able to construe meaningful information exchange is one of assumed trust—trust in the truth of the content, in the intentions behind expressing it, and in the coherence of the code itself: “Our talk exchanges do not normally consist of a succession of disconnected remarks, and [they] would not be rational if they did. They are, characteristically, to some degree at least, cooperative efforts” (Grice 1975, 45). This observation is separate from the question of whether Grice’s Co-operative Principle can and should be interpreted in terms of ‘co-operation’ in communication (e.g. Davies 2007). The matter of importance here is one of communicative etiquette—not so much what your words encode about your perception of the world, as what your decision to use them at all tells me about your perception of me, as your addressee.

There is, as Grice (1975) proposes, an inherent assumption of socially-defined rationality, which manifests as assumed relevance. "As far as the Hearer is concerned, the Speaker providing an uninterpretable (meaningless) utterance would be pointless, and therefore irrational" (Davies 2007, 2324), so that "cooperation is the realisation of rationality applied at the level of discourse, and is explicitly identified as being part of the process" (*Ibid*).

Pragmatics kicks in at the point when a statement appears irrelevant and thus carries the potential of being construed as uninterpretable. It is made meaningful by assuming that there must be a rational drive underneath it. But in the context of AD, assuming relevance may be more painful to the caregiver than assuming that the person with AD no longer operates within the normal pragmatic rules of communication.

If, in producing the utterances, the speaker is following the behavioural norms underlying Grice's Cooperative Principle and the conversational maxims, rather than deliberately flouting them in order to be annoying or disruptive, then the repeated questions and statements must be relevant to the interaction at some level, even if the encoding of the message is not optimal. They could be worthy of direct interpretation, as an honest attempt to gain information that has been forgotten. They could require interpretation at a less literal level, because a different message lies behind the words—as with Meg, in David Clegg's (2010) collection, who used a range of personal formulas, "you're a nice lady . . . I'll write to you privately. You're my brother. Will you see me home now?" to express thanks to him for freeing her fingers from some apron strings" (p.xix-xx). Or the repetitions could indicate a deliberate attempt to annoy—which would place the interpretation outside the bounds of the Cooperative Principle.

It would be appropriate for a caregiver to examine potential interpretations along all three lines. However, all three offer up scenarios that are likely to make the caregiver feel powerless. If the information has been forgotten, then there is an endless cycle of question/answer that the caregiver's previous answers have been impotent to break. This indicates to the caregiver a lower achievement of agency than desired. If the message encoded is different from the one presented, then the caregiver has to try and read between the lines, but has very little basis on which to do so, which will also instil a sense of impotence. And if the speaker is being deliberately annoying, it suggests that the caregiver is not valued.

When a caregiver feels that her best investments of time and effort have been useless or have been rejected, a logical reaction is to modify the operational environment to one in which future insults are less likely, or are less hurtful. One way to do that is to withdraw cognitively. Cognitive withdrawal can be achieved using the same linguistic mechanisms that have led to the problem in the first place. Using formulaic, repetitive language that requires little cognitive effort to produce will enable the caregiver to go through the motions of interaction without actually investing much. This then becomes the 'reason' or justification for why so little recognition is received (Wray 2011). Some of the formulaic linguistic behaviour observed in professional care may be explained in this manner. It is functional and appears adequate on the surface—turns are exchanged that are relevant to the context—but it is empty. Example (9) from Clegg (2010, xxiii) illustrates this:

(9)	Daisy	are you my mother
	Nurse	(without turning round) no Daisy I'm not your mother
	Daisy	I'm your daughter (.) say I'm pretty
	Nurse	You're pretty

Wray (2011, 2012) points out that this sort of emotional and cognitive detachment is dehumanising for both parties, and creates a vicious circle of impoverished communication based on formulaicity.

The alternative is to cease interpreting the language of the person with AD as fundamentally cooperative—that is, to reject the assumption of relevance, or, in Shakespeare's (1998) terms, to view the speaker as a *less-than-full member* of the group of social interactants. It is then possible to uncouple the pragmatics entirely. The caregiver need no more feel assaulted by the repetition than she would by that of a parrot. However, if we accept that there is a "universal cognitive tendency to maximise relevance" driven by the imperative to manipulate the thoughts and actions of others (Wilson and Sperber 2002, p.254; compare Wray 2002), then there is a direct connection between the pursuit of relevance, founded on the assumption of rationality, and our perception of the interlocutor. As Wilson and Sperber observe (p.254-5), the attribution of human-like rationality to one's addressee is sewn into the fabric of inferential communication, because of the need to ensure the observer recognises one's intention. Therefore, to deny rationality is to deny fundamental humanness.

The caregiver, then, is backed into one of two corners. Either allow that the input from the person with AD is rational, and, in order to handle the blows to self-esteem, identity and agency consequent upon that, develop defensive strategies that minimise cognitive engagement. Doing so will co-create with the person with AD a type of superficial communication that is devoid of real meaning. Or cease to view the input as rational and no longer seek real meaning in it, with the onward implication that the speaker is not behaving in a humanlike way. Either choice runs a substantial risk that the person with AD will be treated in a somewhat dehumanised manner—that is, without the level of compassion that society might like to see.

In recent years, increasing attention has been paid to the use of empathy to facilitate compassion (see section 7). However, empathy may bring its own challenges. Empathy entails the emotional capacity sufficiently to align with the other to understand how it might feel to be them—although Mercer and Reynolds (2002) identify four components to effective empathy in the clinical setting: emotional, moral, cognitive and behavioural, they recognise that the emotional element is the determining one. Alzheimer's Disease is a progressive deterioration of cognitive functions that, in its early and mid-stages at least, is in many regards an exaggerated version of what everyone sometimes experiences. You do not need to have AD, or indeed Mild Cognitive Impairment, for an appointment to slip your mind, to forget what you went upstairs for, or to struggle to recall someone's name. As noted earlier, the condition of Mild Cognitive Impairment affects many more people than develop AD. However, as also noted there, MCI is rather easily labelled as the marker of early-stage AD. Inevitably, then, any caregiver is likely to become hypersensitive to anything in her own behaviour that resembles an AD symptom. As a result, empathy itself adds a level of peril to an already perilous environment. The caregiver does not want to understand what it is like to be someone with AD, because that is a frightening thing to contemplate. Schrauf et al (2012) show how people from three different cultures in the US construct the person with AD as 'other', as a means of protecting their own sense of integrity as a normal person.

Thus we see that there are very powerful drives in the AD care environment that are likely to make it difficult for caregivers to exercise compassion (Figure 1). The process by which caregivers detach themselves and create the context for uncompassionate care is similar to what Cameron (2012) terms 'dyspathy': the construction of a barrier between self and the other.

Caregivers will experience extreme stress in the face of these drives because they create dissonances with their underlying commitment to care. That is, the caregiver observes the unkindness of her behaviour (see web-posting, earlier) and is shocked and disappointed by it—yet finds that every available alternative, including empathy, carries negative consequences. To attempt to be kinder entails adopting an assumption of pragmatically rational linguistic behaviour and resisting the urge to detach cognitively as a defence. The result is a direct assault on the caregiver's sense of usefulness and worth, given the implications of the repetitive linguistic behaviour towards them. To uncouple again the assumption of rationality leaves the caregiver no basis on which to interpret the input, and thus no cognitive engagement with it is possible.

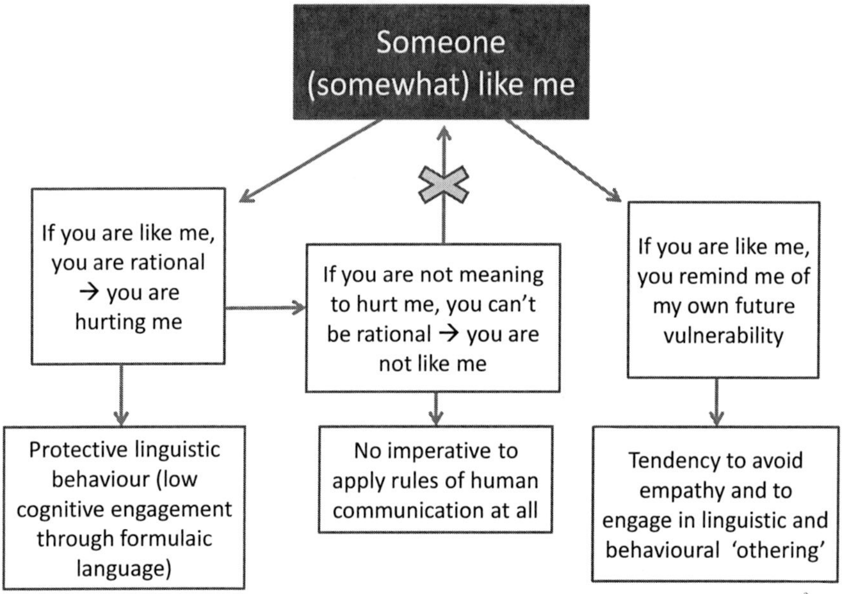

Figure 1: The drives away from compassion

Section 7: Towards a solution

The advice of the Alzheimer's Society (2012, 8) for dealing with repetition is as follows:

> *Look for a reason behind the repetition*: Try to find out if there is a specific cause or trigger for the behavior.
> *Focus on the emotion, not the behaviour*: Rather than reacting to what the person is doing, respond to how he or she is feeling.
> *Turn the action or behavior into an activity*: If the person is rubbing his or her hand across the table, provide a cloth and ask for help with dusting.

Stay calm, and be patient: Reassure the person with a calm voice and gentle touch.

Provide an answer: Give the person the answer that he or she is looking for, even if you have to repeat it several times. It may help to write it down and post it in a prominent location.

These guidelines are offered in the recognition that caregivers need strategies for avoiding negative reactions. Clearly, some caregivers do manage to respond constructively and sustain compassion without undue stress, so how do they manage it? Under what circumstances, or for which sorts of personality, can compassion survive and be nurtured? One focus of interest has been that of operationalising empathy through meditation and mindfulness practices. These approaches seem to offer a firm basis for inculcating a type of compassion that is more cognitive than purely emotional (e.g. Blane and Mercer 2011, Cole-King and Gilbert 2011, Mercer and Reynolds 2002). Mindfulness and meditation have been found to reduce stress in caregivers (Lavretsky et al. 2013, Oken et al. 2010, Waelde et al. 2004), and, as a result, these practices are relevant to initiatives aiming to train caregivers in how to behave compassionately (Chambers and Ryder 2011, Cole-King and Gilbert 2011).

Mindfulness appears to enable the caregiver to pay attention to her own self as a resilient core resource, separate from the ego that is under attack both directly from the apparently unfeeling language of the person with AD and also from the caregiver's own vulnerable sense of esteem, identity and agency. Such a capacity seems to be important in ensuring that the emotional element of empathy does not draw the caregiver into an excessive co-experience of AD (Mercer and Reynolds 2002). The mechanisms by which mindfulness creates a pathway to compassionate care are complex, because they entail a resituating of 'ego' (e.g. Leary 2004) and the management of powerful evolutionary drivers (Gilbert 2009). These mechanisms, and the role of language in achieving them (e.g. Pounds 2010, Pounds 2012) are explored further in Wray (in press).

References

Abraham, A. (2011). *Care and compassion? Report of the Health Service Ombudsman on ten investigations into NHS care of older people.* London: Her Majesty's Stationery Office, http://www.ombudsman.org.uk/__data/assets/pdf_file/0016/7216/Care-and-Compassion-PHSO-0114web.pdf, Accessed: 14.07.13

ADERC (2011). The changing brain (Alzheimer's Disease Education and Referral Center). http://www.nia.nih.gov/alzheimers/publication/part-2-what-happens-brain-ad/changing-brain-ad. Accessed: 14.07.13

Aijmer, K. (1996). *Conversational routines in English*. Harlow: Longman.

Allan, K. and Killick, J. (2008). Communication and relationships: an inclusive social world. In M. Downs and B. Bowers (Eds.), *Excellence in Dementia care: principles and practice*. Maidenhead: Open University Press, 212-229.

Alzheimer's Association (2012). *Behaviors: How to respond when dementia causes unpredictable behaviors.* http://alzheimers.about.com/gi/o.htm?zi=1/XJ&zTi=1&sdn=alzheimers&cdn=health&tm=18&f=00&su=p284.13.342.ip_&tt=13&bt=7&bts=7&zu=http%3A//www.alz.org/national/documents/brochure_behaviors.pdf Accessed: 14.07.13.

Alzheimer's Society (2010). *Mild Cognitive Impairment*. Factsheet 470, http://www.alzheimers.org.uk/site/scripts/documents_info.php?documentID=120 Accessed: 14.07.13

—. (2012). *Dealing with guilt*. Factsheet 516. http://www.alzheimers.org.uk/site/scripts/download_info.php?fileID=1802 Accessed 14.07.13

Asp, E. D., Cloutier, F., Fay, S., Cook, C., Robertson, M. L., Fisk, J., Dei, D.-W. and Rockwood, K. (2006). Verbal repetition in patients with Alzheimer's disease who receive donepezil. *International Journal of Geriatric Psychiatry,* 21, 426-431.

Asp, E. D. and de Villiers, J. (2010). *When language breaks down.* Cambridge: Cambridge University Press.

Austin, J. (1962). *How to do things with words*. Oxford: Clarendon Press.

Backhaus, P. (Ed.). (2011). *Communication in elderly care: crosscultural perspectives.* London/New York: Continuum.

Ballenger, J. F. (2006). *Self, senility and Alzheimer's Disease in modern America.* Baltimore: John Hopkins Press.

Bayles, K. A. and Kaszniak, A. W. (1987). *Communication and cognition in normal aging and dementia.* Boston: College-Hill Press/Little Brown.

Beatty, W., Rogers, C., Rogers, R., English, S., Testa, J., Orbelo, D., Wilson, D., and Ross, E. (1999). Piano playing in Alzheimer's disease: longitudinal study of a single case. *Neurocase* 5: 459-69.

Blane, D. and Mercer, S. W. (2011). Compassionate healthcare: is empathy the key? *Journal of Holistic Healthcare,* 8(3), 18-21.

Brereton, D. (2012) *Caring for caregivers: Supporting the wellbeing of Britain's hidden vulnerable.* Paper presented at Improving care, Improving Lives Conference, Manchester, December

Brown, M and Clegg, D. (2010). *Ancient Mysteries.* Trebus Project. www.trebusprojects.org.

Cameron, L. (2012). Dyspathy: the dynamic complement of empathy *Living with Uncertainty Working paper* 5 http://www.open.ac.uk/researchprojects/livingwithuncertainty/pics/d134491.pdf.

Chambers, C. and Ryder, E. (2011). Excellence in compassionate nursing care: leading the change. *Journal of Holistic Healthcare,* 8(3), 46-49.

Clark, H. H. (1992). *Arenas of language use.* Chicago: University of Chicago Press.

Clegg, D. (Ed.). (2010). *Tell Mrs Mill her husband is still dead.* Trebus Project. www.trebusprojects.org.

Cole-King, A. and Gilbert, P. (2011). Compassionate care: the theory and the reality. *Journal of Holistic Healthcare,* 8(3), 29-37.

Corrigan, R., Moravcsik, E. A., Ouali, H. and Wheatley, K. M. (Eds.). (2009a). *Formulaic language. Vol 2: acquisition, loss, psychological reality, and functional explanations.* Amsterdam: John Benjamins.

Corrigan, R., Moravcsik, E. A., Ouali, H. and Wheatley, K. M. (Eds.). (2009b). *Formulaic language. Vol 1: distribution and historical change.* Amsterdam: John Benjamins.

Coste, J.K. (2003). *Learning to speak Alzheimer's.* London: Vermilion.

Coupland, N., Coupland, J., Giles, H. and Henwood, K. (1988). Accommodating the elderly: invoking and extending a theory. *Language in Society,* 17, 1-41.

Cullen, B., Coen, R.F., Lynch, C.A., Cunningham, C.J., Coakley, D., Robertson, I.H., and Lawlor, B.A. (2005). Repetitive behaviour in Alzheimer's disease: description, correlates and functions. *International Journal of Geriatric Psychiatry*, 2005(20), 686–693.

Davies, B. L. (2007). Grice's Cooperative Principle: meaning and rationality. *Journal of Pragmatics,* 39, 2308-2331.

Ekman, S., Norberg, A., Viitanen, M. and Winblad, B. (1991). Care of demented patients with severe communication problems. *Scandinavian Journal of Caring Sciences,* 5(3), 163-170.

Gilbert, P. (2009). *The compassionate mind: coping with the challenges of living.* London: Constable Robinson.

Goffman, E. (1961). *Asylums: Essays on the social situation of mental patients and other inmates.* New York: Anchor.

Goodrich, J. and Cornwell, J. (2011). Seeing the person in the patient: the King's Fund Point of Care programme. *Journal of Holistic Healthcare,* 8(3), 10-12.

Granger, S. and Meunier, F. (Eds.). (2008). *Phraseology: an interdisciplinary perspective.* Amsterdam: John Benjamins.

Grice, H. P. (1975). Logic and conversation. In P. Cole and J. L. Morgan (Eds.), *Syntax and Semantics, vol. 3.* . New York: Academic Press, 41-58.

Guardian, 2013. Caregivers should be monitored or mental health problems, warn doctors. *The Guardian*, Saturday 11 May 2013.

Hamilton, H. (1994). *Conversations with an Alzheimer's patient.* Cambridge: Cambridge University Press.

Hampel, H., Bürger, K., Teipel, S. J., Bokde, A. L. W., Zetterberg, H. and Blennow, K. (2008). Core candidate neurochemical and imaging biomarkers of Alzheimer's disease. *Alzheimer's and Dementia,* 4(1), 38-48.

Hoadley, J. (2008). Caregivers: dealing with repeated questions. AlzCareBlog. http://www.alzcareblog.com/2008/06/05/dealing-with-repeated-questions-blog/ Accessed: 14.07.13

Kitwood, T. (1997). The experience of dementia. *Aging and Mental Health,* 1(1), 13-22.

Kuiper, K. (1996). *Smooth talkers: the linguistic performance of auctioneers and sportscasters.* Mahwah, NJ.: Lawrence Erlbaum.

Lavretsky, H., Spel, E., Siddarth, P., Nazarian, N., St Cyr, N., Khalsa, D., Lin, J., Blackburn, E. and Irwin, M. (2013). A pilot study of yogic meditation for family dementia caregivers with depressive symptoms: effects on mental health, cognition and telomerase activity.[preprint]. *International Journal of Geriatric Psychiatry* 28(1), 57-65.

Leary, M. R. (2004). *The curse of the self: self-awareness, egotism and the quality of human life.* New York: OUP.

Levinson, S. (1983). *Pragmatics.* Cambridge: Cambridge University Press.

Lilly, M., Robinson, C., Holtzman, S. and Bottorff, J. (2012). Can we move beyond burden and burnout to support the health and wellness of family caregivers to persons with dementia? Evidence from British Columbia, Canada. *Health and Social Care in the Community,* 20(1), 103-112.

Lord, A. B. (2000). *The singer of tales.* 2nd, Cambridge, MA: Harvard University Press.

Mercer, S. W. and Reynolds, W. J. (2002). Empathy and quality of care. *British Journal of General Practice,* 52(Supplement), S9-13.

Meunier, F. and Granger, S. (2008). *Phraseology in foreign language learning and teaching.* Amsterdam: John Benjamins.

Milwain, E. (2000). Mild cognitive impairment: further caution. *The Lancet,* 355(9208), 1018.

National Institute on Aging (2009). Understanding Stages and Symptoms of Alzheimer's Disease.
http://www.nia.nih.gov/Alzheimers/Publications/stages.htm. Accessed: 14.07.13

NHS Confederation (2012). Delivering Dignity: Securing dignity in care for older people in hospitals and care homes.
http://www.nhsconfed.org/Documents/dignity.pdf. Accessed: 14.07.13.

Nussbaum, J. F. and Coupland, J. (Eds.). (2004). *Handbook of communication and aging research.* 2nd edition., London: Routledge.

Oken, B., Fonareva, I., Hass, M., Wahbeh, H., Lane, J., Zajdel, D. and Amen, A. (2010). Pilot controlled trial of mindfulness meditation and education for dementia caregivers. *Journal of Alternative and Complementary Medicine,* 16(10), 1031-1038.

Orange, J. B. and Purves, B. (1996). Conversational discourse and cognitive impairment: implications for Alzheimer's Disease. *Journal of Speech-Language, Pathology and Audiology,* 20(2), 139-150.

Pounds, G. (2010). Empathy as 'appraisal': a new language-based approach to the exploration of clinical empathy. *Journal of Applied Linguistics and Professional Practice,* 7(2), 139-162.

Pounds, G. (2012). Enhancing empathic skills in clinical practice: a linguistic approach. *International Journal of Work Organisation and Emotion,* 5(2), 114-131.

Prince, M. and Jackson, J. (2009). *World Alzheimer's Report.*
http://www.alz.co.uk/research/worldreport/ Accessed: 14.07.13.

Raupach, M. (1984). Formulae in second language speech production In H. Dechert, D. Möhle and M. Raupach (Eds.), *Second language productions.* Tübingen: Gunter Narr, 114-137.

Sabat, S. R. (2001). *The experience of Alzheimer's disease: life through a tangled veil.* Oxford: Blackwell.

Schrauf, R. W., Iris, M., Navarro, E. and Smotrova, T. (2012). How to construct a case of Alzheimer's disease in three languages: case-based reasoning in narrative gerontology. *Ageing and Society,* DOI: 10.1017/S0144686X12000979, (preview) 1-30.

Segalowitz, N. (2010). *Cognitive bases of second language fluency.* London: Routledge.

Shakespeare, P. (1998). *Aspects of confused speech.* Mahwah, NJ: Erlbaum.

Tannen, D. (1989). *Talking voices: repetition, dialogue and imagery in conversational discourse.* Cambridge: Cambridge University Press.

Tappen, R. M., Williams-Burgess, C., Edelstein, J., Touhy, T. and Fishman, S. (1997). Communicating with individuals with Alzheimer's Disease: examination of recommended strategies. *Archives of Psychiatric Nursing,* 11(5), 249-256.

Waelde, L., Thompson, L. and Gallagher-Thompson, D. (2004). A pilot study of a yoga and meditation intervention for dementia caregiver stress. *Journal of Clinical Psychology,* 60(6), 677-687.

Wilson, D. and Sperber, D. (2002). Relevance theory. *UCL Working Papers in Linguistics,* 14, 249-290. http://www.ucl.ac.uk/psychlangsci/research/linguistics/publications/wpl/02papers/wilson_sperber. Accessed: 14.07.13.

Wray, A. (2002). *Formulaic language and the lexicon.* Cambridge: Cambridge University Press.

Wray, A. and Grace, G. W. (2007). The consequences of talking to strangers: evolutionary corollaries of socio-cultural influences on linguistic form. *Lingua,* 117(3), 543-578.

Wray, A. (2008). *Formulaic language: pushing the boundaries.* Oxford: Oxford University Press.

—. (2009). Identifying formulaic language: persistent challenges and new opportunities. In R. Corrigan, E. Moravcsik, H. Ouali and K. Wheatley (Eds.), *Formulaic Language: Vol 1: Structure, Distribution and Historical Change.* Amsterdam: John Benjamins, 27-51.

—. (2010). We've had a wonderful, wonderful thing: formulaic interaction when an expert has dementia. *Dementia: The International Journal of Social Research and Practice,* 9(4), 517-534.

—. (2011). Formulaic language as a barrier to effective communication with people with Alzheimer's Disease. *Canadian Modern Language Review,* 67(4), 429-458.

—. (2012). Patterns of formulaic language in Alzheimer's disease: implications for quality of life. *Quality in Ageing and Older Adults,* 13(3), 168-175.

—. (in press). Formulaic language and threat: the challenge of empathy and compassion in Alzheimer's Disease interaction. In Schrauf, R. and Mueller, N. (eds.) *Dialogue and Dementia: Cognitive and Communicative Resources for Engagement.* New York: Psychology Press.

Youngson, R. (2011). Compassion in healthcare: the missing dimension of healthcare reform? *Journal of Holistic Healthcare,* 8(3), 6-9.

Zigmond, D. (2011). Five executive follies: how commodification imperils compassion in personal healthcare. *Journal of Holistic Healthcare,* 8(3), 13-17.

CHAPTER SIX

DISCOURSE IN LEWY BODY SPECTRUM DISORDER

ANGELA ROBERTS AND J. B. ORANGE
WESTERN UNIVERSITY

Introduction

Lewy Body Spectrum Disorder Defined

The newly developed term Lewy Body Spectrum Disorder (LBSD) refers to a group of disorders including Parkinson disease (PD), Parkinson disease dementia (PDD) and dementia with Lewy bodies (DLB) (Lippa et al. 2007). The term was established to link conceptually similar conditions along a spectrum consisting of common neuropathological, neuromotor, neurophysiological, and cognitive neuroscience features. Within this spectrum, the diagnostic criteria for each of the disorders (i.e., PD, PDD, and DLB) are well defined (See Table 1). PD is defined by characteristic motor symptoms including bradykinesia (e.g., slowed and reduced amplitude of movement) and rigidity (Gelb, Oliver, and Gilman 1999). The diagnoses of PDD and DLB are determined clinically, in part and not exclusively, by the onset of dementia relative to the timing of motor symptom onset. The diagnosis of PDD is established "when dementia develops within the context of established PD" (Emre et al. 2007, 1690). At the other end of the spectrum, DLB occurs when the "diagnosis of dementia precedes or coincides within 1 year" of the development of parkinsonian motor symptoms (e.g., bradykinesia, rigidity) (Emre et al. 2007).

Table 1: Summary of diagnostic features of Parkinson disease (PD), Parkinson disease dementia (PDD), and Dementia with Lewy bodies (DLB)

<table>
<tr><th></th><th>PD
(Gibb and Lees 1988)</th><th>PDD
(Goetz, Emre, and Dubois 2008)</th><th>DLB
(McKeith and Mosimann 2004)</th></tr>
<tr><td>Core Features</td><td>Bradykinesia[1]

Plus at least one of the following:
Rigidity
■ 4 – 6 Hz rest tremor
■ Postural instability[2]</td><td>■ Diagnosis of PD
■ Dementia (slow, insidious, progressive) developing in the context of established PD (usually of duration > 12 months)</td><td>■ Dementia with fluctuating cognition
■ Recurrent visual hallucinations</td></tr>
<tr><td>Supporting Features</td><td>■ Unilateral onset
■ Tremor present only or more prominently with limbs at rest
■ Progressive disorder (clinical course ≥ 10 years)
■ Persistent asymmetry in motor symptoms
■ Excellent motor symptom improvement (70-100%) with levodopa
■ Motor symptoms responsive to levodopa ≥ 5 years
■ Hyposmia
■ Visual hallucinations
■ Chorea induced by levodopa</td><td>■ Attention deficits: (may fluctuate day to day)
■ Executive function deficits
■ Visual spatial deficits: perception and construction
■ Memory deficits: Responds to cuing; Recognition better than recall
■ Word retrieval and sentence comprehension deficits may be present but core language functions relatively preserved
■ Apathy
■ Personality and mood changes
■ Daytime somnolence
■ Hallucinations
■ Delusions</td><td>■ Motor parkinsonism
■ Repeated falls
■ Syncope
■ Transient loss of consciousness
■ Neuroleptic sensitivity
■ Hallucinations
■ REM behavior sleep disorder
■ Depression</td></tr>
</table>

[1] Bradykinesia = Slowness of movement and progressive decrement of amplitude of movement during repetitive motor tasks such as foot tapping, finger tapping or hand opening and closing

[2] Postural instability = not resulting from vestibular, neuropathy or other medical causes

Lewy body dementia (LBD), not to be confused with the term dementia with Lewy bodies (DLB), is a superordinate category title that refers to both PDD and DLB as a combined subgroup within LBSD (Lippa et al. 2007). Throughout this chapter, we refer primarily to DLB as a single disorder. The construct of Parkinson disease with mild cognitive impairment (PD-MCI) is useful within a discussion of LBSD (Caviness et al. 2007), however, there is ambiguity concerning the specific diagnostic criteria of PD-MCI (Martinez-Horta and Kulisevsky 2011). We acknowledge that PD-MCI likely falls between PD and PDD. The focus of this chapter is to describe the published literature on the spoken discourse performance of LBSD vis-à-vis its constituent subgroups. While the authors acknowledge the presence of PD-MCI, it is not specifically discussed in the current chapter because of the weaker diagnostic criteria and the lack of published literature on spoken discourse in PD-MCI.

Common neuropathology features in LBSD include the prominent presence of Lewy bodies and Lewy neurites in brain stem structures, in cortical regions, and in the limbic system (McKeith et al. 2004; Troster 2008). Amyloid plaques and neurofibrillary tangles are common to the disorders within LBSD and overlap with the neuropathology observed in Alzheimer's disease (AD) (McKeith et al. 2004; Troster 2008). Lewy bodies and Lewy neurites are abnormal formations of protein (i.e., largely comprised of alpha-synuclein) found in the neurons (and other cells) of individuals with PD, PDD, and DLB (Troster 2008). While Lewy bodies were first discovered in the early 1900s it was not until the mid-twentieth century that their relationship to cognitive decline in PD was established (Goedert et al. 2013; Troster 2008). Further, the association of Lewy bodies to specific dementias associated with parkinsonism was not realized until the 1960s (Goedert et al. 2013; Troster 2008). The full recognition of DLB occurred only in the early 1990s (McKeith 2004). As such, our understanding of the development, nature, and progression of cognitive decline across LBSD and the downstream effects on language and discourse remains relatively underdeveloped in comparison to other dementias such as dementia Alzheimer's type (DAT).

Cognitive, Language, and Speech Changes in Lewy Body Spectrum Disorders

While our knowledge of the cognitive, language, and spoken discourse consequences of LBSD is in its early development, research on this topic holds great importance given the emerging incidence and prevalence data. According to the Parkinson Disease Foundation, 7 to 10 million people worldwide are living with PD. Point prevalence data indicate that the cumulative prevalence of PDD is as high as 78% at 8 years post-onset of PD (Aarsland et al. 2003). The relative risk of developing dementia is 4 to 6 times higher for individuals with PD compared to community dwelling healthy adults (Emre et al. 2007). PDD is associated with older age of disease onset, increased falls, increased gait and balance instability, and REM behavior sleep disorder (Emre et al. 2007). Given these alarming statistics, the potential impact of PD and more importantly PDD on health resources and quality of life is immense. Recent literature suggests that DLB pathology is second only to DAT in its prevalence among dementias occurring in 22 to 25% of older adults (Levy and Chelune 2007; McKeith 2004).

As in other degenerative cognitive-linguistic disorders (e.g., DAT, frontotemporal dementia (FTD), amyotrophic lateral sclerosis with FTD), the cognitive deficits in LBSD likely have downstream effects on language and discourse. While investigators have explored the effects of cognition on discrete language tasks in PD, very few published studies have specifically examined this relationship in PDD and DLB. Complicating the understanding of how cognitive and language impairments affect discourse in LBSD is the cardinal finding of parkinsonian motor features, including a high prevalence of motor speech changes. It is beyond the scope of this chapter to review the wide-ranging cognitive, language, and motor speech changes associated with LBSD. However, a brief summary of this literature is provided to contextualize the more complete discussion of the discourse impairments in LBSD.

Cognitive Changes in LBSD

Cognitive changes can be present early in PD and can exist in the absence of dementia (i.e., PD-MCI) (Aarsland, Beyer, and Kurz 2008; Aarsland et al. 2010; Benito-Leon et al. 2011; Elgh et al. 2009). Cognitive changes may be present at the time of diagnosis in as many as 30% of PD cases (Elgh et al. 2009). There is a large body of literature relative to cognitive impairments in PD without dementia. The more consistently reported domains of impairment include: 1) impaired verbal fluency for semantic categories, phonemes and action words (Benito-Leon et al. 2011; Green et al. 2002; Elgh et al. 2009; Henry and Crawford 2004; Muslimovic et al. 2005; Pagonabarraga and Kulisevsky 2012; Rodriguez-Ferreiro et al. 2010) 2) impaired attention (e.g., activation, sustained, set-shifting) (Elgh et al. 2009; Green et al. 2002; Muslimovic et al. 2005; Pagonabarraga and Kulisevsky 2012), 3) impaired working memory

(Muslimovic et al. 2005) 4) impaired psychomotor speed (Elgh et al. 2009; Muslimovic et al. 2005) 5) impaired verbal and visual memory (Benito-Leon et al. 2011; Bohlhalter et al. 2009; Elgh et al. 2009; Ivory et al. 1999; Muslimovic et al. 2005; Pagonabarraga and Kulisevsky 2012) and 6) impaired visual construction/visual perceptual skills (Pagonabarraga and Kulisevsky, 2012). The cognitive impairments observed in PDD and DLB are similar to those reported in PD except that they are more ubiquitous and more severe in impairment. The unique cognitive profile of mild-moderate DLB is characterized by deficits in attention particularly for more challenging visual search and attention allocation tasks (Emre et al. 2007). While fluctuations in attention lasting hours to days are common in both PDD and DLB, attention fluctuations are more salient among individuals with DLB (42%) vs. PDD (28%) (Ballard and McKeith 1998; Emre et al. 2007). Although the profile of memory impairment is similar for both PDD and DLB, the incidence of reported memory complaints is higher in DLB vs. PD (Emre et al. 2007). Moreover, the presence of prominent and early executive function deficits is an important marker and in PD may be a harbinger of dementia (Troster 2008).

Language Changes in LBSD

Language impairments in persons with PD, while not pervasive, are frequently reported in the literature. Language problems in PD include disrupted word retrieval in verbal fluency (Henry and Crawford 2004) and impaired confrontation naming (Cotelli et al. 2007; Herrera, Rodriguez-Ferreiro, and Cuetos 2012; Rodriguez-Ferreiro et al. 2009). Researchers suggest that individuals with PD exhibit a specific deficit in word retrieval for verbs vs. nouns (Cotelli et al. 2007; Fernandino et al. 2012; Herrera, Rodriguez-Ferreiro, and Cuetos 2012). One of the more extensively explored areas of language in PD is the impaired processing of syntax and grammar. Multiple investigators demonstrated that individuals with PD are less accurate and/or less efficient vs. controls on tasks requiring extraction of information and decoding of syntax from complex sentences that either are heard or are read (Colman et al. 2011; Grossman et al. 1991; 1992; 1993; 1999; Grossman 1999; Hochstadt et al. 2006; Hochstadt 2009; Natsopoulos et al. 1991; 1993; Skeel et al. 2001; Ye et al. 2012). Moreover, individuals with PD show consistent impairments in comprehension of sentences resulting from impaired processing of semantic ambiguities (For a review see Chenery, Angwin, and Copland 2008). Compared to the comprehension domain, there is scant published literature on syntax production in PD. The few published findings on syntax production in PD generally come from the discourse studies that are reviewed later in this chapter.

Few published studies have specifically addressed language changes in PDD. The presence of verbal fluency impairments (i.e., phonemic and category) is certainly a more consistent finding and is more severely impaired in PDD vs. PD (Henry and Crawford 2004). Individuals with PDD consistently present with impaired confrontation naming of nouns, impaired comprehension of complex syntax forms, and reduced volume of information in spontaneous speech (Emre 2003). The general consensus from the literature is that language functions are less impaired in PDD and DLB vs. in DAT in which language is commonly and prominently impaired (Emre 2003; Emre et al. 2007; Troster 2008). The distinct language impairments in DLB vs. those in PDD have been reported more extensively in the literature. Williams et al. (2007) and Johnson, Morris, and Galvin (2005) reported that individuals with DLB performed significantly better than those with DAT on the *Boston Naming Test*. However, individuals with DLB showed a unique pattern of perceptually based errors (e.g. visual confusion errors) (Williams et al. 2007). Laws et al. (2007) reported that individuals with DLB were significantly more impaired vs. controls on both confrontation naming and on naming to description tasks. Similarly, those with DLB demonstrated a significant category specific deficit for living items vs. non-living items (Laws et al. 2007). Moreover, Ralph et al. (2001) reported that individuals with DLB demonstrated word retrieval deficits reflecting impaired access to the semantic system. Syntax comprehension deficits also are present in DLB for sentences that are longer, contain embedded clauses, require noun phrase movements, and contain syntactic ambiguities generated by semantic incongruity between the verb and the object clause (Gross et al. 2012; Grossman et al. 2012). Collectively, these findings show that the cognitive and language impairments observed in individuals with LBSD can have potentially substantial effects on their discourse performances.

Speech Changes in LBSD

The possible impact of cognitive and language impairments on discourse in LBSD is complicated further by the prominent presence of motor speech problems. While 100% of individuals with PD and PDD will present with motor parkinsonism, the presence of motor parkinsonism is not universal in DLB with 80 to 100% of individuals presenting with motor symptoms (McKeith and Mosimann 2004). When motor symptoms are present, their severity is fairly equivalent across the conditions within

LBSD (McKeith and Mosimann 2004). While motor speech impairments associated with PD are commonly reported in the literature, the authors were unable to find any published studies specifically exploring the epidemiology or characteristics of dysarthria in DLB. However, the underlying commonality of parkinsonism features across disorders in LBSD suggest that the three subgroups would have similar motor speech profiles. Upwards of 90% of individuals with PD will develop articulation and/or voice changes in PD (Ramig, Fox, and Sapir 2004). Changes such as reduced precision of sound articulation, changes in speaking rate (i.e., either increasing or decreasing rate), reduced loudness, and breathy/hoarse voice quality can affect communication at the discourse level in PD (Darley, Aronson, and Brown 1969; 1975; Ramig, Fox, and Sapir 2004). However, more importantly other communication-related changes in PD such as reduced pitch variability, reduced stress patterns, and reduced emotional expression via vocal and facial channels can interact substantially with the ability to convey meaning through language in discourse (Darley, Aronson, and Brown 1969; 1975; Ramig, Fox, and Sapir 2004; Pitcairn et al. 1990; Pell, Cheang, and Leonard 2006). The disruptions in prosody are not limited to the production domain in PD but also are present in the comprehension domain, which can reduce the effectiveness of individuals in their roles of speaker and listener (Monetta, Cheang, and Pell 2008). The motor speech problems in PD negatively affect conversational discourse by altering listeners' perceptions of speakers with PD wherein listeners rate persons with PD as less interested, less involved, less happy, less friendly, and more anxious (Pitcairn et al. 1990; Jaywant and Pell 2010). While investigators have not explored specifically the phenomenon of motor speech problems in PDD and DLB, there is evidence to suggest that worsening motor impairment, including declining motor speech performance, is associated with risk of developing cognitive decline or dementia in PD (Burn et al. 2003; 2006; Elgh et al. 2009; Gago et al. 2009; Green et al. 2002; Verbaan et al. 2007; Locascio, Corkin, and Growdon 2003; Sollinger et al. 2010).

Summary

Taken as a whole the cognitive, language, and motor speech deficits reported in the literature on individuals with LBSD underscore the importance of studying the impact of these deficits on their discourse. The need to complete such research is supported by the results from a series of survey studies completed in the United Kingdom in which investigators reported that the phenomenon of everyday communication challenges in

PD was not limited to motor speech problems but also included cognitive-linguistic changes such as difficulty finding words and difficulty maintaining the train of one's thoughts (Miller et al. 2008; 2011). Given the complexity of cognitive, language, motor speech, and gestural challenges in LBSD the study of discourse production is ideal for revealing the potential interactions among and the functional impact of these changes.

Discourse Studies in Lewy Body Spectrum Disorders: Monologic Discourse

Monologic Discourse Defined

The term monologic discourse refers to structured tasks designed to solicit samples of expressive language. Monologic discourse tasks are not, by their nature, interactional. Unlike conversational discourse, monologic discourse tasks do not per se engage an individual in the active, dynamic, and dyadic exchange of novel information where partners have potentially equal roles in the exchange. Furthermore, some monologic discourse tasks, while representative of everyday language, often do not serve the purpose of building or maintaining relationships, as is the case with conversational discourse. However, the structures and functions of monologic discourse tasks make them uniquely valuable for the study of the interactions among cognition, language, and motor speech components of communication; giving monologic discourse tasks special relevance for the assessment and interpretation of discourse performances among persons with LBSD.

Commonly used monologic discourse tasks include picture description, narrative generation, narrative retelling, procedural and personal narratives including topic guided/directed interviews. Each of these tasks entails a unique set of cognitive and linguistic demands (e.g., memory, personal relevance, linguistic specificity, syntactic complexity, etc.) that are reflected in a person's discourse performance (Shadden 1998a). The use of monologic discourse tasks is well established in the literature in cognitive-communication disorders resulting from neurodegenerative processes (Ash et al. 2006; Orange and Kertesz 2000; Roberts-South et al. 2012; Zraick et al. 2011). For example, monologic discourse tasks can reveal subtle changes in cognitive-linguistic functions in mild cognitive impairment (Fleming and Harris 2008). Multiple monologic discourse tasks also can be used to reveal participants' abilities and impairments in cognition, language, and motor speech production as a function of the intrinsic demands of the task (Shadden 1998a). Given the complex nature of both cognitive-linguistic changes in LBSD (e.g., reduced word retrieval, reduced verbal fluency, reduced syntax processing/production) and its parkinsonian features (e.g., reduced speech loudness, reduced facial expression, altered speech rate, reduced speech articulation), a combination of monologic discourse tasks is ideal for researchers and clinicians to evaluate interactions among cognitive, language, and motor variables in the onset and progression of LBSD.

At present, there are only a handful of published studies on the spoken monologic discourse performance of individuals with LBSD. The majority of these studies explored spoken discourse performance in individuals with PD who showed no cognitive impairment, those who exhibited MCI, or those who were rated with relatively mild disease severity. Few published studies to date have addressed spoken discourse performances in individuals with PD with cognitive impairment, PDD or DLB. Moreover, the majority of published studies have explored only a single spoken discourse genre and have not explored, within the same group of participants, variations in discourse performance as a function of task demands.

Coelho (2007) categorized the analysis procedures for monologic discourse as: 1) microlinguistic (i.e., within-sentence level analyses), 2) microstructural (i.e., across-sentence level analyses), 3) macrostructural (i.e., analyses of thematic unity within the narrative and 4) superstructural (i.e., story grammar level analyses). Coelho's outline structure is used herein as a framework within the discussion of the literature on monologic discourse in LBSD. Within the published discourse literature in LBSD, all of the analyses methods described are categorized as either microlinguistic or macrostructural. Details of each study including the discourse elicitation task and relevant demographic data for the participant groups are presented in Table 2.

Table 2: Summary of Published Discourse Production Studies in Lewy Body Spectrum Disorder

Study	Discourse Genre/Analyses	Participants
Alpert, Rosen, Welkowitz, and Lieberman (1990)	• Structured interactional discourse between participant and researcher using topic directed interview format to solicit personal experiences of the speaker • Analyses: Conversation pause and turn-taking behaviours	• N = 10 PD with mild to moderate dementia • Mean age = 77 years • Mean disease duration = 6.3 years • Range Hoehn and Yahr(/5) = 3 - 4 • Descriptives for motor severity, speech intelligibility and cognitive measures not provided
Ash, McMillan, Gross, Cook, Morgan, Boller, Dreyfuss, Siderowf, and Grossman (2011)	• Narrative discourse (story generation) using the wordless picture book Frog Where Are you? by Mercer Mayer • Analyses: Microlinguistic, macrostructural	• N = 32 LBSD (n = 14 PDD/DLB; n = 18 PDND) and N = 16 HC • Mean age = 71.9(8.5) LBSD; 68.6(6.8) HC • Mean MMSE (/30) = 20.9(4.7) PDD/DLB; 27.9(1.5) PDND; 29.1(1.2) HC • Mean disease duration = 6.6(2.3) PDD/DLB; 6.1(3.2) PDND • Mean UPDRSm (/56) = 24.1(13.3) PDD/DLB; 20.9(9.1) PDND • Mean Hoehn and Yahr (/5) = 2.7(0.6) PDD/DLB; 2.2(0.7) PDND • Speech intelligibility data not provided

Study	Discourse Genre/Analyses	Participants
Ash, McMillan, Gross, Cook, Gunawardena, Morgan, Boller, Siderowf, and Grossman (2012)	• Narrative discourse (story generation) using wordless picture book Frog Where Are You? by Mercer Mayer • Analyses: Microstructural	• N = 35 LBSD (n = 14 PDD/DLB; n = 21 PDND) and N = 16 HC • Mean age = 72(8.4) LBSD; 68.6(6.8) HC • Descriptives for PDD/DLB and HC groups identical for Ash et al. (2011). See above. • Mean MMSE (/30) = 27.4(2.0) PDND • Mean disease duration = 6.0(3.1) PDND • Mean UPDRSm (/56) = 21.7(9.0) PDND • Mean Hoehn and Yahr (/5) = 2.2(0.6) PDND • Speech intelligibility data not provided
Bayles (1990)	• Immediate story-retelling • Analyses: Macrostructural	• N = 12 PDND; 32 HC • Mean age = 68(9.7)PDND; 70.25(8.66)HC • Cognitive assessment = Mental Status Questionnaire (Goldfarb and Antin). PDND and HC all scored between 8 - 10/10 reported as 'normal' cognition by author • Descriptives for motor severity, disease duration, disease staging, speech intelligibility not provided

Study	Discourse Genre/Analyses	Participants
Godbout and Doyon (2000)	• Procedural discourse • Analyses: Macrostructural	• N = 16 PDND; 16 HC • Mean age = 59(5.6) PDND; 54.3(13.7) HC • PD subtype = 6 akinetic rigid; 2 tremor; 8 mixed • Cognitive assessment = C.E.R.A.D protocol of neuropsychological measures (Morris et al., 1989). Authors report as normal for PDND group. • Mean MMSE (/30) = 28.34(1.04) PDND; No score provided for HC • Range disease duration = 1 - 21 years • Range Hoehn and Yahr (/5) = 1 - 3 • Descriptives for motor severity, speech intelligibility not provided
Griffiths, Barnes, Britten, and Wilkinson (2012)	• Unstructured conversation of PD+familiar conversation partner dyads recorded at home • Analyses: conversation analyses procedures focussing on turn-taking, overlap talk and repair sequences	• N = 13 PD+familiar partner dyads • Age range = 64 - 86 PD; HC ages not provided • Range disease duration = 3.5 - 20 years • Range Hoehn and Yahr (/5) = 2 - 5 • Speech intelligibility scores using standardized measures are reported in the article • Descriptives for motor severity, cognitive measures, demographics for HC not provided in article

Study	Discourse Genre/Analyses	Participants
Hall, Ouyang, Lonnquist, and Newcombe (2011)	• Structured interactional discourse between participant and researcher using interview format • Analyses: rating of verbal and non-verbal conversation behaviours using a 40-point standardized rating scale *Chicago's Rating Scale of Pragmatic Communication* (Halper, Cherney, and Burns 1996)	• N = 17 PD; 17 HC • Mean age = 60.9(12.5) PD; 59.3(11.0) HC • Mean disease duration = 8.4(6.0) • Mean UPDRS (/108) = 26.1(10.8) • Hoehn and Yahr (/5) = 2.5(0.4) • Descriptives for cognitive measure, speech intelligibility not provided
Holtgraves, McNamara, Capaert, and Durso (2010)	• Personal narrative discourse using topic directed interview format • Analyses: Microlinguistic via unbiased computer-based analysis software: Linguistic Inquiry and Word Count Program (Pennebaker et al., 2007)	• N = 31 PD • Mean age = 69.87(11.54 PD • Mean UPDRSm (/52)= 9.74(3.51) • Mean Hoehn and Yahr (/5) = 2.57(0.63) • Cognitive function = reported to exclude participants with co-existing Alzheimer's like dementia but criteria used not specified. • Descriptives for speech intelligibility, disease duration, cognitive screening measures not provided
Huber and Darling (2011)	• Expository discourse speaker's topic of choice • Analyses: Microlinguistic, motor speech X discourse interactions	• N = 14 PD; 14 HC • Mean age = 69 PD women; 76 PD men; 71 HC women; 72 PD men • Range disease duration = 1 - 10 years • Range Hoehn and Yahr (/5) = 2 - 3 • Perceptual ratings of speech severity made by trained (SLP) listeners provided in article • Descriptives for motor severity and cognitive measures not provided

Study	Discourse Genre/Analyses	Participants
Illes, Metter, Hanson, and Iritani (1988)	• Personal narrative discourse using topic directed interview format • Analyses: Microlinguistic; motor speech X discourse interactions	• N = 10 PD (all men); 10 HC • Disease severity reported by *Webster 30-point Scale of Parkinsonian Disability* n = 5 mild severity; n = 5 moderate severity • Mean disease = 4.6 years mild group; 10 years moderate group • Cognitive function = self-report of no issues • Descriptives for age, Hoehn and Yahr, speech intelligibility not provided
Illes (1989)	• Personal narrative discourse using topic directed interview format • Analyses: Microlinguistic	• N = 10 PD; 10 HD; 10 DAT; 10 HC (all men) • Participants stratified into early or middle stages for respective diseases n= 5 mild; 5 moderate per subgroup • PD stratified based on Webster scale used in Illes et al. (1988) • Mean age = 56.4 PD early; 66.0 PD middle • Cognitive function = self/care provider report of no issues • Descriptives for disease duration, motor severity, speech intelligibility not provided
Jaywant and Pell (2010)	• Picture description stimuli from *Discourse Comprehension Test* (Brookshire and Nicholas 1997) • Analyses: Microlinguistic; Macrolinguistic (listener perceptions of content); listener perceptions of non-verbal and verbal components of discourse production	• N = 18PD; 17 HC • Mean age = 60.28(7.26) PD; 61.29(9.29) HC • Mean disease duration = 3.57(1.84) • Mean UPDRSm (/56)= 13.67(7.3) • Mean Hoehn and Yahr (/5) = 1.75(0.46) • Mean Mattis Dementia Rating Scale (/144) = 141(2.12) PD; 142.41(1.87) HC • Descriptives for speech intelligibility not provided

Study	Discourse Genre/Analyses	Participants
McNamara, Obler, Au, Durso, and Albert (1992)	• Picture description Cookie Theft stimuli from *Boston Diagnostic Aphasia Exam* (Goodglass and Kaplan, 1983) • Analyses: Microlinguistic; self-monitoring and repair strategies	• N = 178; n = 22 PD; 15 DAT; 141 HC intentionally sampled from 4 age groups (30's to 70's). The 37 participants in the 60's group corresponded in age to the PD group • Mean age = 61.3(2.9)PD; 64.4(2.9) 60's HC • Range Hoehn and Yahr (/5) = 2 - 3 • Cognitive assessment = reported as non-demented by authors; metric not provided • Descriptives for motor severity, disease duration, speech intelligibility and cognitive measures not provided
McNamara and Durso (2003)	• Structured interactional discourse between participant and researcher using interview format • Analyses: rating of verbal and non-verbal conversation behaviours using a standardized measure; *Pragmatic Protocol (Prutting and Kirchner 1987)*	• N = 20 PD; 10 HC • Mean age = 71.5 PD; 48.4 HC • Mean disease duration = 8.8 • Cognitive assessment = reported as non-demented based on non-specified clinical exam and DSM-III criteria • Descriptives of motor severity, Hoehn and Yahr, speech intelligibility not provided

Study	Discourse Genre/Analyses	Participants
Murray (2000)	• Picture description (2 discourse samples) Cookie Theft stimuli from the *Boston Diagnostic Aphasia Exam* (Goodglass and Kaplan 1983) and Grocery Scene (Helm-Esabrooks 1992) • Analyses: Microlinguistic; macrostructral	• N = 10 PD; 10 HD; 18 HC (9 matched to the HD group and 9 matched to the PD group) • Mean age = 70.1(8.8); 67.89(6.13) PD-HC • Mean disease duration = 6.4(2.91) • Mean Hoehn and Yahr (/5) = 3 • Mean Mattis Dementia Rating Scale (/144) = 132.7(6.82)PD; 138.67(3.35) PD-HC • Speech intelligibility scores using standardized measures are reported • Descriptives of motor severity not provided
Murray and Lenz (2001)	• Personal narratives using topic directed interview format • Analyses: Microlinguistic	• N = 10 PD; 9 HD; 17 HC (9 matched to the HD group and 8 matched to the PD group) • Mean age = 70.1(8.8); 68.9(5.7) PD-HC • Mean disease duration = 6.4(2.9) • Mean Mattis Dementia Rating Scale (/144) = 132.8(6.8) PD; 139.0(3.4) PD-HC • Speech intelligibility scores using standardized measures are reported in the article • Descriptives of motor severity, Hoehn and Yahr not provided

Study	Discourse Genre/Analyses	Participants
Rousseaux, Sève, Vallet, Pasquier, and Mackowiak-Cordoliani (2010)	• Structured interactional discourse between participant and researcher using interview format • Analyses: rating of verbal and non-verbal conversation behaviours using a standardized measure; *Lille Communication Test* Rousseaux et al. (2001)	• N = 13 DLB; 29 DAT; 16 FTD; 47 HC • Mean age = 71 DLB; 68 HC • Mean MMSE(/30) = 24 DLB; 29 HC • Dementia Rating Scale (/144) = 123 DLB; 137 HC • Descriptives of motor severity, Hoehn and Yahr, speech intelligibility, disease duration not provided
Whitworth, Lesser, and McKeith (1999)	• Unstructured conversation of PDD/DLB+care partner dyads recorded at home • Interview of perception of conversation impairment with care partner • Analyses: analyses of conversation behaviours focussing on initiation, turn-taking, repair, topic management, use of strategies using a standardized measure; *Conversation Analysis Profile for People with Cognitive Impairment* (Perkins, Whitworth, and Lesser 1998)	• N = 6 PDD+care partner dyads; 6 DLB+care partner dyads • Mean age = 72; PDD; 68 DLB • Range disease duration = 3 - 10 PDD; 4 - 19 DLB • Mean MMSE (/30) = 27.5 PDD; 23.8 DLB • Descriptives of motor severity, Hoehn and Yahr, speech intelligibility not provided

Study	Discourse Genre/Analyses	Participants
Zanini, Tavano, and Fabbro (2010)	• Personal narratives using topic directed interview format • Analyses: Microlinguistic; compared across languages spoken	• Bilingual PD (Friullian and Italian) • N = 9 PD; 9 HC • Mean disease duration = 3.67(2.18) • Mean UPDRS (/108) = 11.22(4.6) • Mean MMSE (/30) = 26.33(2.06) • Descriptives of age, Hoehn and Yahr, speech intelligibility not provided

Note: Age and duration data are presented in years. PD = Parkinson disease assumed or reported as having no dementia. PDD = Parkinson disease dementia. DLB= Lewy body dementia. LBSD = Lewy body spectrum disorder comprised of individuals with PD, PDD, DLB. HC = Health controls assumed to be age-matched to disease group unless otherwise indicated. DAT = dementia Alzheimer's type. HD = Huntington's disease. UPDRS = Unified Parkinson Disease Rating Scale (introduced in 1987 (Fahn et al.) with a more recent version revised by the Movement Disorders Society in 2007 (higher scores represent greater motor impairment). UPDRSm = the shortened version of the UPDRS containing motor testing items only (items 18-31; higher scores represent greater motor impairment). MMSE = Mini Mental Status Examination (lower scores represent greater likelihood of cognitive impairment). Mattis Dementia Rating Scale = lower scores represent greater cognitive impairment. Hoehn and Yahr = measure of symptom staging in Parkinson disease. Higher scores represent greater disease severity

Microlinguistic Analyses

Productivity

Productivity measures in discourse reflect generally the amount and efficiency of language produced in a sample. These measures are influenced highly by cognitive impairments, language disorders, and motor speech problems, Jaywant and Pell (2010), using a picture description task, reported that individuals with PD produced samples that were significantly shorter in duration vs. healthy controls (HC) (PD M = 28.03 sec., SD = 11.35 vs. HC M = 50.33 sec., SD = 31.43). Using a similar picture description task McNamara and colleagues (1992) also showed that individuals with PD produced significantly fewer words vs. HC from a matched age group (PD M = 57.8, SD = 25.4 vs. HC M = 88.5, SD = 64.2). McNamara et al. (1992) also reported that individuals with PD produced significantly fewer words vs. individuals with DAT (M = 102.7, SD = 78.2).

However, the finding of reduced verbal output in persons with LBSD is not a consistent finding in the literature. Murray (2000) reported no differences in total words or total utterances between persons with PD vs. those with Huntington's chorea on a picture description task. Similar findings were reported by Ash et al. (2011) and Ash et al. (2012) using narrative discourse samples generated via a wordless picture book (*Frog, Where Are You?* Mayer 1969). In both studies, the researchers reported significant differences in total words for controls vs. individuals with PDD/DLB but not for controls vs. individuals with PD (Ash et al. 2011; 2012). Similarly, in a personal narrative task that addressed emotional experiences, Crucian et al. (2001) reported no significant differences in total words produced or total duration of discourse for individuals with PD vs. controls. Collectively these results indicate that the total verbal output of discourse in LBSD (i.e., productivity) varies depending on demands of the discourse task and the cognitive status of the participants. More importantly, these findings suggest that the productivity of verbal output is highly variable across LBSD likely as a function of factors such as cognitive decline, language changes, discourse task, and disease progression/severity.

The efficiency of verbal output also has been explored in the LBSD literature as a reflection of productivity. Ash et al. (2011; 2012) reported significantly reduced efficiency of verbal output (words/minute) for PDD/DLB but not PD vs. controls. In contrast, Huber and Darling (2011) reported that only during an expository discourse task, and not during a reading task, did individuals with PD exhibit significantly faster verbal rates (i.e., words/minute) vs. controls. There were no differences in verbal efficiency for the reading task (Huber and Darling 2011). In contrast, Illes et al. (1988) (using discourse samples elicited from personal narratives) showed that individuals with PD were less efficient, producing fewer words/minute. While Illes (1989) reported no group differences for verbal output efficiency among those with PD, Huntington's disease (HD), DAT, and controls persons with PD were significantly less efficient for speaking rate (i.e., total words/minute) vs. verbal rate (i.e., total words/minute after extraction of unfilled pauses > 2 seconds). Interestingly, Illes (1989) found that the presence of verbal disruptions in the form of unfilled pauses > 2 seconds duration interacted with measures of verbal output efficiency in the discourse of individuals with LBSD. Consistent with this finding, once Ash et al. (2012) extracted unfilled pauses > 2 seconds from their narrative samples, the speech rate differences (words/minute) reported for the PDD/DLB subgroup were reduced in magnitude resulting in the absence of statistically significant differences in the verbal rate for individuals with PDD/DLB (M = 115; SD = 47) vs. controls (M = 146; SD = 19). This finding is consistent with Illes et al. (1988) who also reported that verbal rates were equivalent between individuals with PD (M = 169.10; SD = 54.20) and controls (M = 154.50; SD = 25.50).

Taken as a whole the findings on changes in discourse productivity in LBSD, including measures reflecting amount and efficiency, suggest that the changes may be due to the presence of unfilled pauses. Discussed in more detail later in this section, the presence of long unfilled pauses (i.e., > 2 seconds) in the discourse of individuals with LBSD represents a large source of the verbal disruptions in individuals with PD. Further long, unfilled pauses become even more problematic during interactional discourse tasks (i.e., conversation) also discussed in more detail later in this paper. Across studies, the majority of researchers concluded that the reduced output in LBSD is not accounted for solely by bradykinetic (i.e., slowed) motor speech movements associated with LBSD and that cognitive and linguistic changes (e.g., reduced processing time, language formulation deficits) likely contribute to the discourse productivity impairments (Illes et al. 1988; Illes 1989; McNamara et al. 1992).

Syntax

Measures of syntactic complexity, accuracy, and diversity appear frequently in the literature on discourse in LBSD. For example, syntax processing is reduced in LBSD suggesting that syntax impairments may be a potential barrier for communication even in language production (Berg et al. 2003; Colman et al. 2011; Grossman et al. 1991; Grossman et al. 1992; Grossman 1999; Grossman et al. 2002; Grossman et al. 2012; Hochstadt 2009; Lieberman, Friedman, and Feldman 1990; Lieberman et al. 1992; Natsopoulos et al. 1991; Skeel et al. 2001; Walsh and Smith 2011; Ye et al. 2012). The valuable role of contextual information in sentence production underscores the importance of using monologic discourse tasks to understand syntax production (Spivey-Knowlton, Trueswell, and Tanenhaus 1993; Vigliocco 2000; Vigliocco and Hartsuiker 2002), especially in those with LBSD.

Utterance length is one measure used by discourse scholars to evaluate syntactic complexity. Investigators reported generally that the mean length of utterance (MLU) measured in words is not affected significantly for individuals with LBSD. Ash et al. (2011) found that their participants with LBSD presented with equivalent MLU performance vs. controls during narrative generation tasks. Similarly Murray and Lenz (2001) reported that the differences between PD vs. controls for MLU in personal narratives (i.e., topic directed interview) only approached significance ($p = 0.08$). Moreover, Murray (2000) found equivalent performances for MLU between PD vs. controls on a picture description task. Interestingly Huber and Darling (2011), using syllables vs. words as the metric for utterance length, reported that individuals with PD produced significantly shorter utterances vs. controls. These data suggest that syllable level vs. word level analyses possess greater sensitivity to the syntactic complexity changes seen in LBSD. Alternatively, these data may also indicate that the length of an utterance, a marker of linguistic complexity, varies as a function of task difficulty given that the expository discourse task used by Huber and Darling posed fewer semantic, memory and syntactic demands compared to the discourse types reported by other researchers (Ash et al. 2011; Huber and Darling 2011; Murray 2000; Murray and Lenz 2001). However, task complexity alone may not fully explain the variability in utterance length observed in LBSD. Holtgraves, McNamara, Cappaert, and Durso (2010) studied the effects of motor asymmetry in PD on discourse performance using a personal narrative task. By its definition, PD is an asymmetrical motor disease meaning that at onset of motor symptoms one side of the body is more affected than the other (See Table 1). As the disease progresses, this asymmetry generally persists. Holtgraves et al. (2010) reported that individuals with PD with greater left side motor symptoms produced significantly shorter sentences compared to those with greater right side motor symptoms. These findings suggest that in addition to task complexity side of motor symptom presentation, and by extension potentially greater impairment in contralateral brain regions, in LBSD may affect some discourse performance variables (Holtgraves et al. 2010).

Syntactic level analyses using a range of measures have been conducted in LBSD across multiple discourse genres. Murray and Lenz (2001) reported no significant differences between PD vs. controls during topic directed interviews for proportion of grammatical sentences, proportion of complex sentences, number of embeddings per utterance, or proportion of verbs inflected. However, they did find strong and robust correlations for the PD group between a global measure of aphasia and MLU and also between the global measure and the proportion of complex sentences produced (Murray and Lenz 2001). Robust correlations also were reported among performances on a global measure of cognition and MLU, proportion of complex sentences used, and embeddings per utterance (Murray and Lenz 2001). Moreover, Murray and Lenz (2001) reported strong correlations between speech intelligibility and MLU, proportion of complex utterances, and number of embeddings per utterance.

While Murray and Lenz (2001) reported no significant differences on measures of syntax in a personal narrative discourse task, Murray (2000) did find significant differences in proportion of grammatical sentences produced using a picture description task for PD (M = .73; SD = .12) vs. controls (M = .92; SD = .08). No significant group differences were reported for other measures of syntax complexity (i.e., proportion of simple sentences or embeddings per utterance) (Murray 2000; Murray and Lenz 2001). Consistent with the Murray and Lenz's (2001) data from personal narratives, Murray (2000) reported significant correlations among measures of language, cognition, and discourse using picture description tasks. These correlations suggested that length of utterance shortened and syntax become less complex as a function of more impaired performance on cognitive and language tasks. Collectively, the studies of Murray (2000) and Murray and Lenz (2001) suggest that in keeping with the finding that measures of syntax production correlate robustly with standardized measures of cognition and language, syntax accuracy and complexity are potentially more impaired in those discourse genres with greater semantic and linguistic constraints and lower personal saliency.

Illes et al. (1988) and Illes (1989) used a syntactic scoring system, based on complexity of clausal structures within sentences (embedded vs. non-embedded), to analyze syntax complexity for personal narratives in persons with PD. Illes et al. (1988) reported a significant difference in syntactic complexity as a function of PD severity. Overall, her participants with PD did not differ significantly from controls in syntax complexity.

However, Illes et al. (1988) reported that within the PD group individuals with mild PD produced sentences with a significantly higher degree of syntactic complexity (i.e., more embedded clauses) vs. those with moderate PD severity. In addition, the syntax complexity scores correlated significantly and robustly with measures of disease severity (Illes et al. 1988). With increased disease severity, the PD participants from Illes et al. (1988) and Illes (1989) produced longer sentences that were not per se more syntactically complex (i.e., did not contain more embedded clauses). Illes et al. (1988) observed that sentences produced by individuals with more severe PD contained strings of open class phrases organized in a list-like fashion (vs. embedded clauses) resulting in longer sentences with reduced syntactic complexity. Below is an excerpt from Illes et al. (1988) illustrating this discourse feature in an individual with PD. The speaker produced five open class phrases (e.g., content word phrases) in a list-like fashion all modifying the main clause "I worked". Each open class phrase is underlined:

> I worked *for thirty-two years for the [the] Department of Water and Power*, first *as a [a] /m/ [/m - m/] mechanic*, then *a [a] lead man*, then finally *as a /f/ [/f/] foreman.*
>
> (Illes et al. 1988, 156)

The findings from Illes et al. (1988) and Illes (1989) indicate that individuals with PD demonstrate lower syntax complexity as disease severity worsens.

The results from Ash et al. (2011), in which she and her colleagues used a narrative generation task, are in general agreement with those of Illes et al. (1988) and Illes (1989). In Ash et al. (2011) the percentage of well-formed utterances (i.e., utterances containing a subject and a verb clause, free of grammatical errors, and correct to the story) and the percent of utterances with complex structures (i.e., dependent clauses and phrasal adjuncts) did not differ between individuals with PD vs. controls. However, the measures of syntactic complexity did differ significantly for individuals with PDD/DLB vs. controls (Ash et al. 2011). Furthermore, the individuals with PDD/DLB produced discourse samples containing less syntactic complexity vs. PD (Ash et al. 2011). The percentage of well-formed utterances differed significantly between individuals with PDD/DLB (M = 77, SD = 24) and both controls (M = 99, SD = 2) and PD (M = 95, SD = 6) (Ash et al. 2011). However, the percentage of utterances with complex structures differed significantly only between individuals with PDD/DLB (M = 24, SD = 16) and controls (M = 36, SD = 11) (Ash et al. 2011).

In a follow-up study Ash et al. (2012), using the identical discourse elicitation procedure as Ash et al. (2011), evaluated the complexity of sentence structure between individuals with LBSD vs. controls. The researchers designed a composite score of grammatical complexity comprised of 1) presence of a well-formed and accurate sentence, 2) presence of complex structures in the sentence and 3) proportion of nouns with a determiner when one was required. This yielded a scores ranging from 0 to 3 with a score of 0 representing a lower degree of grammatical complexity and a score of 3 representing a higher degree of grammatical complexity (Ash et al. 2012). Ash et al. (2012) reported that individuals with PD (M = 2.27, SD = .19) did not differ significantly from controls (M = 2.35, SD = .26) for grammatical complexity. However, individuals with PDD/DLB (M = 1.91, SD = .46) did differ significantly from controls for grammatical complexity (Ash et al. 2012). Ash et al. (2012) noted that the grammar errors produced by individuals with PDD/DLB included predominately incomplete sentences, omission of determiners, and omission of the verb clause. The omission of the verb clause is particularly intriguing given the research demonstrating verb-specific deficits in word retrieval in PD even in the absence of dementia (Bertella et al. 2002; Boulenger et al. 2008; Colman et al. 2009; Cotelli et al. 2007; Crescentini et al. 2008; Herrera, Rodriguez-Ferreiro, and Cuetos 2012; Peran et al. 2003; Peran et al. 2009; Rodriguez-Ferreiro et al. 2009).

Collectively, the findings from studies on syntactic analyses in LBSD suggest that syntactic impairments in discourse are not uniform across LBSD. In addition, findings indicate that syntactic abilities decline with worsening disease severity (Illes et al. 1988; Illes 1989) and deteriorating cognitive-linguistic performances (Ash et al. 2011; Ash et al. 2012; Murray 2000; Murray and Lenz 2001). Finally, findings show that the demands of the discourse genre may interact with syntax production abilities in LBSD (Murray 2000; Murray and Lenz 2001).

Lexicon

The choice, accuracy, and diversity of words are important measures of monologic discourse performance in adults with progressive neurological disorders affecting cognition and language. In LBSD, lexical skills interact and overlap with cognitive processes, syntax use and structure, semantic access and errors, coherence and cohesion processes, accuracy of conveying information, verbal disruptions, and motor components of speech programming. Research in LBSD suggests that word retrieval impairments and 'tip of the tongue' phenomenon are considerable (Bertella et al. 2002;

Boulenger et al. 2008; Cotelli et al. 2007; Herrera, Rodriguez-Ferreiro, and Cuetos 2012; Matison et al. 1982; Peran et al. 2009; Rodriguez-Ferreiro et al. 2009). Within this body of literature a lexicality effect emerges suggesting that individuals with LBSD have greater deficits retrieving verbs vs. nouns (Bertella et al. 2002; Boulenger et al. 2008; Colman et al. 2009; Cotelli et al. 2007; Crescentini et al. 2008; Herrera, Rodriguez-Ferreiro, and Cuetos 2012; Peran et al. 2003; Peran et al. 2009; Rodriguez-Ferreiro et al. 2009). Consequently, studying lexical diversity in LBSD within discourse paradigms is warranted because such analyses are likely to reveal word retrieval challenges that are not apparent in standardized language testing.

Ash et al. (2011) and Ash et al. (2012) reported no significant differences in the proportion of open class words (i.e., content words; nouns, verbs, adverbs, and adjectives) used between individuals with LBSD vs. controls during a story generation narrative discourse task. All groups (i.e., PD, PDD/DLB and controls) produced approximately 40% open class words (Ash et al. 2011; Ash et al. 2012). Similarly, Murray and Lenz (2001) reported no significant differences between individuals with PD vs. controls in the proportion of closed class words (i.e., non-content conveying words; prepositions, determiners, conjunctions, pronouns) with both groups producing approximately 50% closed class words.

In contrast, Illes et al. (1988) and Illes (1989) analyzed the personal narratives of individuals with PD for the proportion of open class phrases vs. closed class phrases. Individuals with PD produced a significantly higher proportion of open class and open class optional phrases vs. controls (Illes et al. 1988). Illes (1989) reported similar results with significantly higher use of open class phrases by individuals with PD mild disease severity (72.4%) and individuals with PD moderate disease severity (73.2%) vs. controls (62.4%) . In keeping with the previous studies by Illes and colleagues, Holtgraves, McNamara, Cappaert and Durso (2010) reported that individuals with PD and greater left side motor symptoms use fewer verbs and fewer closed class words (i.e., function words). Moreover, the side of motor asymmetry (left vs. right) accounted for 20% of the variance for number of verbs produced and 13% of the variance for number of closed class words produced (Holtgraves et al. 2010). Holtraves et al. (2010) reported that side of motor asymmetry is the greatest predictor of linguistic performance in discourse more so than any of the cognitive tasks administered (i.e., Stroop performance, category fluency, autobiographical memory). The finding of reduced frequency of closed class words is in keeping with the findings from Illes et al. (1988) and Illes (1989) demonstrating an increased proportion of open class phrases vs. closed class phrases. More importantly, these finding suggest that in addition to considering the influence of cognitive-linguistic abilities and general motor/disease severity on discourse performance, that predominant side of motor symptom presentation also should be considered.

There is a relative paucity of data on lexical diversity in discourse production in LBSD compared to other areas of discourse analyses reported in the literature. The data that are available suggest that discourse genre may play an important role in the lexical diversity profiles demonstrated in LBSD. Discourse genres such as personal narratives that focus on sharing a personal recount of information or life events may offer opportunities for participants to generate more of the syntax structures described by Illes et al. (1988). That is, individuals with PD often string together events in a list-like sequence affecting lexical diversity by increasing the number of open class clauses and hence open class words. While Murray and Lenz (2001) used a similar discourse task and found no significant group differences, this may be the effect of disease severity (Murray and Lenz 2001). Illes et al. (1988) and Illes (1989) intentionally sampled participants with a greater variability of disease severity. Conversely story generation paradigms such as those utilized by Ash and colleagues (2011) and Ash et al. (2012) are governed more by the knowledge of story grammar and scripts. Such tasks possess the potential to facilitate the selection of syntax structures not bound by open class words that can yield a normalized distribution of lexical diversity. The available data on lexical diversity in the discourse of individuals with LBSD also suggest that broader lexical measures such as open class vs. closed class words are not sufficient for analyzing lexical diversity in LBSD. Given the current literature suggesting an effect of grammatical class (e.g., verbs more challenging than nouns) and semantic meaning (e.g., degree and type of movement features) on word retrieval in LBSD, analysis measures such as Type-Token Ratio (Templin 1957) may be a more sensitive measure in analyzing lexical diversity in the discourse of individuals with LBSD.

Verbal Disruptions

Verbal disruptions (i.e., disruption in the fluent and fluid output of information) within discourse can result from a host of cognitive and linguistic motor speech sources. For example verbal disruptions in monologic discourse, such as pauses, can result from additional time required to process information, increased time required for planning thoughts or utterances or additional time for retrieving and selecting words. Repetitions of sounds, syllables or words also can reflect cognitive, linguistic or motor speech challenges in planning and execution at phonological or lexical levels. Verbal disruptions such as reformulations or revisions can reveal deficits in word retrieval or syntax.

Huber and Darling (2011) conducted linguistic and motor speech analyses on expository discourse and on oral reading samples of participants with PD and normal controls. While both groups produced significantly more formulation errors (i.e., abandoned utterances, revised phrases, phrase repetitions) in the discourse task vs. oral reading, individuals with PD produced significantly more formulation errors than controls for both tasks (Huber and Darling 2011). In contrast, individuals with PD produced significantly fewer filled pauses (e.g., pauses denoted with a verbal filler such as "um" or "uh") vs. controls during the discourse task (Huber and Darling 2011). During the oral reading task, the proportion of filled pauses was equivalent between PD and controls (Huber and Darling 2011). While both groups produced more disfluencies in the discourse task vs. oral reading, no significant differences were reported for proportion of disfluencies (e.g., repetitions of sounds, single words, or syllables) between the groups during expository discourse (Huber and Darling 2011).

Similarly, using procedural narratives, Illes et al. (1988) reported that the number of unfilled pauses > 2 seconds duration/minute was significantly higher for individuals with PD (M = 1.41) vs. controls (M = 0.03). Importantly, the presence of unfilled pauses > 2 seconds (i.e., silent hesitations) was one of four variables reported to separate individuals with PD vs. controls (Illes et al. 1988). Moreover, the researchers reported that the long unfilled pauses occurred most commonly at the beginning of sentences and at the boundaries between mandatory and optional phrases within the sentence (Illes et al. 1988). In contrast, Illes et al. (1988) reported that the number of filled pauses/minute (e.g., "uh", "uhm") did not differ between individuals with PD vs. controls. These findings suggest that the presence of unfilled pauses may be a salient feature of verbal disruptions in the discourse of individuals with LBSD. More importantly, the location of unfilled pauses suggests an interaction between this form of verbal disruption and language formulation in LBSD.

Illes (1989) investigated the profile of verbal disruptions during a personal narrative discourse task in a group of individuals with PD who were divided into mild and moderate disease severity groups. The moderate severity PD participants produced significantly more unfilled pauses > 2 seconds duration vs. controls (Illes 1989). Individuals in the moderate severity PD group performed similarly to a comparator group of participants with moderate severity DAT relative to the proportion of long pauses (Illes 1989). However, no differences were observed in the PD group with mild disease with respect to unfilled pause duration (Illes 1989). This finding is in agreement with Jaywant and Pell (2010) who reported no significant differences in either mean duration of pause or mean percent pause time on a picture description task for individuals with mild PD severity vs. controls. Illes (1989) also reported that the frequency of aborted phrases (i.e., false starts not corrected), the mean number of words per filled pause, mean number of phonemic approximations and frequency of modalizations and interjections did not differ as a function of PD severity (i.e., mild and moderate disease severity). Further Illes and her colleagues (1988) reported that the occurrence of filled pauses separated the mild vs. the moderate disease severity participants within the PD group, wherein participants in the mild severity group produced significantly more filled pauses vs. the moderate severity group.. Elaborating on the nature of verbal disruptions in LBSD, Illes (1989) reported that the occurrence of interjections (i.e., exclamatory phrases in the stream of language production) and modalizations (i.e., comments made by the speaker about the task or about their performance) were significantly higher for controls (more than twice that of PD). Interestingly, the proportion of semantic paraphasias, neologisms, and phonemic paraphasias that can disrupt output were not significantly different between the PD and control participants (Illes 1989).

Ash et al. (2011) using a narrative generation paradigm reported on the proportion of phonemic errors and phonetic errors produced by individuals with LBSD vs. controls. Ash et al. (2010) defined phonemic errors as speech production errors that result in a word containing sound(s) that are "well-formed" for the language but not "intended or anticipated by the listener" (e.g., "coming out of the gar" for 'coming out of the jar'(Ash et al. 2010, 14). Phonetic errors were defined as speech production errors that result in a word containing a "sequence of sounds" that are "not possible" in the speaker's spoken language (e.g., reduced articulation force/pressure on a target consonant such as softening the /g/ in "dog" resulting in a sound distortion that does not represent an English sound) (Ash et al. 2010, 14). Ash et al. (2011) reported no significant difference between individuals with PD vs. controls in either phonetic or phonemic errors. However, individuals with PDD/DLB produced significantly more phonetic and phonemic errors/100 words than either the PD or control groups (Ash et al. 2011).

Using the same discourse elicitation paradigm Ash et al. (2012) calculated a composite variable they termed "articulation errors" comprised of: 1) proportion of phonetic or phonemic errors, 2) proportion of false starts (i.e., incomplete words subsequently abandoned), 3) proportion of filled pauses (i.e., defined as hesitation markers and editing breaks and 4) proportion of disfluent words (i.e., self-corrected words, word revisions). Verbal disruptions were calculated as a proportion of errors per 100 words. Individuals with PDD/DLB produced significantly more errors (M = 17.3; SD = 11.9) vs. controls (M = 5.9, SD = 6.0). However, no differences were reported between individuals with PD (M = 6.4, SD = 5.0) vs. controls (Ash et al. 2012). Ash et al. (2012) also explored the presences of pauses as a measure of verbal disruption in LBSD. In Ash et al. (2012) pauses exceeding 2 seconds in duration were calculated as a proportion of the total narrative duration. The proportion of verbal disruption pauses was significantly higher for both the DLB/PDD subgroup (M = 37.3, SD = 17) and PD subgroup (M = 13.1, SD = 14.3) vs. controls (M = 4.6, SD = 6.0) (Ash et al. 2012).

Collectively, findings from these studies suggest that a substantial source of verbal disruptions in LBSD are pauses of > 2 seconds in duration. They further support the assertion that measures exploring unfilled pauses or silent hesitations greater than 2 seconds are an important component of discourse analyses in LBSD across discourse genres. The ambiguous findings across studies in the proportion and profile of verbal disruptions may reflect the cognitive-linguistic demands of the particular discourse task reported. Additionally, the disease severity, motor speech severity, and cognitive-linguistic abilities (particularly for the PD groups) were highly variable across studies. These variations in participant features indicate strongly that such variables along with discourse genre task play substantial roles in influencing the profile of verbal disruptions in LBSD.

Additional sources of verbal disruptions in discourse production can occur as a speaker attempts to correct an error in speech or language production. These repair attempts can result in verbal disruptions such as disfluencies, revisions or reformulations at the sound, syllable, word, or phrase level. McNamara et al. (1992) explored the ability of individuals with PD, DAT and controls to self-monitor and correct language errors during picture description. Individuals with PD had significantly more undetected language errors (75%) vs. age-matched control participants (18%) (McNamara et al. 1992). The percentage of undetected errors in a cohort of individuals with PD without dementia was consistent with the undetected error rates of the DAT group (76%) (McNamara et al. 1992).

These findings are consistent with Illes (1989) who reported a high prevalence of self-correction verbal disruptions in DAT and HD, but minimal use of self-correction verbal behaviours (i.e., reformulations, revisions) in the PD group. McNamara et al. (1992) also explored the types of repair strategies applied within discourse. Only 14% of language errors were corrected using a reformulation strategy (i.e., multiword correction where a new constituent is added) in the PD group vs. age-matched controls who used reformulation strategies to repair detected errors 35% of the time (statistically significant) (McNamara et al. 1992). Similarly, individuals with PD used significantly fewer lemma repair strategies (i.e., correction where an error is replaced by a single word) vs. controls with 11% of total errors and 47% of total errors respectively (McNamara et al. 1992).

The data from McNamara et al. (1992), plus the results from the Ash et al (2011, 2012) and Illes (1989) and colleagues (1988) studies, among others, suggest that understanding verbal disruptions in LBSD is complex. While verbal disruptions can reflect language and word retrieval errors in discourse, the frequency of verbal disruptions (i.e., particularly reformulations and revisions) may not be an accurate representation of potential errors in language production in discourse in LBSD. In LBSD, particularly for PD, the rate of undetected errors and the failure to apply repair strategies (i.e., reformulation and lemma) reported by McNamara et al. (1992) suggest that many errors are potentially made in the discourse of LBSD that are not signalled with the occurrence of a verbal disruption. Collectively, this body of literature underscores the value of verbal disruption analyses particularly the quantification of unfilled pauses and the linguistic context of verbal disruptions in the study of discourse in LBSD.

Macrostructural Analyses

Local and Global Coherence

Few studies have explored the discourse of individuals with LBSD from the perspective of creating and maintaining unifying themes within narratives. Cohelo (2007) defined local coherence as “the relationship of the meaning or content of an utterance to that of the preceding utterance” (Cohelo 2007, 124). He further defined global coherence as “the relationship of the meaning or content of an utterance to the general topic of the story” (Coelho 2007, 124). Given the frequency of higher-level language impairments (i.e., figurative language), working-memory impairments, and executive function impairments reported in LBSD it is reasonable to expect impairments in local and global coherence (Berg et al. 2003; Farag et al. 2010).

Only one published study to date has explored the local and global coherence production abilities in individuals with LBSD. Ash et al. (2011) used a narrative generation task and a scoring system to evaluate the events produced by participants with LBSD for: 1) local connectedness (i.e., event presented related to preceding material established via linguistic connecting devices), 2) accurate identification and maintenance of the central theme of the story and 3) global connectedness (i.e., identifying the correct resolution of a problem in the story and linking back the resolution to the main theme and the initiating event). Ash et al (2011) found a main effect of group for both local and global connectedness with the LBSD group who performed significantly worse than controls on measures of local connectedness, identification/ maintenance of theme and global connectedness. A subgroup analysis revealed that the PDD/DLB group was more impaired than the PD group on the measures of local and global connectedness. Ash et al. (2011) reported that while individuals with PD performed worse than controls on all measures of local and global coherence, these differences failed to reach statistical significance. However, significant differences were observed for all measures of local and global coherence between individuals with PDD/DLB vs. controls and vs. PD (Ash et al. 2011). Individuals with PDD/DLB had significantly lower local connectedness scores (M = 16.5, SD = 8.7) vs. controls (M = 27.9, SD = 2.5) and vs. PD (M = 25.9, SD = 4.6). Additionally individuals with PDD/DLB (M = 1.1, SD = 1.50) had lower scores on identifying and maintaining the central theme of the story vs. controls (M = 4.0, SD = 0.0) and vs. PD (M = 3.3, SD = 1.4) (Ash et al. 2011). Similarly, fewer individuals with PDD/DLB (M = 29%, SD = 47) were able to establish global connectedness vs. controls (M = 100%, SD = 0.0) and vs. PD (M = 82%, SD = 39) (Ash et al. 2011). Ash et al. (2011) reported that measures of local connectedness within the PDD/DLB subgroup correlated robustly with motor severity (r = -.69), disease staging (r = -61), and verbal output productivity (words/minute) (r = -.72). In addition, they found that measures of local connectedness correlated robustly and positively with measures of executive function (i.e., reverse digit span, phonemic fluency, and semantic fluency) ranging from r = .61 to r = .70. In contrast, measures of global connectedness correlated significantly only to disease staging (Hoehn and Yahr) r = .70 (Ash et al. 2011). The accurate identification and maintenance of the central theme of the story correlated with verbal output productivity (r = .67) (Ash et al. 2011). They also found that thematic identification and maintenance correlated significantly with phonemic fluency ($r = .60$), semantic fluency ($r = .64$), and Stroop Color Word testing ($r = -.70$) (Ash et al. 2011). The findings of Ash et al. (2011) suggest that while individuals with PD performed worse than controls on measures of local and global coherence, these differences reached statistical significance only for those individuals within LBSD who suffered from dementia. As expected, measures of local connectedness and identification/maintenance of the story theme correlated robustly with measures of executive resources and speech rate suggesting an interaction among cognition-linguistic functions, verbal productivity and discourse structure in LBSD especially in cases progressing to dementia (Ash et al. 2011).

Informativeness

The degree of informativeness in expressive discourse often is measured along the dimensions of the amount, quality, and efficiency of information exchange from the speaker to the listener (Shadden 1998c). Given that one of the primary goals of communication is to convey information, measures of informativeness are a critical component of understanding discourse abilities (Shadden 1998c). While disruptions in discourse informativeness are well documented in the literature for many progressive degenerative neurological cognitive-communication disorders such as DAT, amyotrophic lateral sclerosis, acquired brain injury, Huntington's disease, and frontotemporal dementia (Coelho 2007; Fleming and Harris 2008; Jensen, Chenery, and Copland 2006; Murray 2000; Orange and Kertesz 2000; Roberts-South et al. 2012; Zraick et al. 2011), few studies have explored measures of informativeness in LBSD.

McNamara et al. (1992) investigated the amount and the efficiency of information conveyed using a picture description task in LBSD. The authors identified a priori seven possible units of information. Individuals with PD produced a comparable number of units of information as age-matched controls. However, they produced significantly fewer words per information unit (8.4 words) vs. controls (15.2 words) (McNamara et al. 1992). These findings suggest that while the amount of information conveyed by individuals with LBSD did not differ from controls, the efficiency of information transfer was significantly different from controls (McNamara et al. 1992). Conversely, Murray (2000) who also used picture description tasks to evaluate informativeness in discourse in LBSD, reported that the presence of PD does affect discourse informativeness. She reported that individuals with relatively mild-moderate PD without dementia produced significantly lower percent CIUs (i.e., correct information units) (*M* = 76.69, *SD* = 10.91) vs. controls (*M* = 89.73; *SD* = 5.24) (Murray 2000). Moreover, individuals with PD produced a significantly lower percentage of informative utterances (i.e., complete utterances that communicate accurate and novel information relative to the picture) (*M* = .85, *SD* = .12) vs. controls (*M* = .96, *SD* = .04) (Murray 2000). Methodological differences in the analyses of informativeness likely contribute to the differences seen across these two studies. Further, the ability to generate main ideas/themes from the picture (i.e., content units) may not be as sensitive as percent CIUs or percent informative utterances for revealing impairments in word retrieval, semantics and the ability to generate novel information.

The narrative-retelling task used by Bayles (1990) contained 25 possible a priori units of information. On the whole, individuals with PD did not differ significantly in the amount of information produced vs. controls. However, significant differences were found when Bayles allocated the participants (i.e., both PD and controls) into either a high-normal cognition group or a low-normal cognition group based on scores from a measure of global cognition. In her sub-analysis, the high-normal cognition group, independent of having PD, produced significantly more units of information vs. the low-normal cognition group (Bayles 1990). Bayles's findings, interpreted with caution given the use of arbitrary cut-off points to divide the high-normal vs. low-normal cognition groups, suggest that cognitive status and not the presence of PD per se influenced the amount of information produced in a high declarative memory loaded discourse genre such as narrative-retelling (Bayles 1990).

The ability to generate the required number and correct sequence of steps/units of information for a specified procedure (i.e., procedural discourse) is critical in everyday activities. Godbout and Doyon (2000) explored the performances of PD and control groups on a series of procedural discourse tasks requiring both forward and backward generation of scripts. Their analyses focussed on the amount of and the quality of information conveyed within the contexts of a high degree of sequencing and a high degree of procedural memory constraints. Godbout and Doyon (2000) reported no significant differences between PD vs. controls for the total units of information produced in either the forward or the backward conditions. However, there were differences in the quality of information between the PD and control groups. In both the forward and the backward conditions, individuals with PD produced significantly more errors in sequencing the order of information required to perform the targeted procedure (Godbout and Doyon 2000). In the forward condition,

12/16 individuals with PD produced sequencing errors compared to 1/16 controls (Godbout and Doyon 2000). Performance declined further in the backward condition with 13/13 individuals with PD producing information out of correct sequence vs. 4/16 of the controls (Godbout and Doyon 2000). For 3 of the 16 participants with PD, the procedural narratives in the backward condition were so impaired that they could not be scored at all. These findings suggest that individuals with PD have challenges in sequencing information in spoken procedural narratives even when the amount of information is sufficient. Godbout and Doyon (2000) suggested that the challenges faced by individuals with PD in procedural discourse result from an impaired ability to order events temporally in episodic memory.

Godbout and Doyon (2000) also noted that the differences in quality of information produced in the procedural narratives of individuals with PD extend beyond event sequencing and into the semantic value of the information provided. They used normative data collected in a previously published study of control participants (Godbout 1994) to categorize the actions produced by individuals with PD vs. controls into three categories: 1) Major actions (i.e., actions produced by > than 65% of participants from Godbout 1994), 2) Minor actions (i.e., actions produced by 45-64% of participants from Godbout 1994) and 3) Trivial actions (i.e., actions produced by 25-44% of participants from Godbout 1994) (Godbout and Doyon 2000). Actions produced by participants in Godbout and Doyon (2000) that were not produced by a minimum of 25% of participants in Godbout (1994) (e.g., information of low semantic value) were categorized as intrusions. Intrusions were further classified into relevant (i.e., correct for the target procedure) or irrelevant (i.e., incorrect for the target procedure). Godbout and Doyon (2000) reported a significant interaction of group (i.e., PD vs. controls) x category (i.e., Major, Minor, Trivial actions). Post-hoc testing for the forward condition suggested that controls generated significantly fewer major actions compared to either minor or trivial actions. In contrast individuals with PD generated significantly fewer minor actions vs. either major or trivial actions in the forward condition. The authors interpreted the reduced retrieval of minor actions as a PD-specific impairment in accessing the contextual information that contributes to the richness of scripts associated with procedural narratives (Godbout and Doyon 2000).

The PD participants in Godbout and Doyon (2000) also produced perseveration errors (i.e., repeating information already provided) in both the forward (5/16 participants) and backward (8/16 participants) conditions. In contrast, controls did not produce any perseveration errors.

The authors noted that this finding suggests that individuals with PD have more challenges vs. controls in attention processes (i.e., set-shifting) during procedural discourse (Godbout and Doyon 2000). The authors also reported that their participants with PD produced significantly more irrelevant units of information (e.g., information not correct to the targeted procedure) vs. controls in both the forward and backward conditions (Godbout and Doyon 2000). They stated that this finding indicates that individuals with PD have a specific impairment in maintaining scripts in memory during procedural discourse tasks with a resulting negative impact on informativeness. Moreover, their findings show that while the amount of information produced in spoken procedural discourse is not compromised in individuals with PD, the quality of information produced is reduced in a discourse task with high sequencing demands, high episodic memory demands and high procedural memory demands (Godbout and Doyon 2000).

Collectively, the findings from studies on the informativeness of spoken discourse of individuals with LBSD reveal that their output is less informative, is reduced in its efficiency of information transfer, contains more errors than that of controls, and contains information that is irrelevant, less novel, and repetitive. The semantic constraint of the task plays a substantial influence relative to the amount, the efficiency, and the quality of information. The existing literature suggests that discourse genres with a high degree of semantic or memory demands may be more susceptible to the deficits observed in LBSD.

Summary

In summary, the findings from the literature on the monologic spoken discourse of individuals with LBSD reveal consistent patterns of performance across a range of discourse genres. Findings show that individuals with LBSD vs. controls generally use fewer words, are less informative, are less efficient in conveying content, use less complex syntactic structures, show more verbal disruptions, are less coherent locally and globally, and often do not include or mis-sequence crucial pieces of information. Their spoken discourse output is influenced by cognitive status (i.e., presence of cognitive impairment or dementia), disease severity, motor speech disturbances, side of predominant motor symptoms, and functioning of important cognitive domains that support discourse such as memory, attention, and executive system processes. Caveats concerning the overall robustness of future studies on the discourse of individuals with LBSD will be minimized by investigators who conduct longitudinal prospective designs, who control for cognitive status, disease severity variables, motor speech severity, and who use multiple tasks within a range of different discourse genres to cross-reference performance and to isolate performance variables. Further, the length of discourse samples obtained for study is an important variable that has not been considered consistently as a contributor to discourse performance in the LBSD literature. Both length of discourse sample and discourse task used for elicitation of the language sample are important variables in the reliability, type, and accuracy of data generated from discourse (Brookshire and Nicholas 1994; Doyle, Goda, and Spencer 1995; Shadden et al. 1991).

Moreover within LBSD, most prominently reported for individuals with PD and PDD, medication status (e.g., amount and optimal dosing of dopaminergic medications; use of cholinergic or anticholinergic medications) can contribute to both cognitive and language performances (Bohnen et al. 2006; Gotham, Brown, and Marsden 1988; Ehrt et al. 2010; Kulisevsky et al. 1996; Poletti and Bonuccelli 2013) and may subsequently affect discourse performance. For example, individuals with PD have been shown to have worse performances on tasks of word retrieval (Boulenger et al. 2008; Fernandino et al. 2012) and sentence comprehension (McNamara et al. 1996; Skeel et al. 2001) when levodopa (i.e., a critical dopaminergic medication for management of PD related motor symptoms) is withdrawn intentionally. Conversely, these same participants demonstrated improved performances when levodopa dosing was restored. To date, few studies (Ash et al. 2011; Ash et al. 2012; Holtgraves et al. 2010) have considered the role of medication (i.e., total amount and type of medication(s) taken daily; on vs. off status) on discourse performance in LBSD. Holtgraves et al. (2010) found no significant effect of total dopaminergic medication taken daily on microlinguistic variables of discourse performance. Overall, the body of research using monologic discourse tasks in LBSD would benefit from consideration of these multiple contributing variables in order to ensure rigorous study designs. Collectively these existing studies suggest that discourse abilities are an important area of study in LBSD. However, this literature also highlights the fact that there is still much to explore in the domain of monologic discourse in LBSD via well-controlled and systematic studies.

Discourse Studies in Lewy Body Spectrum Disorders: Interactional Discourse

Interactional Discourse Defined

The fundamental element of communication is its dyadic interactional component. Speakers/writers/gesturers interacting with listeners/readers/ viewers form the minimal dyadic unit. Within the context of interactional discourse, investigators can examine how dyadic partners function and respond to each others actions and reactions. For individuals with LBSD, interactional discourse tasks function to provide researchers with unique and valuable insights on the interplay among cognitive factors, language status, motor speech influences, neurological degeneration, and sociolinguistic forces such as relationships (spouse, relative, unfamiliar partner, etc.) and communicative intent. The published literature on interactional discourse and LBSD is sparse but informative. The reader is directed to Table 2 for a comprehensive summary of the studies covered in this section including participant demographics.

Pauses and Turn-Taking Analyses in Interactional Discourse

Alpert and colleagues (1990) explored the presence of pauses and turn-taking in individuals with mild and moderate PDD during a topic-directed interactional discourse task. The investigators were especially interested in the relationships of pauses and turn-taking behaviours with measures of cognition, depression, and apathy/motivation. They reported multiple significant correlations among the standardized measures of dementia, depression, and motivation/apathy and the frequency and duration of pauses. Specifically, Alpert et al. (1990) noted that dementia measures correlated robustly with the frequency of episodes of simultaneous spoken language (i.e., talking by a speaker who does not have the 'floor'). They also reported that measures of depression correlated significantly with duration of speaking turn. Their findings are the first to show the high risk and significant influence of cognitive impairments, depression and apathy in LBSD on conversation.

Alpert et al. (1990) also stated that participants with mild PDD vs. those with moderate PDD produced pauses of a shorter duration signalling an intention to continue a speaking turn thus reducing the possibility that the conversation partner might misread the pause as signal to yield the 'floor'. Further, those with mild dementia produced more instances of cross-over, simultaneous talking which interrupted their conversational partner. The investigators concluded that the increase in simultaneous speaking indicated that individuals with mild PDD showed increased engagement with the topic and their conversational partners. Conversely, Alpert et al. (1990) noted that use of interruptive talking may reflect merely the increased presence of overlapping talk vs. increased engagement, a phenomenon explored further by Griffiths and colleagues (2012) and discussed later in this section.

Alpert et al. (1990) also reported that individuals with mild PDD vs. those with moderate PDD assumed the role of speaker for significantly longer durations. They interpreted this as an indicator that individuals with mild PDD produced longer and more complex utterances vs. those with moderate PDD. However, the work of Illes et al. (1988) reviewed earlier in this chapter shows that longer durations of speaking turn do not equate to increase syntax or linguistic complexity.. In contrast, the moderate PDD group assumed the role of speaker for shorter durations with a greater tendency to produce monosyllabic utterances (Alpert et al. 1990).

Alpert et al. (1990) observed that the turn-taking exchange between speaker and listener was less fluid among those participants with moderate PDD for two reasons. Firstly, longer pause durations, especially within noun and verb phrases and in concert with obvious word finding problems, can be an ambiguous turn-taking signal. Secondly, conversation partners had longer response latencies when interacting with those with moderate dementia suggesting they had challenges in reading turn-taking signals. Interestingly, participants with moderate PDD produced fewer occurrences of simultaneous and interruptive talking vs. those with mild PDD. This finding may reflect decreased engagement with the topic/speaker as Alpert et al. (1990) suggested. It also may reflect increasing difficulties with concept formulation and language planning as a result of increased cognitive impairment. One potential consequence of these challenges is that individuals with LBSD are excluded from the turn-taking sequence of the conversation and play a minimal role as a contributing member of the dyad. Collectively, the findings reported by Alpert et al. (1990) underscore the importance of understanding the nature, linguistic context, and role of pauses and simultaneous talking in conversational discourse in LBSD.

Griffiths et al. (2012) investigated the role of pauses, turn-taking and overlapping talk relative to conversational repair in individuals with PD. Using interactional non-topic guided conversations recorded in the homes of individuals with PD, the investigators reported that instances of overlapping talk were caused by impairments either in speech initiation or by cognitive processing speed. Possible sources of overlap talk that the authors identified include delays in either initiating the speech response or delays in processing the conversation partner's conveyed information. According to the investigators, these delays can result in a disruption of the fluidness of conversation turn-taking and can result in overlapped talking. As illustrated in the examples presented by Griffiths et al. (2012), the overlapped talking produced by their participants with PD that is off-topic can result in the signalling of repair as initiated by the conversation partner. However, as pointed out by Griffiths et al. (2012), the repairs by the persons with PD are not always successful. This can lead to a deletion of the PD speaker's turn resulting in the perception that he/she is not engaged fully in the conversation. Griffiths et al. (2012) concluded that two major issues are at stake with the overlap talk in the conversations of individuals with PD. Firstly, the overlapping talk, while normal and potentially appropriate, often is mistimed and occurs part-way through the PD speaker's turn resulting in overlap. Secondly, when overlapping talk occurs there is a greater likelihood of it resulting in a repair sequence because of the cognitive, language and motor speech problems common in the spoken output of individuals with PD.

In concert with the findings of Alpert et al. (1990), the frequency and duration of pauses in the spontaneous speech of individuals with PD also present potential sources for overlapping talk (Alpert et al. 1990; Griffiths et al. 2012). Griffiths et al. (2012) concluded that the potential cognitive and language impairments in PD can lead to challenges in "self-retrieving the elements of their talk that has been overlapped by other speakers" (Griffiths et al. 2012, 40-41). The poor retrieval or self-monitoring of their comments may trigger the need for further repair signalling and repair attempts (i.e., stacked repair sequences). The most significant consequence of overlapping talk is a failed repair cycle that leads to the deletion of the speaking turn for the person with PD. The investigations of Alpert et al. (1990) and Griffiths et al. (2011, 2012) highlight the communication value of conversation analyses in LBSD. Further, such analyses expand the knowledge of how conversations involving individuals with LBSD break down and are repaired, information that is critical from a clinical intervention perspective. Most importantly, however, such studies capture unique interactional elements and provide potential explanations for the commonly voiced frustrations by individuals with LBSD that they are often 'left out of conversations' or that the conversation 'moves on without them'.

Standardized Measures in the Analyses of Interactional Discourse

Several researchers have used standardized assessment protocols of conversation and analyses of pragmatics in the study of interactional discourse in LBSD. In fact, a review of the literature on interactional discourse in LBSD reveals that the most commonly applied methodology is the use of standardized measures or rating scales to quantify impairments in pragmatics in conversational discourse. Whitworth, Lesser, and McKeith (1999) used the *Conversation Analysis Profile for People with Cognitive Impairment* (CAPPCI) (Perkins, Whitworth, and Lesser 1998) to explore conversation abilities of individuals with LBSD (i.e., using a conversation sample recorded in the home) and caregivers' perspectives of conversational challenges (i.e., using an interview process). Whitworth, Lesser, and McKeith (1999) reported that for both individuals with PDD and those with DLB, the most problematic areas of conversational discourse were challenges in initiation, topic maintenance, and turn-taking including (1) response failures to initiation attempts by their partner, (2) response delays, (3) reliance on minimal acknowledgments, (4) reduced frequency (i.e., not absent) of topic initiation, (5) reduced topic maintenance, and (6) reduced ability to create context or to orient partner to new topics. The presence of response delays are consistent with the work of Alpert et al. (1990) and are also consistent with the presence of long pauses reported in the monologic discourse literature described previously. Also consistent with Alpert et al. and Griffiths et al. (2012), are the findings showing that the participants with PDD exhibited simultaneous or overlapping talk resulting in violations of their conversation partner's speaking turn. Whitworth, Lesser, and McKeith (1999) reported that the participants with DLB presented with the unique feature of initiating topics that were hallucinatory in topic nature and that they persevered on preferred/favourite topics.

Whitworth, Lesser, and McKeith (1999) also showed conversational impairments in their LBSD participants relative to poor use of repair strategies, the influences of memory and attention on conversational performance, including (1) reduced self-monitoring for errors, (2) reduced initiation of repair sequences, (3) decreased abilities to retain instructions and (4) repetitive question asking and repetitive comments. Their finding of poor self-monitoring is consistent with the results reported by McNamara et al. (1992) in monologic discourse.

The CAPCCI (Perkins, Whitworth, and Lesser 1998) used by Whitworth, Lesser, and McKeith (1999) also captures conversational discourse information pertaining to language abilities, articulation and prosody. Participants in both the PDD and DLB groups showed word retrieval failures, circumlocutions, reduced voice volume loudness/control, reduced prosody and reduced articulatory precision (Whitworth, Lesser, and McKeith 1999). The investigators also noted comprehension problems for the DLB participants during conversations and their poor use of prosody to convey word meaning via sound and syllable stress. Similarly, participants in both the PDD and the DLB groups displayed fluctuations in conversational ability where those with DLB exhibited more frequent fluctuations (Whitworth, Lesser, and McKeith 1999).

Rousseaux et al. (2010) used a standardized measure of interactional discourse, the *Lille Communication Test* (Rousseaux et al. 2001), to compare and to contrast verbal and non-verbal features of conversation of individuals with DAT, frontotemporal dementia and DLB vs. controls. Surprisingly, the only areas in which individuals with DLB differed significantly from controls included fluent speech production, word retrieval difficulties and gestural communication. It is likely that methodological differences between the discourse assessment measures (*Lille Communication Test vs. CAPCCI*) and conversation elicitation methods (e.g., structured conversation sample with a researcher vs. naturally occurring conversation samples with a caregiver recorded in the home environment) account for some of the disparities in findings between Rousseaux et al. (2010) and Whitworth, Lesser, and McKeith (1999). However, the differences in the results of these two studies may reflect differences in the relative severity of conversational difficulties experienced by individuals with PDD who were included in the Whitworth, Lesser, and McKeith (1999) study but not in Rousseaux et al. (2010) vs. individuals with DLB suggesting that individuals with PDD may present with a greater magnitude of conversation impairment compared to DLB.

Hall, Ouyang, Lonnquist and Newcombe (2011) used the *Rehabilitation Institute of Chicago's Rating Scale of Pragmatic Communication* RSPCS (Halper, Cherney, and Burns 1996) to rate conversational interactions between individuals with PD and an unfamiliar conversation partner and then to compare their performances with conversations between control participants and their unfamiliar partners. The conversation abilities of individuals with PD were rated as significantly more impaired in both verbal and non-verbal features vs. controls. The investigators reported that individuals with PD were specifically impaired in intonation, facial expression, eye contact, gestural use, proxemics (i.e., observing physical space boundaries in conversation), topic initiation, turn-taking, and response length.

In keeping with other researchers who have used standardized protocols McNamara and Durso (2003) used the *Prutting Pragmatic Protocol* (Prutting and Kirchner 1987) to rate 10 to 15 minute conversation samples, generated using a semi-structured interview protocol, between individuals with PD/controls and a researcher interlocutor. The *Prutting Pragmatic Protocol* like the RSPCS (Hall et al. 2011), the *Lille Communication Test* (Rousseaux et al. 2010), and the CAPCCI (Whitworth et al. 1999) measures a wide range of verbal and non-verbal communication behaviours in the context of conversation. The authors reported a significant difference between PD (M = 20.4%; SD = 18) and controls (M = 3.8%; SD = 11) for the percentage of 'inappropriate' behaviours (e.g., violations of acceptable conversation behaviours such as failure to observe turn-taking rules, maintain eye contact, etc.). In addition, McNamara and Durso (2003) collected a comprehensive battery of cognitive measures. While there were no significant differences reported between PD and controls on a general measure of cognition (See Table 2) or on phonemic fluency, there was a significant difference reported between the two groups (i.e., PD more impaired) on a design fluency task, a measure of executive function. Moreover, the percentage of 'inappropriate' behaviours correlated significantly with other tasks of attention and frontal lobe processes (i.e., Stroop and Tower of London tasks). In other words, as performance on cognitive tasks worsened participants were rated as more 'inappropriate' in their conversational behaviours (McNamara and Durso 2003). These findings underscore the important potential contributions of cognition on discourse performance in LBSD and the need to characterize carefully cognitive and language abilities in participants in discourse studies beyond cognitive or dementia screening measures.

While conversational discourse performances in LBSD remain a relatively unexplored area of investigation, collectively the extant literature confirms that disruption in interactional discourse is prevalent across the spectrum of the three disorders comprising LBSD. Moreover, the findings from the published studies suggest, as did the results from studies on monologic discourse in LBSD, that the disruption in interactional discourse in LBSD results largely from interactions among problems in cognition, language and motor speech. Further, many of the deficits reported in monologic discourse (e.g., word retrieval, verbal disruptions, reduced response length/output) are manifest in interactional discourse. Most importantly, the data from interactional discourse in LBSD replicates and expands the findings from monologic discourse analyses and supports the importance of understanding cognitive operations, linguistic processes and motor speech formulation demands relative to discourse competence in LBSD.

Interlocutor Perceptions of Interactional Discourse

As a unique dimension to their seminal work Whitworth, Lesser, and McKeith (1999) explored the strategies that caregivers of individuals with LBSD use to prevent breakdown andor to initiate repairs during conversational interactions. The most commonly reported facilitative strategies (59.2%) included: 1) allowing more response time, 2) use of alternate modalities to facilitate output, 3) repeating information with altered input including reduced rate, rephrasing, stressing key words, 4) encouragement, 5) reality orientation in the cases of hallucinatory topics and 6) filling in the correct response/information for the person with LBSD. Other strategies used included acceptance strategies (22%), confrontational strategies (12.6%), avoidance strategies (5.2%), and emotive responses (e.g., yelling, comments of annoyance) (1%). Overall, there was relatively strong agreement between the perception of conversational impairments by the caregivers and the researcher-observed impairments in the dyad conversation samples with 69.2% agreement for the PDD group and 65.7 % agreement for the DLB group. These figures suggest that the caregivers of individuals with LBSD are reliable in identifying impairments in interactional discourse.

To date Whitworth, Lesser, and McKeith (1999) is the only published study to examine caregivers' perceptions of the conversational discourse performances of individuals with LBSD. Recent data collected by the authors of this chapter expands on the findings of Whitworth, Lesser, and McKeith (1999) in their exploration of the conversational difficulties in PDD from the perspectives of five members of a nuclear family (i.e., a wife and four adult children of a gentleman with PDD) (Roberts and Orange, submitted). Two of the adult children lived at home with their parents < 50% of the time and the other two children lived at home > 50% of the time. The impact of conversation difficulties on family members was measured using the Perception of Conversation Index-Dementia Alzheimer's Type (PCI-DAT) (Orange et al. 2009) measure. The PCI-DAT is a pen and paper questionnaire containing 74 questions divided into 5 sections. It contains a 7-point scale designed to measure family members' perceptions of conversation difficulties including: 1) nature of conversation difficulties exhibited by the person with DAT, 2) helpfulness of actions used by family members to signal and to repair conversation problems, 3) helpfulness of actions the person with DAT uses to signal and to repair conversation problems, 4) emotional responses to conversation difficulties, and 5) social consequences faced by family members as a function of conversation difficulties. Overall, the results suggest that the PDD substantially affected conversation effectiveness for all five family members. Data showed that the impact of conversation difficulties differ widely across family members and across PCI-DAT sections. Interestingly, and perhaps not surprisingly, despite relatively unified views regarding the nature of conversation difficulty and effective strategies, the emotional and social burden of conversation difficulties varied substantially across family members. Such a finding is in keeping with the outcomes reported by Purves and Phinney (2013), which show unique family member-specific responses top the conversational discourse problems exhibited by individuals with DAT and progressive nonfluent aphasia (Purves and Phinney 2013).

In the Roberts and Orange study, the spouse of the participant with PDD experienced the greatest degree of emotional burden vs. her four children. The burden associated with social challenges or lifestyle changes resulting from conversational discourse difficulties was felt relatively equally by the two adult children who lived with their parents. The eldest child, who no longer lived at home, reported no emotional impact of conversation difficulties and reported no substantial effect on lifestyle challenges. Collectively, these data are in agreement with those from the literature, which shows that the understanding of impairments in conversational discourse is greatly enhanced by obtaining the perspective of multiple family caregiver conversational partners (Orange 1991; Purves 2011; Purves and Phinney 2013). Particularly when designing treatment and intervention approaches designed to facilitate conversation in LBSD, the vantages of multiple communication partners are critical to ensuring comprehensive, uniquely tailored and likely successful programs. More importantly, recent work in this area suggests that in LBSD, as in DAT, collecting the perspectives of multiple family communication partners offers valuable insights into not only the nature of conversation impairments and effective strategies but also into the coping mechanisms of the family unit as a result of changes in communication. This insight is critical in treatment and intervention within these disorders.

Summary

The current literature on interactional discourse in individuals with LBSD is less extensive than that which addresses monologic discourse. Nonetheless findings show that LBSD affects negatively and with great impact the objective and perceived interactional discourse skills of individuals with LBSD. Findings on conversational discourse in LBSD replicate, in part, and expand in new areas the findings from monologic discourse studies in which individuals with LBSD show shorter responses and lengths of conversational turns, problems signalling turn-taking and understanding turn-taking signals, difficulties maintaining conversational topics, and poor signalling and repairing of conversational problems.

As with the literature on monologic discourse in LBSD, the current literature on interactional discourse is challenging to synthesize and to apply confidently in clinical domains. The challenges arise, in part, from the methodological differences (e.g., structured conversation tasks recorded in the research setting vs. unstructured in-home recordings), philosophical approaches (e.g., conversation analysis methods vs. standardized assessment tools), and variable participant populations (e.g. variable cognitive impairment, disease severity, sex, age, etc.) across studies. Specifically, in the interactional discourse literature insufficient reporting of participant characteristics presents challenges in generalizing findings within clinical settings. As Table 2 summarizes, while 3/6 studies on interactional discourse provide a gross measure of disease staging (Hoehn and Yahr score), only one study presented data on the motor severity of participants (Unified Parkinson Disease Rating Scale scores) which is the more classic clinical scale used to describe motor impairment in individuals with LBSD. Only three studies provide data on cognitive screening results and only one study provided information on speech intelligibility. Moreover, unlike in the monologic discourse literature, only one group of researchers to date (McNamara and Durso 2003) explored the relationships among interactional discourse impairments and performance on discrete cognitive tasks (e.g., executive function). To date, no published studies within the interactional discourse literature have investigated the relationship between medication status and conversation abilities. Finally, and critical to optimizing conversation abilities in clinical practice, few investigators have explored how conversation ability differs between the person with LBSD and multiple different interlocutors. Preliminary research demonstrates that caregivers of persons with LBSD, particularly family members, each are affected differently by their relative's conversational problems, much like family caregivers of individuals with other types of dementia.

Also of great importance is the perspective of individuals with LBSD regarding conversational impairments. To date the perspectives of conversation challenges from the perspective of individuals with LBSD have been explored minimally. A recent study published by Miller, Noble,

Jones, Allcock, and Burn (2008) using a communication questionnaire administered to 140 individuals with PD reported that individuals with PD rated all markers/feelings of communication success as significantly worse post-disease onset (Miller et al. 2008). Among numerous markers of communication difficulty sampled, individuals with PD reported significantly more challenges post-disease onset in the ease of getting a message across, feeling equal in communication exchanges, and being sociable (Miller et al. 2008). Future studies on the interactional discourse of individuals with LBSD are warranted, particularly with respect to illuminating the differential effects of cognition, language and motor speech problems. Further, the multiple influential dynamics on and perceptions of interactional discourse from the perspective of persons with LBSD, family caregivers and professional caregivers are of paramount importance in understanding the clinical relevance of potential intervention strategies for optimizing conversational interactions in LBSD.

Summary of Discourse Changes in LBSD and Future Research Needs

LBSD is a constellation of neurodegenerative diseases that results in deleterious consequences on the monologic and interactional discourses of those with LBSD and on those who care for them. Published studies on the discourse of individuals with LBSD have documented myriad effects including, but not limited to, reduced verbal output, disrupted syntactic production and comprehension, word retrieval errors, poor turn-taking and conversational topic maintenance, moderately impaired conversational problem signalling and repair, and multiple differential influences of discourse disruption on family caregivers. Future research would benefit from exploring the phenomenon of discourse production and comprehension across a spectrum of discourse genres (e.g., picture description, procedural, conversation) within the same cohort of individuals with LBSD in order to evaluate discourse performance within the context of differing cognitive and language demands posed by varying discourse tasks. Furthermore, as in other disorders (e.g., traumatic brain injury, aphasia post stroke) the current literature reveals the need for developing a consistent set of valid and sensitive measures for specifically evaluating discourse performance in LBSD in order to optimize the potential for discourse analyses in the diagnosis, characterization and ultimately therapeutic planning for deficits within this spectrum. For example, it is possible that particular discourse impairments such as the pattern of verbal disruptions or the frequency, type, and location of pausing may be specifically characteristic of LBSD. Moreover, findings reported by Ash et al. (2011; 2012) suggest that patterns of discourse impairment may be sensitive for separating the disorders within LBSD. The sensitivity of discourse measures for detecting nuances of cognitive-linguistic changes in the presence of neurodegenerative disorders and the potential for such data to inform directly the clinical practice of individuals working to optimize communication in LBSD underscore the importance of the study of discourse in this population.

A careful review of the current literature on discourse in LBSD reveals that future research studies should thoughtfully consider the variables that can influence discourse performance in LBSD. These variables include a careful characterization of the motor symptoms (e.g., lateralization) and disease staging using clinically accepted measures. Pharmaceutical contributions to performance, particularly dopaminergic and cholinergic medications, also should be considered. Moreover, given the prominence of motor speech disorders in this population, future discourse studies would benefit from characterizing the motor speech abilities of participants and considering the possible contribution to discourse performance. Furthermore, the relationships among cognition, language and discourse performance suggest that studies exploring discourse in LBSD would benefit from quantification of some of these variables and the potential influence on discourse performance.

As in other neurodegenerative diseases, the current LBSD literature suggests that the assessment of discourse may inform clinical practice. Given the consistency of findings that suggest challenges in pausing, turn-taking, repair behaviours and informativeness, individuals with LBSD would benefit potentially from social based treatments used in aphasia including PACE (Promoting Aphasics' Communicative Effectiveness (Davis 2005), Response Elaboration Training (Kearns 1985), and supportive conversation techniques (Kagan et al. 2001). Finally, it is most critical that future research focus on the effects of discourse impairments on the relationships and conversation effectiveness between individuals with LBSD and their respective conversation partners in order to develop effective interventions for optimizing communication and quality of life in LBSD. Given the magnitude of these disorders within our health system focussing on this area of research is of foremost importance.

Acknowledgment

The authors wish to acknowledge Mrs. Bracia Eaton for her assistance in preparing and formatting the manuscript.

References

Aarsland, Dag, K. Bronnick, C. Williams-Gray, D. Weintraub, K. Marder, and J. Kulisevsky. 2010. Mild cognitive impairment in Parkinson disease: A multicenter pooled analysis. *Neurology* 75 (12): 1062-1069.

Aarsland, Dag, and M.K. Beyer, and M.W. Kurz. 2008. Dementia in Parkinson's disease. *Curr Opin Neurol* 21 (6): 676-682.

Aarsland, Dag, and Kjeld Andersen, Jan P. Larsen, and Anette Lolk. 2003. Prevalence and characteristics of dementia in Parkinson disease: An 8-year prospective study. *Archives of Neurology* 60 (3): 387-392. Doi:10.1001/archneur.60.3.387.

Alpert, M., A. Rosen, J. Welkowitz, and A. Lieberman. 1990. Interpersonal communication in the context of dementia. *J Commun Disord* 23 (4-5): 337-346.

Ash, S., C. McMillan, R.G. Gross, P. Cook, D. Gunawardena, B. Morgan, A. Boller, A. Siderowf, and M. Grossman. 2012. Impairments of speech fluency in lewy body spectrum disorder." *Brain Lang* 120 (3): 290-302.

Ash, S., and C. McMillan, R.G. Gross, P. Cook, B. Morgan, A. Boller, M. Dreyfuss, A. Siderowf, and M. Grossman. 2011. The organization of narrative discourse in lewy body spectrum disorder. *Brain Lang* 119 (1): 30-41.

Ash, S., and C. McMillan, D. Gunawardena, B. Avants, B. Morgan, A. Khan, P. Moore, J. Gee, and M. Grossman. 2010. Speech errors in progressive non-fluent aphasia. *Brain Lang* 113 (1): 13-20.

Ash, S., and P. Moore, S. Antani, G. McCawley, M. Work, and M. Grossman. 2006. Trying to tell a tale: Discourse impairments in progressive aphasia and frontotemporal dementia. *Neurology* 66 (9): 1405-1413.

Ballard, C., and Ian McKeith. 1998. Psychiatric features in diffuse lewy body disease. *Neurology* 50 (2): 573

Bayles, Kathryn A. 1990. Language and Parkinson disease. *Alzheimer Dis Assoc Disord* 4 (3):171-180.

Benito-Leon, J., E. Cubo, and C. Coronell. 2011. Impact of apathy on health-related quality of life in recently diagnosed Parkinson's disease: The ANIMO study. *Mov Disord* 27 (2): 211-218.

Berg, E., C. Bjornram, L. Hartelius, K. Laakso, and B. Johnels. 2003. High-level language difficulties in Parkinson's disease. *Clin Linguist Phon* 17 (1): 63-80.

Bertella, L., G. Albani, E. Greco, L. Priano, A. Mauro, and S. Marchi. 2002. Noun verb dissociation in Parkinson's disease. *Brain Cogn 48* (2-3): 277-280.

Bohlhalter, S., E. Abela, D. Weniger, and B. Weder. 2009. Impaired verbal memory in Parkinson disease: Relationship to prefrontal dysfunction and somatosensory discrimination. *Behav Brain Funct* 5: 49-59.

Bohnen, N.I., D.I. Kaufer, R. Hendrickson, L.S. Ivanco, B.J. Lopresti, and G.M. Constantine. 2006. Cognitive correlates of cortical cholinergic denervation in Parkinson's disease and parkinsonian dementia. *Journal of Neurology* 253 (2) 242-247.

Boulenger, V., L. Mechtouff, S. Thobois, E. Broussolle, M.Jeannerod, and T.A. Nazir. 2008. Word processing in Parkinson's disease is impaired for action verbs but not for concrete nouns. *Neuropsychologia* 46 (2): 743-756.

Brookshire, R.H., and L.E. Nicholas. 1994. Speech sample size and test-retest stability of connected speech measures for adults with aphasia. *Journal of Speech, Language and Hearing Research* 37 (2): 399.

Burn, D.J., E.N. Rowan, L.M. Allan, S. Molloy, J.T. O'Brien, and I. McKeith. 2006. Motor subtype and cognitive decline in Parkinson's disease, Parkinson's disease with dementia, and dementia with lewy bodies. *J Neurol Neurosurg Psychiatry* 77 (5): 585-589.

Burn, D.J., and E.N. Rowan, T. Minett, J. Sanders, P. Myint, J. Richardson, A. Thomas, J. Newby, J. Reid, J.T. O'Brien, and I. McKeith. 2003. Extrapyramidal features in Parkinson's disease with and without dementia and dementia with lewy bodies: A cross-sectional comparative study. *Mov Disord* 18 (8): 884-889.

Caviness, J.N., E. Driver-Dunckley, D.J. Connor, M.N. Sabbagh, J.G. Hentz, B. Noble, V.G. Evidente, H.A. Shill, and C.H. Adler. 2007. Defining mild cognitive impairment in Parkinson's disease. *Mov Disord* 22 (9): 1272-1277.

Chenery, H. J., A.J. Angwin, and D.A. Copland. 2008. The basal ganglia circuits, dopamine, and ambiguous word processing: A neurobiological account of priming studies in Parkinson's disease. *J Int Neuropsychol Soc* 14 (3): 351-364.

Coelho, C.A. 2007. Management of discourse deficits following traumatic brain injury: Progress, caveats, and needs discourse analyses and dementia. *Semin Speech Lang Brain Lang* 28 (2): 122-135.

Colman, K. S., J. Koerts, L.A. Stowe, K.L. Leenders, and R. Bastiaanse. 2011. Sentence comprehension and its association with executive functions in patients with Parkinson's disease. *Parkinsons Dis*: 1-15. Doi:10.4061/2011/213983.

Cotelli, M., B. Borroni, R. Manenti, M. Zanetti, A. Arevalo, and S.F. Cappa. 2007. Action and object naming in Parkinson's disease without dementia. *Eur J Neurol* 14(6): 632-637.

Crucian, G.P., L. Huang, A.M. Barrett, R.L. Schwartz, J.E. Cibula, J.M. Anderson, W.J. Triggs, D. Bowers, W.A. Friedman, M. Greer, and K.M. Heilman. 2001. Emotional conversations in Parkinson's disease. *Neurology* 56 (2): 159-165.

Darley, F. L., A.E. Aronson, and J.R. Brown. 1969. Differential diagnostic patterns of dysarthria. *Journal of Speech, Language and Hearing Research* 12 (2): 246-269.

Darley, F. L., and A.E. Aronson, and J.R. Brown. 1975. *Motor Speech Disorders*. Saunders Philadelphia.

Davis, G.A. 2005. PACE revisited. *Aphasiology* 19 (1): 21-38.

Doyle, P.J., A.J. Goda, and K.A. Spencer. 1995. The communicative informativeness and efficiency of connected discourse by adults with aphasia under structured and conversational sampling conditions. *American Journal of Speech Language Pathology* 4 (4): 130-134.

Ehrt, U., K. Broich, J.P. Larsen, C. Ballard, and D. Aarsland. 2010. Use of drugs with anticholinergic effect and impact on cognition in Parkinson's disease: A cohort study. *Journal of Neurology, Neurosurgery & Psychiatry* 81 (2): 160-165.

Elgh, E., M. Domellof, J. Linder, M. Edstrom, H. Stenlund, and L. Forsgren. 2009. Cognitive function in early Parkinson's disease: A population-based study. *Eur J Neurol* 16 (12): 1278-1284.

Emre, M. 2003. Dementia associated with Parkinson's disease. *The Lancet Neurology* 2 (4): 229-237.

Emre, M., and D. Aarsland, R. Brown, D.J. Burn, C. Duyckaerts, Y. Mizuno, G.A. Broe, J. Cummings, D.W. Dickson, S. Gauthier, J. Goldman, C. Goetz, A. Korczyn, A. Lees, R. Levy, I. Litvan, I. McKeith, W. Olanow, W. Poewe, N. Quinn, C. Sampaio, E. Tolosa, and B. Dubois. 2007. Clinical diagnostic criteria for dementia associated with Parkinson's disease. *Mov Disord* 22 (12): 1689-1707.

Fahn, S.R.L.E., R.L. Elton, and Committee, U. P. D. R. S. D. 1987. Unified Parkinson's disease rating scale. *Recent Developments in Parkinson's Disease* 2: 153-163.

Farag, C., V. Troiani, M. Bonner, C. Powers, B. Avants, J. Gee, and M. Grossman. 2010. Hierarchical organization of scripts: Converging evidence from FMRI and frontotemporal degeneration. *Cereb Cortex* 20 (10): 2453-2463.

Fernandino, L., L.L. Conant, J.R. Binder, K. Blindauer, B. Hiner, and K. Spangler. 2012. Parkinson's disease disrupts both automatic and controlled processing of action verbs. *Brain Lang: 1-10.*

Fleming,Valarie B., and Joyce L. Harris. 2008. Complex discourse production in mild cognitive impairment: Detecting subtle changes. *Aphasiology* 22 (7-8): 729-740.

Gago, Miguel, M. Garrett, M. Fonseca, M. Rosas, M. Simoes, S. Vieira, and F. Botelho. 2009. How do cognitive and axial motor signs correlate in Parkinson's disease? A 6-year prospective study. *Journal of Neurology* 256 (10): 1655-1662.

Gelb, D.J., E. Oliver, and S. Gilman. 1999. Diagnostic criteria for Parkinson disease. *Arch Neurol* 56 (1): 33-39.

Gibb, W.R., and A.J. Lees. 1988. The relevance of the lewy body to the pathogenesis of idiopathic Parkinson's disease. *J Neurol Neurosurg Psychiatry* 51 (6): 745-752.

Godbout, L., and J. Doyon. 2000. Defective representation of knowledge in Parkinson's disease: Evidence from a script-production task. *Brain Cogn* 44 (3): 490-510.

—. 1994. Représentation mentale d'activités familières (scripts) chez des patients porteurs de lesions. Corticales circonscrites ou atteints de la maladie de Parkinson Unpublished Doctoral Dissertation: Université Laval, St-Foy, Québec, Canada.

Goedert, M., M.G. Spillantini, K. Del Tredici, and H. Braak. 2013. 100 years of lewy pathology. *Nat Rev Neurol* 9 (1): 13-24.

Goetz, C.G., M. Emre, and B. Dubois. 2008. Parkinson's disease dementia: Definitions, guidelines, and research perspectives in diagnosis. *Ann Neurol* 64: S81-S92.

Gotham, A.M., R.G. Brown, and C.D. Marsden. 1988. 'Frontal' cognitive function in patients with Parkinson's disease 'on' and 'off' levodopa. *Brain* 111 (2): 299-321.

Green, J., W.M. McDonald, J.L. Vitek, M. Evatt, A. Freeman, and M. Haber. 2002. Cognitive impairments in advanced PD without dementia. *Neurology* 59 (9): 1320-1324.

Griffiths, S., R. Barnes, N. Britten, and R. Wilkinson. 2012. Potential causes and consequences of overlap in talk between speakers with Parkinson's disease and their familiar conversation partners. *Semin Speech Lang* 33 (1): 27-43.

Griffiths, S., and R. Barnes, N. Britten, and R. Wilkinson. 2011. Investigating interactional competencies in Parkinson's disease: The potential benefits of a conversation analytic approach. *Int J Lang Commun Disord* 46 (5): 497-509.

Gross, R.G., C.T. McMillan, K. Chandrasekaran, M. Dreyfuss, S. Ash, B. Avants, P. Cook, P. Moore, D.J. Libon, A. Siderowf, and M. Grossman. 2012. Sentence processing in lewy body spectrum disorder: The role of working memory. *Brain Cogn* 78 (2): 85-93.

Grossman, M., R.G. Gross, P. Moore, M. Dreyfuss, C.T. McMillan, P.A. Cook, S. Ash, and A. Siderowf. 2012. Difficulty processing temporary syntactic ambiguities in lewy body spectrum disorder. *Brain Lang* 120 (1): 52-60.

Grossman, M., and C. Lee, J. Morris, M.B. Stern, and H.I. Hurtig. 2002. Assessing resource demands during sentence processing in Parkinson's disease. *Brain Lang* 80 (3): 603-616.

Grossman, M. 1999. Sentence processing in Parkinson's disease. *Brain Cogn* 40 (2): 387-413.

Grossman, M., and S. Carvell, and L. Peltzer. 1993. The sum and substance of it: The appreciation of mass and count quantifiers in Parkinson's disease. *Brain Lang* 44 (4): 351-384.

Grossman, M., and S. Carvell, M.B. Stern, S. Gollomp, and H.I. Hurtig. 1992. Sentence comprehension in Parkinson's disease: The role of attention and memory. *Brain Lang* 42 (4): 347-384.

Grossman, M., and P. Crino, M. Reivich, M.B. Stern, and H.I. Hurtig. 1992. Attention and sentence processing deficits in Parkinson's disease: The role of anterior cingulate cortex. *Cereb Cortex* 2 (6): 513-525.

Grossman, M., and S. Carvell, S. Gollomp, M.B. Stern, G. Vernon, and H.I. Hurtig. 1991. Sentence comprehension and praxis deficits in Parkinson's disease. *Neurology* 41 (10): 1620-1626.

Hall, D., B. Ouyang, E. Lonnquist, and J. Newcombe. 2011. Pragmatic communication is impaired in Parkinson disease. *Int J Neurosci* 121 (5): 254-256.

Halper, A., L. Cherney, and M. Burns. 1996. *Clinical Management of Right Hemisphere Dysfunction.* Gaithersburg: Aspen Publications.

Henry, Julie D., and John R. Crawford. 2004. A meta-analytic review of verbal fluency performance following focal cortical lesions. *Neuropsychology* 18 (2): 284-295.

Herrera, E., J. Rodriguez-Ferreiro, and F. Cuetos. 2012. The effect of motion content in action naming by Parkinson's disease patients. *Cortex* 48 (7): 900-904.

Hochstadt, J. 2009. Set-shifting and the on-line processing of relative clauses in Parkinson's disease: Results from a novel eye-tracking method. *Cortex* 45 (8): 991-1011.

Hochstadt, J., and H. Nakano, P. Lieberman, and J. Friedman. 2006. The roles of sequencing and verbal working memory in sentence comprehension deficits in Parkinson's disease. *Brain Lang* 97 (3): 243-257.

Holtgraves, T., P. McNamara, K. Cappaert, and R. Durso. 2010. Linguistic correlates of asymmetric motor symptom severity in Parkinson's disease. *Brain and Cognition* 72 (2): 189-196.

Huber, J.E., and M. Darling. 2011. Effect of Parkinson's disease on the production of structured and unstructured speaking tasks: Respiratory physiologic and linguistic considerations. *J Speech Lang Hear Res* 54 (1): 33-46.

Illes, J. 1989. Neurolinguistic features of spontaneous language production dissociate three forms of neurodegenerative disease: Alzheimer's, Huntington's, and Parkinson's. *Brain Lang* 37 (4): 628-642.

Illes, J., and E.J. Metter, W.R. Hanson, and S. Iritani. 1988. Language production in Parkinson's disease: Acoustic and linguistic considerations. *Brain Lang* 33 (1): 146-160.

Ivory, S. J., R.G. Knight, B.E. Longmore, and T. Caradoc-Davies. 1999. Verbal memory in non-demented patients with idiopathic Parkinson's disease. *Neuropsychologia* 37 (7): 817-828.

Jaywant, A., and M.D. Pell. 2010. Listener impressions of speakers with Parkinson's disease. *J Int Neuropsychol Soc* 16 (1): 49-57.

Jensen, A.M., H.J. Chenery, and D.A. Copland. 2006. A comparison of picture description abilities in individuals with vascular subcortical lesions and Huntington's disease. *J Commun Disord* 39 (1): 62-77.

Johnson, D.K., J.C. Morris, and J.E. Galvin. 2005. Verbal and visuospatial deficits in dementia with lewy bodies. *Neurology* 65 (8): 1232-1238.

Kagan, A. 1998. Supported conversation for adults with aphasia: Methods and resources for training conversation partners. *Aphasiology* 12 (9): 816-830.

Kearns, K.P. 1985. Response elaboration training for patient initiated utterances. *In Clinical Aphasiology Conference: Clinical Aphasiology Conference* (1985: 15th: Ashland, OR: June 2-6, 1985) BRK Publishers(1985): 196-204.

Kulisevsky, J., A. Avila, M. Barbanoj, R. Antonijoan, M.L. Berthier, and A. Gironell. 1996. Acute effects of levodopa on neuropsychological performance in stable and fluctuating Parkinson's disease patients at different levodopa plasma levels. *Brain* 119 (6): 2121-2132.

Laws, Keith R., John R. Crawford, Francesca Gnoato, Giuseppe Sartori, T.A. Ala, L.F. Hughes, G.A. Kyrouac, M.W. Ghobrial, R.J. Elble, and M. Ballmaier. 2007. A predominance of category deficits for living things in Alzheimer's disease and lewy body dementia. *Journal of the International Neuropsychological Society* 13 (3): 401-409.

Levy, James A., and Gordon J. Chelune. 2007. Cognitive-behavioral profiles of neurodegenerative dementias: Beyond Alzheimer's disease. *Journal of Geriatric Psychiatry and Neurology* 20 (4): 227-238.

Lieberman, P., E. Kako, J. Friedman, G. Tajchman, L.S. Feldman, and E.B. Jiminez. 1992. Speech production, syntax comprehension, and cognitive deficits in Parkinson's disease. *Brain Lang* 43 (2): 169-189.

Lieberman, P., and J. Friedman, and L.S. Feldman. 1990. Syntax comprehension deficits in Parkinson's disease. *J Nerv Ment Dis* 178 (6): 360-365.

Lippa, C.F., J.E. Duda, M. Grossman, H.I. Hurtig, D. Aarsland, B.F. Boeve, D.J. Brooks, D.W. Dickson, B. Dubois, and M. Emre. 2007. DLB and PDD boundary issues diagnosis, treatment, molecular pathology, and biomarkers. *Neurology* 68 (11): 812-819.

Locascio, J. J., S. Corkin, and J.H. Growdon. 2003. Relation between clinical characteristics of Parkinson's disease and cognitive decline. *J Clin Exp Neuropsychol* 25 (1): 94-109.

Martinez-Horta, S., and J. Kulisevsky. 2011. Is all cognitive impairment in Parkinson's disease "Mild Cognitive Impairment"? *J Neural Transm* 118 (8): 1185-1190.

Matison, R., R. Mayeux, J. Rosen, and S. Fahn. 1982. "Tip-of-the-tongue" phenomenon in Parkinson disease. *Neurology* 32 (5): 567-570.

Mayer, M. 1969. *Frog, where are you?* The Dial Press: New York.

McKeith, Ian. 2004. Dementia with lewy bodies. *Dialogues Clin Neurosci* 6 (3): 333-341.

McKeith, Ian, and Jacobo Mintzer, Dag Aarsland, David Burn, Helen Chiu, Jiska Cohen-Mansfield, Dennis Dickson, Bruno Dubois, John E Duda, and Howard Feldman. 2004. Dementia with lewy bodies. *The Lancet Neurology* 3 (1): 19-28.

McKeith, Ian, and U. P. Mosimann. 2004. Dementia with lewy bodies and Parkinson's disease. *Parkinsonism & Related Disorders* 10: S15-S18.

McNamara, P., and R. Durso. 2003. Pragmatic communication skills in patients with Parkinson's disease. *Brain Lang* 84 (3): 414-423.

McNamara, P., and M. Krueger, K. O'Quin, J. Clark, and R. Durso. 1996. Grammaticality judgments and sentence comprehension in Parkinson's disease: A comparison with broca's aphasia. *Int J Neurosci* 86 (1-2): 151-166.

McNamara, P.,and L.K. Obler, R. Au, R. Durso, and M.L. Albert. 1992. Speech monitoring skills in Alzheimer's disease, Parkinson's disease, and normal aging. *Brain Lang* 42 (1): 38-51.

Miller, N., S. Andrew, E. Noble, and M. Walshe. 2011. Changing perceptions of self as a communicator in Parkinson's disease: A longitudinal follow-up study. *Disabil Rehabil* 33 (3): 204-210.

Miller, N., and E. Noble, D. Jones, L. Allcock, and D.J. Burn. 2008. How do I sound to me? Perceived changes in communication in Parkinson's disease. *Clin Rehabil* 22 (1):14-22.

Monetta, L., H.S. Cheang, and M.D. Pell. 2008. Understanding speaker attitudes from prosody by adults with Parkinson's disease. *J Neuropsychol* 2 (Pt 2): 415-430.

Murray, L.L. 2000. Spoken language production in Huntington's and Parkinson's diseases. *J Speech Lang Hear Res* 43 (6): 1350-1366.

Murray, L.L., and L.P. Lenz. 2001. Productive syntax abilities in Huntington's and Parkinson's diseases. *Brain Cogn* 46 (1-2): 213-219.

Muslimovic, D., B. Post, J.D. Speelman, and B. Schmand. 2005. Cognitive profile of patients with newly diagnosed Parkinson disease. *Neurology* 65 (8): 1239-1245.

Natsopoulos, D., G. Grouios, S. Bostantzopoulou, G. Mentenopoulos, Z. Katsarou, and J. Logothetis.1993. Algorithmic and heuristic strategies in comprehension of complement clauses by patients with Parkinson's disease. *Neuropsychologia* 31 (9): 951-964.

Natsopoulos, D., and Z. Katsarou, S. Bostantzopoulou, G. Grouios, G. Mentenopoulos, and J. Logothetis. 1991. Strategies in comprehension of relative clauses by parkinsonian patients. *Cortex* 27 (2): 255-268.

Orange, J.B., and A. Kertesz. 2000. Discourse analyses and dementia. *Brain Lang* 71 (1): 172-174.

Orange, J.B., and Rosemary Lubinski, Andrew Johnson, Barbara Purves, and Jeff Small. 2009. Validity analyses of a measure of conversation in dementia. *In Clinical Aphasiology Conference* 39th: Keystone, CO: May 26-30.

Orange, J.B. 1991. Perspectives of family members regarding communication changes. *Dementia and communication:* 168-186.

Pagonabarraga, Javier, and Jaime Kulisevsky. 2012. Cognitive impairment and dementia in Parkinson's disease. *Neurobiology of Disease* 46 (3): 590-596.

Parkinson Disease Foundation. 2013. *Statistics on Parkinson's.* http://www.pdf.org/en/parkinson_statistics.

Pell, M.D., H.S. Cheang, and C.L. Leonard. 2006. The impact of Parkinson's disease on vocal- prosodic communication from the perspective of listeners. *Brain Lang* 97 (2): 123-134.

Peran, P., D. Cardebat, A. Cherubini, F. Piras, G. Luccichenti, and A. Peppe. 2009. Object naming and action-verb generation in Parkinson's disease: A fMRI study. *Cortex* 45 (8): 960-971.

Peran, P., and O. Rascol, J.F. Demonet, P. Celsis, J.L. Nespoulous, and B. Dubois. 2003. Deficit of verb generation in nondemented patients with Parkinson's disease. *Mov Disord* 18 (2): 150-156.

Perkins, Lisa, Anne Whitworth, and Ruth Lesser. 1998. Conversing in dementia: A conversation analytic approach. *Journal of Neurolinguistics* 11 (1): 33-53.

Pitcairn, T. K., S. Clemie, J.M. Gray, and B. Pentland. 1990. Impressions of parkinsonian patients from their recorded voices. *Br J Disord Commun* 25 (1): 85-92.

Poletti, M., and U. Bonuccelli. 2013. Acute and chronic cognitive effects of levodopa and dopamine agonists on patients with parkinson's disease: A review. *Therapeutic Advances in Psychopharmacology* 3 (2) 101-113.

Prutting, C.A., and D.M. Kirchner. 1987. A clinical appraisal of the pragmatic aspects of language. *J Speech Hear Disord* 52 (2): 105-119.

Purves, Barbara A. 2011. Exploring positioning in Alzheimer disease through analyses of family talk. *Dementia* 10 (1): 35-58.

Purves, Barbara A., and Alison Phinney. 2013. Family voices: A family systems approach to understanding communication in dementia. *Canadian Journal of Speech-Language Pathology* 36 (4): 284-300.

Ralph, M.A.L., J. Powell, D. Howard, A.B. Whitworth, P. Garrard, and J.R. Hodges. 2001. Semantic memory is impaired in both dementia with lewy bodies and dementia of Alzheimer's type: A comparative neuropsychology study and literature review. *Journal of Neurology, Neurosurgery and Psychiatry* 70 (2): 149-156.

Ramig, L. O., C. Fox, and S. Sapir. 2004. Parkinson's disease: Speech and voice disorders and their treatment with the Lee Silverman voice treatment. *Seminars in Speech and Language* 25 (2): 169-180.

Roberts-South, A., K. Findlater, M.J. Strong, and J.B. Orange. 2012. Longitudinal changes in discourse production in amyotrophic lateral sclerosis. *Semin Speech Lang* 33(1): 79-94.

Rodriguez-Ferreiro, J., F. Cuetos, E. Herrera, M. Menendez, and R. Ribacoba. 2010. Cognitive impairment in Parkinson's disease without dementia. *Mov Disord* 25 (13): 2136-2141.

Rodriguez-Ferreiro, J., and J., M. Menendez, R. Ribacoba, and F. Cuetos. 2009. Action naming is impaired in Parkinson disease patients. *Neuropsychologia* 47 (14): 3271-3274.

Rousseaux, M., A. Seve, M. Vallet, F. Pasquier, and M.A. Mackowiak-Cordoliani. 2010. An analysis of communication in conversation in patients with dementia. *Neuropsychologia* 48 (13): 3884-3890.

Rousseaux, M., and A. Delacourt, N. Wyrzykowski, and M. Lefeuvre. 2001. *Lille Communication Test.* Isbergues: Ortho Edition.

Shadden, Barbara B. 1998a. Obtaining the discourse sample. *In Analyzing Discourse in Communicatively Impaired Adults, 9-33.* Edited by L. Cherney, B. Shadden, and C. Coelho. Gaithersburg: Aspen Publishers.

—. 1998b. Sentential/surface level analyses. *In Analyzing Discourse in Communicatively Impaired Adults 35-60.* Edited by L. Cherney, B. Shadden, and C. Coelho. Gaithersburg: Aspen Publishers.

—. 1998c. Information analyses. *In Analyzing Discourse in Communicatively Impaired Adults, 85-111.* Edited by L. Cherney, B. Shadden, and C. Coelho. Gaithersburg: Aspen Publishers.

Shadden, Barbara B., and Rhonda B. Burnette, Beverly R. Eikenberry, and R. DiBrezzo. All discourse tasks are not created equal. *In Clinical Aphasiology Conference: Clinical Aphasiology Conference* (1990: 20th: Santa Fe, NM: June 1990) Pro-Ed (1991): 327-342. http://aphasiology.pitt.edu/archive/00000153/

Skeel, R. L., B. Crosson, S.E. Nadeau, J. Algina, R.M. Bauer, and E.B. Fennell. 2001. Basal ganglia dysfunction, working memory, and sentence comprehension in patients with Parkinson's disease. *Neuropsychologia* 39 (9): 962-971.

Sollinger, A. B., F.C. Goldstein, J.J. Lah, A.I. Levey, and S.A. Factor. 2010. Mild cognitive impairment in Parkinson's disease: Subtypes and motor characteristics. *Parkinsonism Relat Disord* 16 (3): 177-180.

Spivey-Knowlton, M. J., J.C. Trueswell, and M.K. Tanenhaus. 1993. Context effects in syntactic ambiguity resolution: Discourse and semantic influences in parsing reduced relative clauses. *Canadian Journal of Experimental Psychology* 47 (2): 276-309.

Templin, M. 1957. *Certain language skills in children: Their development and relationships.* Minneapolis: University of Minnesota Press.

Troster, A.I. 2008. Neuropsychological characteristics of dementia with lewy bodies and Parkinson's disease with dementia: Differentiation, early detection, and implications for "mild cognitive impairment" and biomarkers. *Neuropsychol Rev* 18 (1): 103-119.

Verbaan, D., J. Marinus, M. Visser, S.M. van Rooden, A.M. Stiggelbout, and H.A. Middelkoop. 2007. Cognitive impairment in Parkinson's disease. *J Neurol Neurosurg Psychiatry* 78 (11): 1182-1187.

Vigliocco, G. 2000. The anatomy of meaning and syntax. *Curr Biol* 10 (2): R78-R80.

Vigliocco, G., and R.J. Hartsuiker. 2002. The interplay of meaning, sound, and syntax in sentence production. *Psychological Bulletin* 128 (3): 442-472. Doi: 10.1037/0033-2909.128.3.442

Walsh, B., and A. Smith. 2011. Linguistic complexity, speech production, and comprehension in Parkinson's disease: Behavioral and physiological indices. *J Speech Lang Hear Res* 54 (3): 787-802.

Whitworth, Anne, Ruth Lesser, and Ian McKeith. 1999. Profiling conversation in Parkinson's disease with cognitive impairment. *Aphasiology* 13 (4-5): 407-425.

Williams, V.G, J.M. Bruce, H.J. Westervelt, J.D. Davis, J. Grace, P.F. Malloy, and G. Tremont. 2007. Boston naming performance distinguishes between lewy body and Alzheimer's dementias. *Arch Clin Neuropsychol* 22 (8): 925-931.

Ye, Z., M. Milenkova, B. Mohammadi, K. Kollewe, C. Schrader, and R. Dengler. 2012. Impaired comprehension of temporal connectives in Parkinson's disease: A neuroimaging study. *Neuropsychologia* 50 (8): 1794-1800.

Zanini, S., A. Tavano, and F. Fabbro. 2010. Spontaneous language production in bilingual Parkinson's disease patients: Evidence of greater phonological, morphological and syntactic impairments in native language. *Brain Lang* 113 (2): 84-89.

Zraick, Richard I., Portia B. Carr, Brent A. Gregg, and Laura Smith-Olinde, Courtney Ghormley and Terri J. Hutton. 2011. Information units produced by persons with mild Alzheimer's disease during a picture description task. *Journal of Medical Speech-Language Pathology* 19 (2): 37-45.

CHAPTER SEVEN

CHALLENGES AND OPPORTUNITIES OF GROUP CONVERSATIONS: THE DAY CARE CENTER AS A COMMUNICATION MILIEU

CAMILLA LINDHOLM
UNIVERSITY OF HELSINKI

Introduction

Ferdinand, an elderly man with Alzheimer's disease and hearing impairment, David, an elderly man with vascular dementia, and nurse Rebecka are having a conversation at a day care center in southern Finland for Swedish-speaking elderly people with memory problems. Ferdinand is in the middle of telling about his experiences from World War II, explaining in detail how the soldiers slept in tents, and got cold feet, while their heads were covered with sweat. As a reaction to his telling, Rebecka poses a question: *did you always have as a fire warden someone* (line 1):

(1) FIRE WARDEN

01 Rebecka:	did you always have as a fire warden someone
02	(0.2)
03 Ferdinand:	**what**
04	(0.2)
05 Rebecka:	did you always have someone who sat as a fire warden
06	(0.9)
07 David:	<fire warden>
08	(1.6)
09 Rebecka:	in [ta- in the tent
10 David:	[about that
11 Ferdinand:	**[I don't hear that well**
12	(about [that)

13 Rebecka:	[did you always have someone who sat
14	as a fire warden in the tent
15	(1.0)
16 David:	did someone sit as a <fire warden>
17 Ferdinand:	yes yesyes yesyes (.h) *kipinäkalle*
18 Rebecka:	oh heh heh heh

The English structure is a word-by-word translation of the original Swedish structure; see appendix for the original Swedish transcriptions. Ferdinand's response *what* (line 3) expresses his inability to fully hear or understand Rebecka's question, which renders him incapable of providing an answer. In an attempt to improve Ferdinand's understanding, Rebecka repeats her previous turn (line 5). This time, the word order is changed, but the content is kept intact. Yet Ferdinand does not respond. Instead, David engages in the conversation (line 7). Ferdinand's *what* question does not focus on a specific element of the previous turn but targets the whole turn as the trouble source (cf. Drew 1997). Nevertheless, David repeats the term *fire warden*, thus revealing his interpretation that Ferdinand encountered trouble in grasping this specific word. David speaks very slowly, using exaggerated articulation to resolve a problematic situation.

Ferdinand's next turn, *I don't hear that well*, explicates his problem as a hearing problem. Expressing hearing problems in conversation is a more recurrent practice than referring to comprehension problems, since admitting problems of understanding is usually at least potentially more face-threatening than is expressing trouble in hearing (Svennevig 2008). This problem indicator is followed by repeating Rebecka's original question, with the specifying addition *in the tent* (lines 13–14). David, in his turn, assists Rebecka by reformulating her question, intensifying the articulation of the *fire warden* word, which is uttered slowly and with stress on the first syllable. Finally, their efforts are successful, and Ferdinand gives an answer to Rebecka's question (line 17), using the Finnish word *kipinäkalle*, a playful expression for a fire warden, which may have been used by soldiers during World War II.

In this extract, both Rebecka and David work actively to help Ferdinand when he has trouble following the conversation. In the terminology of Emergent Pragmatics (Perkins 2007), which is the theoretical framework of this study, communication impairment in an individual is said to create a state of intrapersonal imbalance, for which the interlocutors compensate. This happens, for example, when one individual (Ferdinand in this case) has hearing difficulties and the interlocutors (here Rebecka and David) help him or her out by repeating and reformulating the original utterance.

Extract 1 illustrates how a group conversation functions as a system in that language and communication disorders "become common property, rather than solely the problem of an individual" (Perkins 2007, 67). This study, based on a piece previously published in Finnish (Lindholm 2012), analyzes how a group setting at a day care center involves both challenges and opportunities for elderly persons with dementia, and how the group jointly develops strategies for managing the individual communication difficulties arising from dementia.

Emergent Pragmatics

Traditionally, pragmatics has been viewed as a distinct entity. Mainstream pragmatic theories have concentrated on language, seeing pragmatics either as a level of language (like phonology, syntax, or semantics) or as a component of the linguistic system. Clinicians, on the other hand, have stressed the role of cognition, Theory of Mind above all, in pragmatic functioning. These prior approaches have, thus, focused on pragmatics as a distinct entity, existing independently of entities with which it interacts. Emergent Pragmatics (Perkins 2005; 2007, 2008), on the other hand, characterizes pragmatics not as a discrete entity but as the emergent outcome of interactions among cognition, language, and sensorimotor systems. Apart from language and cognition (e.g., memory and executive function), nonverbal entities such as gaze, gesture, and body posture and sensory entities like hearing and vision are included as elements of pragmatics. In Emergent Pragmatics, interactions are seen as taking place both within and between individuals – i.e., in the *intrapersonal* and the *interpersonal* domain.

Emergent Pragmatics sees pragmatics as involving the range of *choices* open to us when we communicate – for example, what is said, where it is said, how it is said, and to whom it is said. These choices are involved at all levels of language processing from discourse down to phonetics. The choices are not exclusively linguistic – in conversation, participants constantly make choices not only about how to use language but also about how to use nonverbal resources such as gaze, gesture, and body posture. Thus, Emergent Pragmatics represents a multimodal approach to communication, suggesting that meaning may be explicit not only through language but also through nonverbal resources. To be qualified as "pragmatic," choices in communication need to be motivated by the requirements of interpersonal communication: "pragmatic choices are those which are made by human beings because they wish or need to communicate with each other, and they involve the use of any resources which may help to do the job" (Perkins 2007, 60). According to this definition of pragmatics as choices, pragmatic impairment is defined as a restriction on the choices available for encoding or decoding of meaning – a person is defined as pragmatically impaired if the range of choices open to him or her is more restricted than the range enjoyed by more typical speakers.

Besides the idea of pragmatics as choices, Emergent Pragmatics suggests that there is no direct link between an underlying deficit and a resulting pragmatic behavior. Pragmatic behavior is viewed as a result of complex interactions among semiotic, cognitive, and sensorimotor elements in the intrapersonal and the interpersonal domain. The elements interacting may constrain or facilitate one another, and any malfunctioning capacity in one domain can create a state of interactional imbalance both within the domain and across domains. This will result in a redistribution of resources, *compensatory adaptation*, in an attempt to maintain equilibrium. Therefore, a distinct pragmatic behavior is perhaps not a direct result of a dysfunction in a discrete mechanism but caused by adaptation in another area. A communicative group is viewed as an organism in the same way as an individual, and unsuccessful intrapersonal compensation creates pressure for interpersonal compensation (as demonstrated in extract 1 above, where Rebecka and David provided compensation for Ferdinand's difficulties).

Emergent Pragmatics provides a holistic approach in that it takes into account both the behavior of the individuals involved in the communication process and the underlying factors that contribute to such behavior. Thereby, Emergent Pragmatics moves beyond the level of description of behavior to providing an explanatory model of the underlying reasons for the behavior. In its aim of explaining pragmatic behavior, Emergent Pragmatics differs from prior interactional models such as Conversation Analysis (CA), which focuses solely on the interaction among the conversation's participants as a collective process in which participants cooperate to produce meaning (Goodwin 2003), not on the individuals. Whereas CA provides a useful tool for highlighting the strategies the impaired individuals and their interlocutors use to compensate for communication problems, Emergent Pragmatics targets both the underlying causes of pragmatic impairment and its behavioral manifestations. In this study, I use the fine-grained inductive approach typical of CA to analyze my data, and I reflect my conversation-analysis-informed discoveries against ideas from Perkins of pragmatic impairment as an emergent phenomenon.

Dementia: problems in understanding, and repair initiators

Dementias are often associated with only memory problems, which, while, of course, the most frequent symptom, do not form the full picture; symptoms displayed in other elements of cognition – for example, in orientation, attention, language, and problem-solving – are required for a diagnosis of dementia. Because dementias are complex conditions that result in neurological symptoms of various types, our point of departure is that both language impairment and other cognitive symptoms affect the communication skills of persons with dementia. In dementia, determining the relationship between a certain pragmatic behavior and an underlying deficit is difficult. Therefore, the model Perkins (2005; 2007; 2008) presents of pragmatics as interactions among linguistic, cognitive, and sensorimotor systems is fruitful for a study of communication involving this group of patients.

This study deals with situations in which the elderly participants' receptive-communication impairment – i.e., problems in hearing and understanding – is revealed. That dementia results in impaired language comprehension has been thoroughly reported in previous literature for Alzheimer's disease (Fromm and Holland 1989; Kempler 1995; Orange and Ryan 2000; Maxim and Bryan 2006), although this may not be the case for other memory disorders. Some studies, such as Grossman et al (1996) show that problems in language comprehension caused by, for example, vascular dementia are reasonably mild. Investigating comprehension problems even in Alzheimer's disease has, however, turned out to be problematic, because these problems are often kept beneath the conversation's surface (cf. Wilkinson 2007). This generates trouble in assessing whether the participants really experience the situation as problematic or whether the analyst is making this interpretation only because of prior knowledge of the situation as involving persons with communication deficits (Hamilton 1994).

To overcome this methodological problem, I have chosen to study situations in which hearing and comprehension trouble are revealed through so-called repair initiators. Repair initiators are turns with which speakers show that they have encountered an interaction problem (as in Ferdinand's turns in extract 1, lines 3 and 11). The repair initiators differ in how much of the previous turn the speaker presents him- or herself as having understood (Schegloff et al. 1977). An open question such as *what* or a meta-comment of the sort *I don't hear that well* targets the whole previous turn as a potential problem, while question words like *who* or *where* focus on a specific unclear element. Taking elderly participants' repair initiators as a point of departure provides an opportunity to focus on such points in conversation, at which the elderly themselves express a problem. This follows the methodological frame of conversation analysis, suggesting that trouble is trouble only if the participants treat it as trouble (Guendouzi and Müller 2006).

Data

The research site is a day care center for Swedish-speaking elderly people in a bilingual area in Finland. The official language at the center is Swedish, and the first language of both the elderly and the carers is Swedish, even if some of the seniors have lived at least at some point in a mostly Finnish-speaking environment. The seniors visited the day care center once or twice a week, for approximately six hours (from 9am to 3pm) at a time. They did not receive long-term institutional care but lived in their own home or with their family.

This study draws on, in total, 30 hours of videotaped data, involving various types of communication situations, such as engaging in small talk at the lunch table and coffee table, playing games (Lindholm 2008; Lindholm and Wray 2012), and reading the day's newspaper as a group activity. Depending on the activity, the number of conversation participants varied between two and six. My initial aim when starting the recordings was to be solely an observer, but taking the position of a bystander turned out to be difficult – in the end, I became more of a participant observer, taking part in the group activities (cf. Antelius 2009, 35). Transcription of the data followed the conventions of conversation analysis (Atkinson and Heritage 1984).

The participants in this study were six elderly persons (David, Ferdinand, Martin, Anna, Irene, and Olga) and three nurses (Giselle, Isabella, and Rebecka). Four of the seniors (Ferdinand, Martin, Anna, and Irene) were diagnosed with Alzheimer's disease and one (David) with vascular dementia. One person, Olga, had no dementia diagnosis. She participated in this group for social stimulation. As a researcher, I sometimes feature in the conversation extracts, where I am denoted as R (for "Researcher"). Since the data were collected in a Swedish-language setting, I have conducted all analyses from the original Swedish data; however, to improve the readability of this article, I have chosen to place the Swedish extracts in an appendix while providing English translations in the body of the piece.

Challenges of group conversations

Following and participating in group conversations can be difficult, especially for persons with language and communication impairment. Bayles and Tomoeda (2007, 196) give the advice to limit the number of conversation partners in order to improve language comprehension, and they suggest that persons with dementia communicate best one on one. There are various reasons for this. First, several participants may compete to take the floor, creating overlapping talk. Situations in which several participants speak simultaneously easily create problems related to hearing and understanding; in fact, Drew (1997, 94) argues that overlapping talk is a "canonical" sequential environment for the occurrence of trouble. This becomes particularly noticeable if one or more participants have communication difficulties. In addition, group conversations with more than three participants readily fragment into several parallel conversations (Egbert 1997). This makes the situation difficult to grasp for elderly people with dementia, since many of them have attention deficits, which render it difficult for them to concentrate on several stimuli at the same time (Collette et al. 1999; Baddeley et al. 2001, Bayles and Tomoeda 2007). Extract 2 shows a case of overlapping talk causing trouble for a person with dementia, related here to illustrate a typical setting in which problems occur:

(2) ROOT VEGETABLE (WINTER VEGETABLE) CASSEROLE

01 Olga:	last time that was good th[at
02 Giselle:	[chicken
03	(0.6)
04 Ferdinand:	((laughs))
05 David:	°or i[f you want me to [take something else°
06 Olga:	[root vegetable casserole
07 Anna:	**[what did you say**
08 Olga:	that last time that was good that root crop
09	casserole

The participants are seated at the coffee table, talking about the day's lunch, when nurse Giselle asks the seniors to choose between two lunch alternatives. Here, Giselle is noting David's choice (*chicken*, line 2) when Olga turns towards Anna and makes a comment on the other lunch option, *last time that was good that* (line 1). So, there are two ongoing, simultaneous conversations: Giselle→David and Olga→Anna. Anna has difficulties in following the conversation, which is exposed by her repair initiator (*what did you say*).

There are various possible reasons for Anna's trouble in fully grasping Olga's utterance: Olga speaks in overlap with Giselle and David, and, further, Olga's utterance is produced in two parts (lines 1 and 6), separated by other participants' contributions. The first part of Olga's utterance (line 1) contains the final demonstrative pronoun *that* (Swedish: *den där*; see appendix), which projects a continuation and clearly marks this utterance as syntactically incomplete. The content-carrying noun (*root vegetable casserole*) is not uttered until later (line 6). Because Anna has Alzheimer's disease, which elicits problems in short-term memory, her understanding may be impaired by the fragmentary nature of Olga's utterance (cf. Bayles and Tomoeda 2007, 197). Previous research (Almor et al. 1999; Orange and Colton-Hudson 1998; Hopper 2001; Bayles 2003; Bayles and Tomoeda 2007) has demonstrated that interpreting pronouns and understanding what these refer to often create difficulties for persons with dementia. Further, people with dementia may have problems in understanding that demonstrative pronouns project – that is, demand – a continuation. Conversations are produced gradually, and persons with dementia may face difficulties in grasping the pieces as parts of the same unit.

Alongside overlapping talk, messages produced simultaneously with other activities are difficult to make out for people with dementia (cf. Bayles and Tomoeda 2007, 172–173 and 182–183). This is illustrated in the next extract, wherein David, nurse Giselle, and the researcher are seated on the terrace. Giselle tells the researcher that she is going to fetch another hat for David, and this creates problems for David, who asks *what was she going to do?*

(3) ANOTHER SUN HAT

01 Giselle:	I'm going to fetch another sun hat for David
02	(.)
03 R:	right
04	(1.8)
05 David:	**what was she going to do**
06	(0.3)
07 R:	fetch another sun hat for [you
08 David:	[*yes* heh heh

There are two potential reasons for David's incapacity to grasp the contents of Giselle's utterance. First, Giselle is walking at the same time as she is producing the utterance in line 1. Thus, a verbal activity overlaps a non-verbal one. Second, Giselle addresses her utterance not to David but to the researcher, so she does not help him to get hold of the conversation by using any specific means.

This is a recurrent pattern in the conversations at the day care center. When the nurses speak to healthy interlocutors, the elderly encounter difficulties in following the conversation. We can think of various possible reasons for the difficulties. For example, when the nurses address healthy co-participants, their speech contains difficult words and/or complex linguistic structures. Further, they do not guide the elderly persons' attention by using such non-verbal resources as gaze and gesture. In the terminology of Emergent Pragmatics (Perkins 2005; 2007; 2008), the interlocutor does not compensate for the communication impairment of the person with dementia, and in such a situation the person with dementia might initiate repair, explicitly expressing the need for compensation. For another example of this pattern, one can consider extract 4, in which Giselle tells a story about her experiences, clearly addressing her talk to a nurse colleague and the researcher.

(4) IT WASN'T THAT BEAUTIFUL
01 Giselle: [...] our chef who then cooked and baked and (.hh)
02 wonderful desserts [...] but anyway
03 I noticed when I tried to put on a
04 skirt for Christmas and (2.0) it wasn't that
05 beautiful then anymore [heh heh
06 David: [a- what came
07 Isabella: [heh heh heh
08 R: [heh heh heh
09 Giselle: I had I had put on so many pounds
10 [when I had had so much dessert
11 David: [yes oh
12 Giselle: our chef on ((X)) had cooked so mu[ch good stuff
13 David: [yes
14 David: w- w- what did you say about the skirt
15 Giselle: it was too tight
16 David: oh ri[ght
17 Isabella: [heh heh heh

David's question *what came* displays that he has problems in understanding Giselle's story. His question is produced at the correct sequential place, immediately after the climactic phrase, *it wasn't that beautiful anymore*, at the point where storyteller Giselle, her colleague Isabella, and the researcher have started laughing. Thus, David apparently identifies the story's climax and his own inability to grasp the culmination of the story. He appears to have a capacity to follow the ongoing conversation but not to comprehend all details. The sequential placement of David's question gives a hint that it probably is targeted at the "punch line" of the story, but it contains no lexical elements connecting it directly to the previous talk. David uses the verb *came*, which does not occur in Giselle's story. In lines 9–10 and 12, Giselle explains the culminating part of the story to David by changing her original, indirect expression (*it wasn't that beautiful then anymore*) into an explicit account (*I had put on so many pounds when I had had so much dessert*). First David responds with brief acknowledgement tokens (lines 11 and 13), but then he poses another question, *what did you say about the skirt*. Thus, the referent *skirt*, which is related to the story's climax, becomes the focus of his question; David wants Giselle to explain this element further. When Giselle tells him that her skirt was too tight, David reacts by saying, *oh right*, showing that this is news to him (see Heritage 1984 on *oh* as a news-receipt marker). Nurse Isabella responds by laughing (line 17), thus showing that she understands Giselle's story to be meant to be funny and entertaining. David's response, on the other hand, does not reveal such an understanding of the meaning of the story as a whole. On the basis of David's behavior in extract 4, we can draw the cautious conclusion that his difficulties probably are related to the indirectness of Giselle's story, either to comprehending her indirect expression containing the punch line (*it wasn't that beautiful anymore*) or to differentiating between a serious and a non-serious mode (Schegloff 1987). We can see Giselle making several attempts to compensate for David's problems, but it remains unclear whether she succeeds.

In the extract above, David used a repair initiator to enter the conversation. By explicitly expressing his inability to follow the conversation, David makes an attempt to initiate compensation to "restore balance to a dysfunctional system" (Perkins 2007, 55). The compensatory behavior is carried out by Giselle in her pursuits of repeating and rephrasing the story's climax. Even if David's repair initiator shows comprehension problems in need of compensation, it also demonstrates his assumption that Giselle has said something worth following up, even at the expense of revealing a failure to understand. David's eagerness to become more actively involved in the interaction, to exchange the participatory role of a bystander and overhearer for that of a ratified recipient (Goffman 1981), indicates traces of intact pragmatics, if we define pragmatics as choices motivated by a need to communicate with other people (Perkins 2007, 60). The next extract provides another example of this behavior.

(5) BLEACHING TEETH
01 Giselle: I have a sister who lives in Stockholm […]
02 now I talked to her on Midsummer and she
03 had now decided that she'll bleach
04 her teeth
05 (1.0)
06 R: *(hh)*
07 (0.5)
08 Isabella: *hh*
09 (1.3)
10 David: ((clears throat)) she'll what ((turns towards Giselle))
11 Giselle: she'll bleach her teeth
12 (0.3)
13 David: *oh*
14 (0.7) ((Giselle shakes her head, looks at Isabella))
15 R: *(h)*
16 (0.5)
17 Isabella: I had a buddy who did who bought just
18 through some TV shop or something

When talking about her sister, Giselle is facing Isabella, gazing at her and apparently treating her as the primary recipient of the utterance (Lerner 2003). Both Isabella and the researcher, who is seated on the other side of the table, start laughing. The healthy co-participants react to Giselle's utterance as a laughing matter, whereas David asks, *she'll what* and turns towards Giselle. He uses both verbal and non-verbal means to show his willingness to engage in an information exchange in which he was not addressed as the primary recipient. As her answer, Giselle repeats the most important content of her previous utterance, *she'll bleach her teeth* (line 11), simultaneously turning towards David, who is seated at her right side.

David's reaction to Giselle's repair turn is brief. He only says, *oh*, smiles, and returns to his prior activity of eating soup. Giselle does not pay further attention to David; instead, she focuses non-verbally on Isabella, smiling and looking at her. We can see Giselle treating David's *oh* as a sufficient response, not engaging in further explanations of the matter of bleaching one's teeth. In cases of this kind, wherein the topic is related to the nurses or the physical environment and in which the people with dementia were not originally addressed as the primary recipients, the nurses are prepared to treat a single news-receipt token as a sufficient response, not as an indication of pragmatic impairment in need of compensation (Lindholm forthcoming). Thus, the potential problem is allowed to "pass" (Firth 1996). The nurses do not ensure the elderly participants' understanding; they are satisfied with maintaining a comfortable atmosphere of small talk.

Varying competence

The varying linguistic and communication skills of the elderly are another element causing communication challenges at the day care center. This variation means that they differ in their opportunities to participate in conversation. The seniors who participated in this study are people living at home or with their families – there are no elderly people with severe memory disturbances in this group. Nonetheless, even mild and moderate memory problems affect communication skills. Besides the memory problems, other factors affect interaction: for example, Ferdinand has a hearing impairment. Olga, in contrast, has no memory problems or other traits weakening her conversation skills. The differences in skills of the participants become visible in all conversations, but they are especially prominent in certain therapeutic activities, such as games.

The following analysis focuses on two situations in which the participants are playing games. My analysis focuses on how Anna (with moderate Alzheimer's disease), Ferdinand (with mild Alzheimer's disease and hearing impairment), and Olga (with no linguistic or cognitive difficulties) have differing points of departure when participating in this activity. In extract 6, Giselle, Ferdinand, Olga, and Anna are playing a therapeutic game in which Giselle reads descriptions aloud and the elderly participants have the task of recognizing a certain word on the basis of the description. The word searched for in the present example is "flogging." Giselle describes this word by saying that she is looking for *another word for spanking and beating*.

(6) ANOTHER WORD FOR SPANKING AND BEATING

01 Giselle:	another word for spanking (0.2) and beating
02	(0.5)
03 Olga:	flogging
04	(0.3)
05 Giselle:	flogging
06 Ferdinand:	**for what:**
07 Olga:	°mh°
08	(0.5)
09 Giselle:	another word for spanking (0.2) and beating
10	(2.5)
11 Ferdinand:	**now I don't catch it your s[po-**
12 Giselle:	[ANOTHER WORD
13	[FOR BEATING

14 Ferdinand:	[yes
15	(0.5)
16 Giselle:	one b- does m: one beats someone
17	(1.0)
18 Giselle:	FLOGGING
19	(0.4)
20 Giselle:	have you heard of FL[OGGING
21 Ferdinand:	[yes yes
22 Ferdinand:	yes yes
23 Giselle:	yes
24	(0.2)
25 Ferdinand:	**beating I didn't catch it oh right**

After a short pause, Olga produces the correct answer (line 3), which is repeated by Giselle. Ferdinand, on the other hand, responds by asking, *for what* Ferdinand thus shows that he heard the preposition *for* and something else, which is targeted as the problem. Giselle, however, repeats the whole previous turn, not only the element targeted by Ferdinand as troublesome. This repair turn, though, does not help Ferdinand, who expresses his hearing problem again, *now I don't catch it*. Giselle takes another repair turn (lines 12–13), in which she repeats the first part of her trouble turn, here with a louder voice, also adding the description *one beats someone* (line 16). When there is no response to this repeated repair turn, Giselle utters the correct answer, *flogging*, at higher volume (line 18). Still, it is not until she poses another question – *have you heard of flogging* – that Ferdinand answers: his acknowledgement tokens in lines 21 and 22 and the elaborated response in line 25 demonstrate that he has grasped the item sought.

We can see how Olga, who has no communication difficulties, is capable of providing the correct answer after only a short time, whereas Ferdinand is able to demonstrate recognition of the searched-for answer only after a long and complicated repair sequence. Both Ferdinand's hearing impairment and the slowness in his language processing caused by Alzheimer's disease have potential to affect his problems: Ferdinand's answer in line 25 does not comment on the expression *flogging* used in Giselle's previous turn, but he uses *beating* from lines 1, 9, and 13. It is possible that Ferdinand's understanding is based not on the prior turn but on the first part of the sequence – language processing just takes him a long time. We cannot be absolutely sure whether the reasons for Ferdinand's difficulties lie in the cognitive or the sensory area or with a combination of the two, but under the Emergent Pragmatics model, this is not so important to know: "pragmatics is not exclusively linked to any single cognitive process, but typically draws on multiple areas of cognition"

(Perkins 2007, 5). What does become evident in the interaction is Giselle's success in compensating for his problems, whatever their causes may be.

In some situations, several participants exhibit delayed reactions to an initiative. This is the case in the next extract.

(7) THE RED FLOWER OF LOVE

01 Giselle:	the red flower of love
02	(0.3)
03 Giselle:	yes that is a,
04 Anna:	rose
05 Giselle:	rose good An[na
06 Anna:	**[see I knew <u>some</u>[thing**
07 Giselle:	[oh yes
08 Anna:	**but one doesn't make it you're too fast**
09 Giselle:	are we <u>fast</u> I'll take it slow[e-
10 Anna:	[no:
11 Giselle:	heh [heh heh
12 Anna:	[(-) you just go on
13	(1.7)
14 Ferdinand:	**was it rose**
15 Giselle:	it was rose
16 Ferdinand:	rose oh

Giselle, Olga, Anna, and Ferdinand are playing a bingo game that uses flowers instead of numbers. Giselle is in charge of the game, and she reads a description of a flower. The other participants guess which flower it is from the description. Each player has a bingo card with pictures of flowers. If this card has a picture of the flower Giselle has described, the player puts a marker on the card. In this game, the elderly practice two skills: working out the name of the correct flower on the basis of a description and recognizing that flower in a picture. Games of this kind do not necessarily work well if the participants' skill levels span a wide range, which is the case in this conversation.

In the extract, nurse Giselle solves this problem by providing Anna with an opportunity to participate. First, she prompts an answer by saying, *yes that is a…* and directing her gaze at Anna. Here, Giselle creates a slot for Anna to fill in, apparently compensating for Anna's problems in language and attention. Anna succeeds in providing the correct response. Still, she seems aware of her limitations. She responds to the other's compliments by saying, *see I knew something* and commenting on the others' fast reactions (line 8). Thus Anna expresses explicitly that the pace of the conversation is unsuitable for her. That Alzheimer's disease causes slowness in processing of information, which, in turn, creates communication difficulties, is well-known in the literature (cf. Bayles 2003). Still, Anna's comments show that she, in spite of her difficulties, is capable of observing, drawing conclusions, and analyzing her participation and her opportunities in this conversation. In the terminology of Emergent Pragmatics, Anna is pragmatically competent and incompetent at the same time: pragmatically compromised since there is a need for compensating behavior on the part of the interlocutors but simultaneously demonstrating pragmatic skills in her capacity to make her communication needs explicit to those interlocutors (Perkins 2007, 56).

Not only Anna but also Ferdinand has problems in following the rapidly proceeding conversation. Even though Anna produced the correct response, *rose*, in line 4, and Giselle repeated it in line 5, Ferdinand asks about it in line 14. Ferdinand's question implies a return to the agenda: Anna's and Giselle's comments (lines 6–12) form a side sequence, which cuts off the current topic. Ferdinand uses the past tense – ***was** it rose* – when he asks about the correct answer. His usage of the past tense shows that his question targets something discussed a while ago; the past tense expresses a distance between the speaker and the matter asked about. The past tense further demonstrates that this is a clarification question, which the speaker uses to ensure that his hearing or understanding is correct. There are at least two possible reasons for the distance between the problem source and Ferdinand's question: Ferdinand's slow language processing and the competition for the floor; Ferdinand simply does not get the opportunity to pose his question earlier. Both of these factors are emphasized in group situations.

Paradoxically, the fact that the day care center provides various types of pastimes and therapeutic activities can cause the participants problems. Some pastimes cause trouble – for example, because they introduce abstract topics – and the elderly participants cannot use the physical context to get help in interpreting these topics. Let us consider how a game using proverbs causes trouble for Irene (who has an Alzheimer's diagnosis). These games are used at the day care center as a memory- and language-stimulating activity. The game material consists of a pack of cards with fixed Swedish-language sayings. In the game, a nurse reads the first part of a proverb aloud, creating a slot that the care recipients are intended to fill in by producing the second part. The nurse reads the relevant card to verify whether the response provided is correct. Sometimes the nurse also refers to the text on the cards as an external source of authority, stating the correct answer. Extract 8 deals with the saying "Rome wasn't built in a day," whose first part Giselle reads aloud in line 1 (See Lindholm and Wray 2012 for another analysis of this example). In this situation, Giselle is in charge of the game, and Irene and Martin are playing. Martin, in contrast, does not participate actively in the game at this point.

(8) ROME WASN'T BUILT IN A DAY

01 Giselle:	Rome wasn't built
02	(2.1)
03 Irene:	**why not**
04	(0.3)
05 Giselle:	in a day
06	(0.2)
07 Irene:	**heh heh heh (0.2) why not**
08	(0.6)
09 Giselle:	y'know it's big [Rome the city is huge
10 Irene:	[heh heh heh
11	(0.5)
12 Giselle:	small children small worries,

Giselle's utterance *Rome wasn't built* is followed by a lengthy pause. Previous research has suggested that pauses occurring after questions can point to two types of problems in conversations involving elderly people with dementia. Either the person with dementia did not comprehend the prior turn or he or she needs more time to process the information provided (Perkins et al. 1998). Irene's question *why not* cannot clearly be categorized as an expression of either problem type. This question could indicate a failure to understand Giselle's previous turn, but another interpretation is that Irene is making a joke, signaling a playful attitude towards the game the group is playing.

It is impossible to determine the speaker's intentions on the basis of what happens in this sequence. We must stick to considering how nurse Giselle reacts to Irene's response. Giselle does not comment on Irene's reply. Instead, she continues to produce the searched-for second part, *in a day* (line 5), perhaps intending to increase Irene's understanding. Irene's next contributions, however, are laughter and a repeated *why* question (line 7). She could be simply continuing with her joke. But it is just as likely that she has not been able to make anything of the proverb completion, failing to understand the utterances in lines 1 and 5 to be parts of the same proverb unit and therefore not gaining increased understanding. Giselle's reaction indicates that she believes this is indeed the case, because she starts explaining why it would be impossible to build such a big city in a day. Still Irene responds with only laughter, not revealing whether she has understood Giselle's explanation (Lindholm 2008). When Giselle continues to the next proverb, in line 12, it is unclear whether Irene has understood anything of the discussion about Rome.

While the sequence analyzed in extract 8 is a dialogue between Giselle and Irene, the problem perceived by Irene might be related to the group setting. It seems unclear whether Irene is aware of the ongoing activity and its rules. One possible reason for this lies in how the activity was introduced in the group setting. When the game started, nobody explained what was going on: Giselle just obtained the game material and referred to it implicitly, by saying, "Here we have this stuff, which Martin is really good at." My assumption is that Giselle's way of introducing the activity, implicitly and addressing only Martin as a recipient, might have influenced Irene's comprehension problems. Irene would have needed another type of introduction than Martin did if she were to be capable of fully attending to the game. This is reminiscent of the examples in which healthy participants spoke to one another and did not compensate for the impairment of other participants; Giselle has solely targeted Martin as a recipient, and, in so doing, she fails to compensate for Irene's difficulties.

Games of various types are activities of a kind that causes the elderly problems, for example, stemming from the frequent topic changes. Further, the topics are abstract and unrelated to the current physical context. The interaction trouble could be remedied if the activity were carefully framed and explained through meta-comments – e.g., if the speaker explicitly announces his or her aim to change the topic (Orange 2001, 239).

Opportunities for group conversations

We have seen that communication and interaction challenges can build up in the group setting at the day care center. The participants can, however, apply certain practices to deal with these challenges. This is the topic of the next section.

The elderly helping each other

As illustrated above, the group situations analyzed here are heterogeneous, involving elderly people with varying competencies. Nonetheless, the group is always a resource, with performance sometimes being further assisted through active interventions from the person in charge of the group, sometimes by interaction between the group's participants. In the following interaction, we can see Olga helping Anna to follow the conversation:

(9) WHAT WAS HER NAME

01 Ferdinand:	a big farm, (0.6) Park Farm
02	(0.8)
03 Ferdinand:	(there) (to-)
04	(2.8)
05 Ferdinand:	(bring-) my my youth so
06	(2.0)
07 Ferdinand:	so it was owned owned by a (0.6) Mrs Wilson (0.2)
08	(mt) (0.8) her husband died
09	(1.7)
10 Anna:	**what did you say [her name was]**
11 Ferdinand:	[and his spouse] wife to[ok his place
12 Olga:	[Wilson
13 Ferdinand:	it was [now
14 Anna:	[(Wilson)

Ferdinand is starting to tell a story from his childhood, about a farm and the people who owned and took care of this farm. Ferdinand is the main speaker, and Giselle, Olga, and Anna are listening. The participants are seated on two couches. In line 10, Anna poses a question about the name of the lady Ferdinand was referring to. Olga, who is seated next to Anna, provides the name Anna asked about, turning towards Anna while answering (line 12). Next, Anna repeats the searched-for element (line 14), showing that repair was successful. Olga responds to Anna's repair turn. According to Egbert (1997), this is a special feature of group conversations: someone other than the one who uttered the problem turn can provide repair. During conversations at the day care center, Olga recurrently teams up with Anna to support her in various situations, as in extract 2, in which Olga provided hints about preferable lunch dishes. Therefore, we can note as a feature of this particular group that Olga has taken on the responsibility of compensating for Anna's difficulties. Over time, certain patterns of interpersonal compensation become inherent features of the group dynamics.

Sometimes Olga selects on her own initiative to provide support, as in the previous extract, but on other occasions, Anna explicitly addresses Olga when asking for help. This happens in the next extract, wherein Anna poses a question directly to Olga. Her behavior illustrates another feature typical of repair in group settings: a participant can initiate repair by expressing a problem in hearing or understanding through addressing of someone else, not the one who produced the problem turn.

(10) WHAT IS HE TALKING ABOUT
01 Anna: but what is the name of this place
02 (0.7)
03 Olga: it belongs to Helsinki
04 (0.4)
05 Anna: oh
06 (3.7)
07 Anna: right
08 (5.9)
09 David: I think I have (1.3) several of my (1.1) children and
10 grandchildren (0.5) here in (0.9) this (-)
11 (0.3)
12 Olga: mm:
13 (2.5)
14 Anna: what do you think he is talking about
15 (3.7)
16 Olga: (mm:)
17 (0.8)
18 Anna: it's not that importan[t
19 Olga: [no:

The elderly people are seated on the terrace of the day care center and talking about the name of the place where they are. Olga responds to Anna's and David's questions by uttering the name of the town where they are situated at the moment. In lines 9–10, David brings up a new topic. His utterance is somewhat difficult to follow, and it might be a case of confabulation – i.e., a false memory, or a pathological report of events that never happened (Tallberg 2001). David typically makes these statements about the here and now, somehow expressing that he is confusing times and places (Lindholm 2011). Certain features of the physical surroundings appear to prompt comments of this kind. My analysis of the elements in David's utterances in lines 9 and 10 as confabulative is tentative and related more to David's way of speaking than to the contents of his utterances; it is, of course, possible that several of his children and grandchildren live in Helsinki. His way of speaking is, however, different than otherwise: he speaks more slowly, with a lower voice, and turns inwards, not actively inviting feedback from the others (Tallberg 2001). Further, his speech is fragmented and contains elements expressing uncertainty, such as the modal verb phrase *I think*. It is on the basis of these features that I have drawn the conclusion that David is confabulating rather than telling the truth about his family.

The other elderly people frequently encounter problems in understanding David when he produces possible confabulations. Here, nobody responds to David's remark about his children and grandchildren. Instead Anna asks Olga for help; she fails to make anything of David's utterance and turns to Olga to get support. Olga, however, responds with only the minimal acknowledgement token *mm*. As a result of this, Anna states, *it's not that important*. By stating an explicit judgment of the topic as not being worth pursuing, Anna could be trying to save face. She has made an attempt to enter the current conversation but has failed. When she realizes that she is incapable of following the conversation, she decides that it is not important for her, so that she won't mind not following it. Simultaneously, Anna appears to be making an excuse for Olga's inability to help her. As I have mentioned above, Olga and Anna usually team up and Olga has taken on the responsibility of helping Anna in varying possibly problematic situations. But here, even when Anna asks Olga for help, Olga is incapable of providing that help. In this situation, neither Olga nor Anna knows what David is talking about, which renders Olga incapable of compensating for Anna's problems.

It is not only a person with no communication problems who can be a resource and help the others. Sometimes elderly people with dementia help each other in group situations. In extract 11, the extract previously analyzed as extract 1 in the introductory section of the paper, nurse Rebecka's question causes Ferdinand problems, which is revealed in line 3.

(11) FIRE WARDEN
01 Rebecka: did you always have a fire warden someone
02 (0.2)
03 Ferdinand: what
04 (0.2)
05 Rebecka: did you always have someone who sat as a fire warden
06 (0.9)
07 David: <fire warden>
08 (1.6)
09 Rebecka: in [ta- in the tent
10 David: [about that
11 Ferdinand: [I don't hear that well
12 (about [that)
13 Rebecka: [did you always have someone who sat
14 as a fire warden in the tent
15 (1.0)
16 David: did someone sit as a <fire warden>
17 Ferdinand: yes yesyes yesyes (.h) *kipinäkalle*
18 Rebecka: oh heh heh heh

Ferdinand's *what* starts a sequence in which David and Rebecka support each other to help Ferdinand grasp the message. Rebecka's first repair turn (line 5) carries the same content as the previous turn, but there is a change in word order. The order is changed to correspond to the written-language grammar. This may be a result of a presupposition that the change would make the message easier to catch. David's repair strategy is different – he concentrates on repeating the most important element of Rebecka's problem turn, *fire warden*, at a slower pace. In doing so, he seems to have interpreted Ferdinand's repair initiator as targeting a certain element.

When Ferdinand makes a second expression of his hearing problems (line 11), Rebecka repeats her previous question again (lines 13–14), and David also formulates his repair turn as a question – *did someone sit as a fire warden* – though exaggerating the articulation of "fire warden." Here Ferdinand finally perceives what the others are talking about and responds by providing the element *kipinäkalle* in Finnish. As in extract 6, above, it is impossible to say whether Ferdinand gains his new understanding as a result of only the previous repair turn or from the combined effect of several repair turns. We can, however, note that Ferdinand apparently is helped by the combination of slower talk and repetitions of previous turns; the compensations provided by several co-participants are successful. Ferdinand is demonstrating both pragmatic ability and disability; his choice to ask "What?" is motivated by his wish to communicate with Rebecka, but he requires input from the interlocutors in order to succeed.

In the previous extract, David participated actively in designing the repair turns. However, his ability to function in group situations is reasonably well preserved, so it is perhaps unsurprising that he is capable of customizing his turn to resolve a problematic situation. In other situations, even Anna, who otherwise is passive in group contexts, helps other participants. This is illustrated in the next extract, with two parallel ongoing conversations. Nurses Giselle and Isabella are setting the table, simultaneously talking about the food (the turns in lines 3, 6, and 9 belong to a conversation between the nurses). Ferdinand, David, and Anna are seated at the lunch table, and Ferdinand introduces a new topic by making a comment about today's weather. David's question *what did you say* is targeted at Ferdinand's previous turn, not at Giselle's turn in line 3.

(12) IT'S A BEAUTIFUL DAY TODAY

01 Ferdinand:	it's a beautiful day today?
02	(1.2)
03 Giselle:	is this now (sauce)
04	(.)
05 David:	**<u>what</u> [did you say**

06 Giselle: [I don't know
07 (2.0)
08 Anna: that it's a [beautiful [day (today)
09 Isabella: [mm
10 Ferdinand: [it's a beautiful
12 day to[day
13 David: [beautiful day today yes

Anna provides an answer to David's question by repeating Ferdinand's original turn (line 8). Her turn is not, however, pure repetition, since she adds the turn-initial conjunction *that*, signaling that she is repeating a turn produced by another speaker. Ferdinand repeats his original question also, in overlap with Anna, and in line 13 we can see David uttering *beautiful day today yes*, thus expressing his awareness of the contents of the previous turns. We must be careful in our interpretation of this sequence – we cannot know with certainty how exactly David solved the problem. The repetition of previous turns seems, nevertheless, to have helped David gain understanding, and the previous extract provides an illustration of how all of the elderly people in the setting participate to compensate for David's difficulties.

The carers supporting the elderly

One of the greatest challenges in group conversations involves encouraging everyone to participate actively and supporting this, especially in situations wherein some of the participants are likely to withdraw from the conversation on account of communication difficulties. At the day care center, the nurses sometimes invite the elderly to participate by addressing questions and comments explicitly to certain people. The next extract provides another illustration of this phenomenon. It is not a coincidence that two of these cases (extracts 7 and 13) illustrate how Giselle provides Anna with support during a game situation. Anna has problems in following the game, and she remains passive during this activity, so this is why Giselle works actively to engage Anna in the conversation, compensating for Anna's difficulties.

(13) AQUAVIT
01 Giselle: what's [that
02 Anna: [I was about to say aquavit
03 Olga: that's aster th[en
04 Anna: [but it did[n't work
05 Giselle: [yes it's aster right
06 Olga: yes

07 Giselle:	**what were you thinking of Anna (.hh) (0.2) aquavit?**
08	(0.2)
09 Anna:	yes
10 Giselle:	[[heh heh[heh
11 Isabella:	[[heh heh[heh
12 Anna:	[*we're talking about* (0.2) *other things here*
13 R:	heh heh heh ((quietly))

The group is playing the same bingo game as in extract 7. Both Olga and Ferdinand have made the guess that the searched-for flower is the amaryllis. Giselle, though, insinuates that their suggestions are wrong, and Olga follows by providing the correct answer, *aster*, in line 3. Before that, Anna, however, has turned towards Olga and said, *I was about to say aquavit* (line 2). Giselle reacts first by confirming Olga's answer (line 5), after which she makes a comment on Anna's playful suggestion (line 7). Giselle uses a question format in *what were you thinking of Anna, aquavit* whose format could refer to a problem in hearing or understanding. Giselle's question is, however, a combination of a general "what" question and a suggested candidate answer, *aquavit* (cf. Linell et al. 2003). Since the focus of the questions is internally narrowed down, Anna's task is to confirm or reject the candidate answer in her response. She provides a confirming response in line 9, and everyone except Ferdinand starts laughing.

Here nurse Giselle succeeds in taking a risk. The risk has to do with her interpretation of Anna's turn in line 2. Anna's turn is complex, since it may refer either to Anna's incapacity of providing the searched-for response or to her playful attitude towards the ongoing activity (cf. the analysis of extract 8, line 3). Anna's use of the past tense in line 2, *I was about to* and her continuation in line 4, *but it didn't work*, however, provide keys to interpreting the meaning of line 2. Here Anna expresses a certain competence: she had considered giving the wrong answer, but she realized that it was wrong. Still, it remains a fact that Anna failed to provide the correct answer. Accordingly, nurse Giselle takes a risk when she focuses on the wrong answer. This had potential to be a face-threatening situation, and some guidelines for dementia communication stress that the healthy co-participant should avoid concentrating on wrong answers. But here the risk-taking is successful: the participants laugh together at Anna's alternative answer, and Giselle manages to engage Anna in the conversation of the whole group.

How did Giselle dare to focus on an incorrect answer, given that doing so might have been a face-threatening activity? Continuity is the key to high-quality care of people with dementia; it is most important that the personnel know the elderly people, their biography, and their traits. As the nurse in charge of the day care center, Giselle knows that Anna appreciates humor and irony, and Anna often makes ironic comments about herself and her behavior. Because Giselle knows this about Anna, she dares to behave in a manner that in another context could have caused an embarrassing situation or perhaps conversation breakdown. Instead, the extract ends with common laughter – the nurses and Anna are laughing together. This extract provides another detail-level illustration of interpersonal compensation: patterns of providing successful interpersonal compensation may develop within groups over time (see extract 9).

Conclusions

The group situations at the day care center easily create interactional challenges. The problems are often caused simply by the fact that there are more than two participants in the conversations, which causes overlapping talk and parallel conversations. Because of the diverse tasks of the health-care personnel, the nurses often have to perform other activities simultaneously while talking to the elderly, and this easily results in hearing and comprehension problems. Of course, it is impossible to avoid these situations completely, but on some occasions the interaction can be improved if the nurses become aware of this. If the nurse, for example, were to stop while talking to the elderly person, the result would probably be better than that of walking from one place to another while talking at the same time, and it would not necessarily require any more time in the end.

Additional challenges are caused by the participants' varying capabilities of functioning in group situations. An ideal group would consist of people with the same abilities and disabilities, but it is not always possible to form homogenous groups. If the group is heterogeneous, the group leader needs to pay attention to the participants as individually as possible – for example, to make it easy for a certain participant to provide a response. Heterogeneous groups require great contributions from the group leader yet still do not acknowledge the individuals' needs as well as more homogenous groups do.

Certain therapeutic activities used at the day care center give rise to problems readily, because they underline the differences in skills and needs of the participants. An elderly person who has difficulties in following the activities may frequently withdraw from the interaction. Planning the activities carefully is important. In the analysis of extract 8, I mentioned that the nurse introduced the proverbs game indirectly, without repeating the rules. When the participants are people with memory disturbances, it would be justifiable to go over the rules every time a new game is started – one cannot assume that the participants are going to remember the rules introduced in a previous game session. Also, even if the rules are introduced at the beginning of the game, repeating them during the game is probably necessary when players display memory problems. The proverbs game is a challenging activity for elderly people with memory problems, for various reasons (Lindholm and Wray 2012). Because of this, the nurses have an important role, as the gatekeepers for this activity. If the game does not work out, it could damage the self-esteem of the seniors instead of activating them, in turn causing frustration and anxiety. Therefore, the nurses need to follow the participants' reactions, so as to evaluate whether they are enjoying the game or, instead, it is causing them problems. In addition, the game material could be used in a more relaxed manner, if the nurses were to abandon the single-minded pursuit of correct responses and instead use the material to stimulate conversation. Obviously, memory-training activities in their own right have potential to trigger joint sequences of laughter, word play, and remembering together, but the nurses should not be too governed by the institutional agenda of keeping the game going.

Regardless of these challenges, the group is always a potential resource – the individual's performance is sometimes aided through active interventions (such as questions and comments addressed explicitly to certain persons) from the nurse in charge of the group (extracts 7 and 13), sometimes via interaction between elderly participants (extracts 9 and 11). If we follow the line of thought of Perkins (2007), the group is a domain wherein linguistic and cognitive resources become common property. And, of course, impairment within one domain (for example, of one individual) can generate problems both within that domain itself and across domains. If we apply this thought to the group setting analyzed in this study, we can say that the more participants there are in the interaction, the more opportunities are created for individual impairments to affect group situations. On the other hand, the group setting also involves many domains in which the problems can be solved. Both healthy and impaired interlocutors engage in mutual work to compensate for the impairments within the individuals. While much of the previous research has suggested that continuity over time is part of high-quality care (van der Steen 2012: 871), this study provides a more detailed picture of how continuity may result in successful compensation behavior in various communication situations (extracts 9 and 13). Traditionally, research has focused on continuity with respect to the carers involved, but the conversations at the day care center demonstrate the equally important role of stable group composition – over time, the elderly participants may take responsibility for compensating for each other's challenges, with this becoming an established pattern in the group interaction.

Transcription symbols

[	beginning of overlap
]	the point at which overlapping utterances stop overlapping
(0.6)	interval in the stream of conversation, given in tenths of a second
(.)	micropause, less than 0.2 seconds
,	continuing intonation
<u>oh</u>	emphasis
°oh°	quiet/muted speech
oh:	prolongation of a sound
#oh#	creaky voice
((laughs))	laughter
(heh)	one laughter particle
oh	"smiling" voice
(.h)	inhalation
(h), (hh)	exhalation
(( ))	description of the speech or of non-verbal activity

References

Almor, Amit, Daniel Kempler, Maryellen C. MacDonald, Elaine S. Andersen, and Lorraine K. Tyler. 1999. "Why Do Alzheimer Patients Have Difficulty with Pronouns? Working Memory, Semantics, and Reference in Comprehension and Production in Alzheimer's Disease." *Brain and Language* 67 (3): 202–227.

Antelius, Eleonor. 2009. *Different Voices – Different Stories: Communication, Identity and Meaning Among People with Acquired Brain Damage*. Linköping, Sweden: Linköping University Press.

Atkinson, Maxwell and John Heritage (Eds.). 1984. *Structures of Social Action: Studies in Conversation Analysis*. Cambridge, UK: Cambridge University Press.

Baddeley, Alan D., Hilary A. Baddeley, Romola S. Bucks, and Gordon K. Wilcock. 2001. "Attentional Control in Alzheimer's Disease." *Brain* 124 (8): 1492–1508.

Bayles, Kathryn A. 2003. "Effects of Working Memory Deficits on the Communicative Functioning of Alzheimer's Dementia Patients." *Journal of Communication Disorders* 36 (3): 209–219.

Bayles, Kathryn A. and Cheryl K. Tomoeda. 2007. *Cognitive-Communication Disorders of Dementia*. San Diego: Plural Publishing.

Collette, Fabienne, Martial van der Linden, Eric Salmon, and Sophie Bechet. 1999. "Phonological Loop and Central Executive Functioning in Alzheimer's Disease." *Neuropsychologia* 37 (8): 905–918.

Drew, Paul. 1997. "'Open' Class Repair Initiators in Response to Sequential Sources of Trouble in Conversation." *Journal of Pragmatics* 28 (1): 69−101.

Egbert, Maria M. 1997. "Some Interactional Achievements of Other-initiated Repair in Multiperson Conversation." *Journal of Pragmatics* 27 (5): 611−634.

Firth, Alan. 1996. "The Discursive Accomplishment of Normality: On 'Lingua Franca' English and Conversation Analysis. *Journal of Pragmatics* 26 (2): 237−259.

Fromm, Davida and Audrey L. Holland. 1989. "Functional Communication in Alzheimer's Disease." *Journal of Speech and Hearing Disorders* 54 (4): 535−540.

Goffman, Erving. 1981. *Forms of Talk*. New York: Pantheon Books.

Goodwin, Charles. 2003. "Introduction." In Charles Goodwin (Ed.) *Conversation and Brain Damage*. Oxford, UK: Oxford University Press: 3−20.

Grossman, Murray, Mark D'Esposito, Elizabeth Hughes, Kris Onishi, Nadia Biassou, Tammy White-Devine, and Keith M. Robinson. 1996. "Language Comprehension Problems in Alzheimer's Disease, Multi-Infarct Dementia, and Frontotemporal Degeneration." *Neurology* 47 (1): 183−189.

Guendouzi, Jacqueline and Nicole Müller. 2006. *Approaches to Discourse in Dementia*. New Jersey/London: Lawrence Erlbaum.

Hamilton, Heidi E. 1994. "Requests for Clarification As Evidence of Pragmatic Comprehension Difficulty: The Case of Alzheimer's Disease." In Ronald L. Bloom, Loraine K. Obler, Susan De Santi, and Jonathan S. Ehrlich (Eds.) *Discourse Analysis and Applications: Studies in Adult Clinical Populations*. Hillsdale, NJ: Lawrence Erlbaum: 185−199.

Heritage, John. 1984. "A Change-of-State Token and Aspects of Its Sequential Placement." In Maxwell Atkinson and John Heritage (Eds.) *Structures of Social Action: Studies in Conversation Analysis*. Cambridge, UK: Cambridge University Press: 299–345.

Hopper, Tammy. 2001. "Indirect Interventions to Facilitate Communication in Alzheimer's Disease." *Seminars in Speech and Language* 22 (4): 305–315.

Kempler, Daniel. 1995. "Language Changes in Dementia of the Alzheimer's Type." In Rosemary Lubinski, Joseph B. Orange, Donald Henderson, and Nancy Stecker (Eds.) *Dementia and Communication.* San Diego / London: Singular Publishing Group: 98−114.

Lerner, Gene H. 2003. "Selecting Next Speaker: The Context-Sensitive Operation of a Context-Free Organization." *Language in Society* 32 (2): 177−201.

Lindholm, Camilla. 2008. "Laughter, Communication Problems and Dementia." *Communication and Medicine* 5 (1): 3−14.

Lindholm, Camilla. 2011. "Responsibility and Narrativity in Conversation – the Case of Confabulations" (paper presented at the 12th International Pragmatics Conference, Manchester, July 8).

—. 2012. "Vuorovaikutuksen haasteita ja mahdollisuuksia – tapaustutkimus muistisairaiden päivätoiminnasta" ["Challenges and Opportunities of Interaction – a Case Study from a Day Care Center"] In Leealaura Leskelä and Camilla Lindholm (Eds.) *Haavoittuva keskustelu. Keskustelunanalyyttisia tutkimuksia kielellisesti epäsymmetrisestä vuorovaikutuksesta* [*Vulnerable Conversation: Conversation Analytic Studies of Linguistically Asymmetric Interaction*]. Helsinki: Opike: 57−98.

—. Forthcoming. "Comprehension in Interaction – Communication at a Day-Care Center." In Jens Brockmeier, Lars-Christer Hydén, and Hilde Lindemann (Eds.) *Beyond Loss: Dementia, Identity, Personhood.* Oxford, UK: Oxford University Press.

Lindholm, Camilla and Alison Wray. 2012. "Proverbs and Formulaic Sequences in the Language of Elderly People with Dementia." *Dementia* 10 (4): 603−623.

Linell, Per, Johan Hofvendahl, and Camilla Lindholm. 2003. "Multi-Unit Questions in Institutional Interactions: Sequential Organizations and Communicative Functions." *Text* 23 (4): 539−571.

Maxim, Jane and Karen Bryan. 2006. "Language, Communication and Cognition in the Dementias." In Karen Bryan and Jane Maxim (Eds.) *Communication Disability in the Dementias.* London: Whurr Publishers: 73–124.

Orange, Joseph B. 2001. "Family Caregivers, Communication and Alzheimer's Disease." In Mary Lee Hummert and Jon F. Nussbaum (Eds.) *Aging, Communication and Health.* Mahwah, NJ: Lawrence Erlbaum: 225−248.

Orange, Joseph B. and Angela Colton-Hudson. 1998. "Enhancing Communication in Dementia of the Alzheimer's Type." *Topics in Geriatric Rehabilitation* 14 (2): 56–75.

Orange, Joseph B. and Ellen Bouchard Ryan. 2000. "Alzheimer's Disease and Other Dementias: Implications for Physician Communication." *Clinics in Geriatric Medicine* 16 (1): 153–167.

Perkins, Lisa, Anne Whitworth, and Ruth Lesser. 1998. "Conversing in Dementia: A Conversation Analytic Approach." *Journal of Neurolinguistics* 11 (1–2): 33–53.

Perkins, Michael. 2005. "Pragmatic Ability and Disability As Emergent Phenomena." *Clinical Linguistics and Phonetics* 19(5): 367–377.

—. 2007. *Pragmatic Impairment*. Cambridge, UK: Cambridge University Press.

—. 2008. "Pragmatic Impairment As an Emergent Phenomenon." In Martin J. Ball, Michael R. Perkins, Nicole Müller, and Sara Howard (Eds.) *The Handbook of Clinical Linguistics*. Oxford, UK: Blackwell: 79–91.

Schegloff, Emanuel A. 1987. "Some Sources of Misunderstanding in Talk-in-Interaction." *Linguistics* 25 (1): 201–218.

Schegloff, Emanuel A., Gail Jefferson, and Harvey Sacks. 1977. "The Preference for Self-Correction in the Organization of Repair in Conversation." *Language* 53 (2): 361–382.

Steen, van der Jenny T. 2012. "Ensuring Continuous High-Quality Care for People with Impaired Condition Including Dementia at the End of Life." *Palliative Medicine* 26 (7): 871–872.

Svennevig, Jan. 2008. "Trying the Easiest Solution First in Other-initiated Repair." *Journal of Pragmatics* 40 (2): 333–348.

Tallberg, Ing-Mari. 2001. "Deictic Disturbances after Right-Hemisphere Stroke." *Journal of Pragmatics* 33 (8): 1309–1327.

Wilkinson, Ray. 2007. "Managing Linguistic Incompetence As a Delicate Issue in Aphasic Talk-in-Interaction: On the Use of Laughter in Prolonged Repair Sequences." *Journal of Pragmatics* 39 (3): 542–569.

Appendix

(1, 11) SATT NÅGON ELDVAKT

01 Rebecka:	hade ni eldvakt allti nån
02	(0.2)
03 Ferdinand:	**va**
04	(0.2)
05 Rebecka:	hade ni allti nån som satt eldvakt
06	(0.9)
07 David:	<eldvakt>
08	(1.6)
09 Rebecka:	i [ta- i tälte
10 David:	[om de
11 Ferdinand:	**[ja har lite dålit me hörseln min**
12	(om [de där)
13 Rebecka:	[hade ni nån alltid som satt eldvakt i tältet
14	(1.0)
15 David:	**satt nån <eldvakt>**
16 Ferdinand:	jo jojo jojo (.h) *kipinäkalle*
17 Rebecka:	jaha heh heh heh

(2) DEN DÄR ROTSAKSLÅDAN

01 Olga:	sist va den god d[en där
02 Giselle:	[broiler
03	(0.6)
04 Ferdinand:	((skrattar))
05 David:	°eller o[m du vill att ja ska [ta nå annat°
06 Olga:	[rotsakslådan
07 Anna:	**[va sa du**
08 Olga:	att sist va den god den där
09	rotsakslådan

(3) EN ANNAN SOLHATT

01 Giselle:	ska gå å ta en annan solhatt åt David
02	(.)
03 R:	jå just de
04	(1.8)
05 David:	**va skulle hon**
06	(0.3)
07 R:	ta en annan solhatt åt [dej
08 David:	[*ja* heh heh

(4) DET VAR INTE SÅ VACKERT

01 Giselle:	[…] kocken som då laga å baka å (.hh)
02	härliga efterrätter […] men i alla
03	fall så märkte ja nä ja sku sätta på mej en

04 såndän kjol ti julen å (2.0) de va int så
05 vackert sen mera [heh heh
06 David: [a- va kom
07 Isabella: [heh heh heh
08 R: [heh heh heh
09 Giselle: ja hade ja hade fått så många kilon till
10 [nä ja hade äti så mycke efterrätt
11 David: [jå aj
12 Giselle: vår kock hade på ((X)) laga så my[cky gott
13 David: [jå:å
14 David: v-v-va sa du om kjolen
15 Giselle: den va för spänd
16 David: aj ja[ha
17 Isabella: [heh heh heh

(5) BLEKA TÄNDER
01 Giselle: ja har en syster som bor i Stockholm [..]
02 nu tala ja på missommarn me henne å hon
03 ha nu besluta sej att hon ska bleka
04 sina tänder
05 (1.0)
06 R: *(hh)*
07 (0.5)
08 Isabella: *mh*
09 (1.3)
10 David: ((harklar sig)) hon ska va ((vänder sig mot Giselle))
11 Giselle: hon ska bleka sina tänder
12 (0.3)
13 David: *aj*
14 (0.7) ((Giselle skakar på huvudet, tittar på Isabella))
15 R: *(h)*
16 (0.5)
17 Isabella: ja hade en kompis som gjo- som köpte just
18 via nån sån hän teveshop eller nånting

(6) ETT ANNAT ORD FÖR SMISK Å STRYK
01 Giselle: ett annat ord för smisk (0.2) å stryk
02 (0.5)
03 Olga: aga
04 (0.3)
05 Giselle: aga
06 Ferdinand: för va:
07 Olga: °mh°
08 (0.5)
09 Giselle: ett annat ord för smisk (0.2) å stryk
10 (2.5)

11 Ferdinand:	**nu uppfattar ja int ditt s[po-**
12 Giselle:	[ETT ANNAT ORD
13	[FÖR STRYK
14 Ferdinand:	[jo
15	(0.5)
16 Giselle:	man s- gör m: man slår nån
17	(1.0)
18 Giselle:	AGA
19	(0.4)
20 Giselle:	ha du hört om A[GA
21 Ferdinand:	[ja ja
22 Ferdinand:	jo jo
23 Giselle:	jå
24	(0.2)
25 Ferdinand:	**stryk ja uppfatta int jaha**

(7) KÄRLEKENS RÖDA BLOMMA

01 Giselle:	kärlekens röda blomma
02	(0.3)
03 Giselle:	ja de är en,
04 Anna:	ros
05 Giselle:	ros bra An[na
06 Anna:	**[sidu att ja kunde nån[ting**
07 Giselle:	[nåjo?
08 Anna:	**men man hinner int ni e så snabba**
09 Giselle:	e vi snabba ja ska ta de långsam[ma-
10 Anna:	[nä:
11 Giselle:	heh [heh heh
12 Anna:	[(-) ni på bara
13	(1.7)
14 Ferdinand:	**va de ros**
15 Giselle:	de va ros
16 Ferdinand:	ros jaha

(8) ROM BYGGDES INTE PÅ EN DAG

01 Giselle:	Rom byggdes inte
02	(2.1)
03 Irene:	**vafför int**
04	(0.3)
05 Giselle:	på en da
06	(0.2)
07 Irene:	**heh heh heh (0.2) varför int**
08	(0.6)
09 Giselle:	de vetdu den e stor [Rom staden e ju jättestor
10 Irene:	[heh heh heh
11	(0.5)

12 Giselle: små barn små bekymmer,

(9) VAD HETTE HON
01 Ferdinand: stor gård, (0.6) Hofgård
02 (0.8)
03 Ferdinand: (där) (till-)
04 (2.8)
05 Ferdinand: (bring-) min min ungdom så
06 (2.0)
07 Ferdinand: så ägdis ägdes den av en (0.6) fru Paerman (0.2)
08 (mt) (0.8) mannen hade dött
09 (1.7)
10 Anna: va sa du [att hon hette]
11 Ferdinand: [å hustrun] frun träd[de i ställe de
12 Olga: [Paerman
13 Ferinand: va [nu
14 Anna: [(Paerman)

(10) VAD BERÄTTAR HAN
01 Anna: men va heter den här platsen
02 (0.7)
03 Olga: de hör ti Helsingfors
04 (0.4)
05 Anna: jaha
06 (3.7)
07 Anna: just så
08 (5.9)
09 David: ja tror ja borde ha (1.3) flera av mina (1.1) barn å
10 barnbarn (0.5) där i (0.9 detta (-)
11 (0.3)
12 Olga: mm:
13 (2.5)
14 Anna: va månne han berättar
15 (3.7)
16 Olga: (mm:)
17 (0.8)
18 Anna: de e int så vikti[t
19 Olga: [nä:

(12) EN VACKER DAG IDAG
01 Ferdinand: de e en vacker dag idag?
02 (1.2)
03 Giselle: e de här nu (sås)
04 (.)
05 David: va [sa du
06 Giselle: [int vet ja

07 (2.0)
08 Anna: att de e [vacker [da (ida)
09 Isabella: [mm
10 Ferdinand: [de e vacker
12 da i[da
13 David: [vacker dag idag jå+å

(13) AKVAVIT
01 Giselle: va e de [där
02 Anna: [ja tänkte säga akvavit
03 Olga: de e aster d[å
04 Anna: [men de pas[sa int
05 Giselle: [aster e de precis jå
06 Olga: jå
07 Giselle: va tänkte du säga Anna (.hh) (0.2) akvavit?
08 (0.2)
09 Anna: jo
10 Giselle: [[heh heh[heh
11 Isabella: [[heh heh[heh
12 Anna: [*vi talar här om* (0.2) *om andra saker*
13 R: heh heh heh ((tyst))

CHAPTER EIGHT

ONLINE ROUNDTABLE SUMMARY: IDENTIFYING NEEDED RESEARCH

BOYD DAVIS
UNIVERSITY OF NORTH CAROLINA-CHARLOTTE
AND J. B. ORANGE
WESTERN UNIVERSITY

Background

On May 15, 2013, the authors held an online roundtable conference, using a conference call system that, while not totally satisfactory, did support commentary from Charlotte, North Carolina, Charleston, South Carolina, University Park, Pennsylvania, and Hammond, Louisiana in the U.S.; Christchurch, New Zealand; Helsinki, Finland; Cardiff, Wales; and London, Canada.. Our objective was to share with each other new needs and constructs that had surfaced during our collaboration, and to identify next steps in research on pragmatics in dementia. The discussion was transcribed, and organized under a summary of main points; we include quotations from the interaction as illustration, and identify participant-speakers by initials. Participants, listed alphabetically by first name, were Alison Wray, Angela Roberts, Boyd Davis, Camilla Lindholm, Charlene Pope, Jacqueline Guendouzi, JB Orange, Julie Cook, Margaret Maclagan and Robert Schrauf.

From the interaction: a major emphasis

The strongest emphasis that emerged from the discussion is that theoretical foundations, novel and current, are needed to help bridge the knowledge gaps among the many disciplinary perspectives on pragmatics in dementia (e.g., social psychology, cognitive neuroscience, sociolinguistics, neurology, neuropsychology, applied linguistics, speech-language pathology, gerontology). The linkages will ensure that we have the best foundations to guide interpretations of conversational data where the conversations include persons with dementia.

> JBO: Because what ends up happening is you end up with, as we have in Canada sometimes, the two solitudes, one not talking to the other. We're aware of the information and wealth of knowledge that can be used, and it informs one another. So, essentially, a double-headed arrow or a back and forth bridge, whatever metaphor you wish to use to ensure that one is learning from the other.

> AW: I'm very concerned that across the different disciplines working in dementia, there are a great many different assumptions, theoretical assumptions, about the nature of grammar and of the word. So, a lot of people who come out of psychology, sociology and coming from neurolinguistics, or neurology, maybe are not using the most up-to-date models of language and, so they're making assumptions about, for example, what it means to not be able to retrieve a word. What is a word? Where does the word start and end? What does it mean to know one? And, so, I just want to see an opportunity to hook back into linguistic theory.

Need for a range of perspectives and approaches

A number of the following theoretical perspectives have been employed in our various chapters:

i. intercultural pragmatics;
ii. intergenerational facets affecting pragmatics;
iii communication accommodation theory as it intersects with pragmatics;
iv. aspects of cognitive neuroscience: memory, attention and executive function systems and processes involved in pragmatics;
v. mental models of what language really means to individual speakers and how concepts are represented in and shared among participants in a conversation;

In addition, there are other approaches which need to be brought into the discussion, such as extended examinations of politeness, (im)politeness, speech acts, implicature, inferentiality, indexicality, narrativity – the list goes on. The exploration of pragmatics in dementia discourse is new.

BD: I hear a very strong desire for interpersonal, intercultural pragmatics, interaction with sociolinguistics: where else are we going, what other theories are we going to need to look at?

JG: I was thinking about some of the social psychology stuff. I was thinking about Howard Giles on speech accommodation. And, there's some interesting links with that.... I recently just was doing a grant proposal for training caregivers, professional caregivers. And I went back to that speech accommodation model because we have ... conversation training programs that speech pathology uses, and even with the neurotypical people, we haven't even gone in and thought about gender, age, different backgrounds. Even before we get to the people with the dementia.

RS: ... There's also a link here to some of the work in linguistic anthropology and indexicality like Silverstein's and how language indexes macro-social identities, and, then, as Charlene was sort of saying, they become ... joined across the conversation. Particularly for a person who might have difficulties in remembering. But what remains unexplored is what the cognitive correlates are of processing the indexical information in that way. . . . [in] current diagnostic practice, and current practice in neuropsychology and cognitive psychology, you get short-term memory, long-term memory and various kinds, you know, of word finding and syntactic complexity and those kinds of things, at a micro-level, and at a macro-level, maybe folk psychology of meditation, but there seems to me there's a meso-level if we rethink what cognition is or what the relevant cognitive abilities are cast as or in a conversation then it involves kind of repackaging of things we think of as cognitive....

JBO: . . . there's going to be some ways of measuring neuronal function as you're doing these various pragmatic functions in an interactive conversational dyadic context. And, that may be one way of looking at how we're going to bridge among a number of different concepts with those that Charlene and Jackie raised in sociolinguistic and cultural stuff, and the stuff you're raising, Bob, relative to sort of cognitive processing elements that, certainly, are driven more by a medical model approach, but nonetheless, is certainly coming out in the literature. At least, in the discourse processing literature.

New questions are needed

Several participants identified a need to examine pragmatics at a meso-level: that is, links among cognitive systems and processes, language systems and processes, and social forces. Within a meso-level context we must focus on questions such as with whom are we interacting, what are his/her social roles and profiles, what are our own social profiles and roles when interacting with persons with dementia, what are newly emerging perceptions (real or based on stigma(s)/myth(s)) of dementia, and our perceptions of what we do in interactions, how we interact and how we use language with others.?

CP: My sense is that socialized identity and its practices that are emergent over time, this goes beyond memory. So, you may not remember a piece of the word, but you know what that kind of person is. … Maybe there's more to social identity than simply overt conscious memory.

BD: It's such a risk for a person with dementia any time to agree to speak with other persons. They don't know who the person is; if they're in an institution, they have the feeling that they need to be nice. They need to say something to who's there in some way, and they need to have some way of finding common ground and they have not the slightest idea of what the other person is bringing to the conversation.

AR: I can only speak a little bit from the work that's been done in Lewy Body Spectrum Disorder. But, one of the things that they have shown is that there seems to be some correlate between the imaging findings and what they're finding in story grammar structures and also those associated with executive function. So, ~~if~~ there does seem to be a least some connection in the middle between some of those more discreet cognitive functions and what is seen on imaging and what correlates with discourse.

Locating translatability

For practical reasons, we identified a need for greater translatability, transparency and transferability of pragmatics theories and approaches and data interpretation: here we move to address the concept of knowledge accessibility and knowledge translation, and finish each other's sentences.

CL: . . . greater emphasis on multimodality

MM:. . . put different [approaches] together

RS: . . . [see] how to repackage our understanding of fundamental cognitive abilities, as tied to conversational tasks.

JG: . . . I tell my students this, we separate these things to study them, but they happen, they just are in an interactive system. They happen all at once.

BD: . . . [it's the] notion of taking what we have found in our research into training models for staff, caregivers, family.

RS: . . . what NIH calls translation research

JBO: . . . It's couched within the concept of evidence-based practice. And, that is that you need to be able to link theoretical elements within the applied domain, and there has to be the seamlessly interwoven connection of your paradigm that really gets translated in measurable outcomes that have real world impact.

Starting to bridge the gaps in discourse research

Finally, we identified the need to understand current and accurate theoretical frameworks and to adapt those consistently in the research on discourse in general and to dementia discourse in particular. Furthermore, we agreed that there is a need to begin to link discourse data to both the neurological underpinnings of these disease state changes and to the clinical applications of discourse data for both assessment and for intervention.

JBO: -- laid on top of the cognitive decisions . . . are the issues around “With whom am I communicating?" "How much can I share with that individual?" "Do I want to reveal how much of a social relationship with that individual that might otherwise allow me to share certain types or not certain types of information or memories of my wedding because this individual is not married or widowed or a widower of some sort.” So, there are these other social linguistic forces that otherwise add another dimension to the multiple layers of decision making that goes about how we actually structure the sentences, let alone the content that goes along with it, or the manner in which we share that information. So, I think it's multiple dimensions of cognitive social forces among others that determine our final output

AS-R: ...we have to be careful as we discuss these patterns of comfort in initiating social discussions or having perspective that we appreciate that the different dementia subtypes may have different issues with that. So, if we relegate our thoughts just to the Alzheimer's dementia domain, some of that is true, but in cases of the more frontal lobe dementias, where they actually reduce inhibition, it may not be as much of an issue in terms of initiating those social interactions as ~~or~~ having, or even making an appreciation of the other person's perspective. . . .

This collection of integrated but wide-raging topics on discourse and dementia, and our discussions of future research needs and directions, as outlined above, are merely the beginning of long but exciting journeys.

CHAPTER NINE

EPILOGUE: READING COMPROMISED AND PRESERVED COGNITION INTO AND OUT OF CONVERSATIONAL DATA

ROBERT W. SCHRAUF
PENNSYLVANIA STATE UNIVERSITY

Introduction

This chapter draws on the data from the various contributors of this volume to address the mutual enrichments of pragmatics and cognitive gerontology/cognitive neuropsychology in understanding the language of persons with dementia. On the one hand, moving *from cognition to conversation*, this epilogue poses the question: how might we interpret the conversational data of persons with Alzheimer's disease in light of the signature cognitive deficits of the disease—severely diminished working memory, impaired executive function, problematic lexical retrieval and degenerating semantic organization? This question begins with cognitive abilities as identified, articulated, and operationalized in cognitive gerontology and the neuropsychology of Alzheimer's disease and then seeks to account for trouble spots in Alzheimer's speech in light of them. On the other hand, moving *from conversation to cognition*, we ask: what cognitive competencies are presupposed by the real-time, naturally-occurring, communicative performances of persons with Alzheimer's disease? This question begins with a pragmatic analysis of actual conversation and seeks to identify (and perhaps construct) candidate cognitive abilities that would account for both impaired and unimpaired speech. Ultimately the goal of the chapter is to show that *re-thinking Alzheimer's disease in terms of conversation re-shapes how we understand both Alzheimer's disease and the underlying architecture of cognition itself.*

These are issues that must be addressed across a variety of disciplines, with their associated methodological practices, underlying assumptions, and current theoretical entertainments. Minimally, these range from the experimental and psychometric disciplines of cognitive gerontology and geriatric neuropsychology, to various fields of applied linguistics including discourse analysis, conversation analysis, pragmatics, clinical linguistics, and speech language pathology. Two rather different paradigms—perhaps complementary, perhaps competing—underlie either end of this disciplinary continuum (for reviews, see Müller and Schrauf *in press*; Potter and Te Molder 2005).

On the one hand, cognitive gerontology and geriatric neuropsychology are largely driven by a cognitivist paradigm with its roots in cognitive psychology and cognitive science. Cognition in this tradition has its source within individual minds where information, in the form of mental representations, is manipulated or processed by well-defined and experimentally constructed cognitive mechanisms. Language is one such mental representation, and communication is the exchange between minds of these representations. On the other hand, the various disciplines of applied linguistics, linguistic anthropology, discursive psychology, etc. are driven by a discursivist paradigm that understands language as talk-in-interaction and cognition as an essentially social process. In this approach, thinking, evaluating, problem-solving and the like are primarily worked out between people in conversation (and often over many conversations), and within-person, intramental occurrences are constituted by these interpersonal processes.

Even within the discursivist literature, the integration of these different views of language and cognition is sometimes considered problematic and sometimes ruled out of court. A sampling of such views can be found in the edited volume entitled *Conversation and Cognition* (Te Molder and Potter 2005), in which the contributors address the issue from conversation analysis, ethnomethodology, and discursive psychology. At one end of the continuum, some researchers suggest that discursivists make covert assumptions about inner psychological states and that the challenge is to "show how an analysis can be developed that does not depend on an inner, psychological notion of motive and to demonstrate the insufficiency of the idea of inner states dictating what is said" (Potter and Te Molder 2005, 38, also see Sanders 2005). At the other extreme, there have been calls in the pragmatics literature to abandon any consideration of the individual (his or her mental states, intentions, goals, etc) and to explain communication as an emergent phenomenon explicable only in terms of the interactional phenomena themselves (Arundale 2008; Haugh 2008, 2009, but see Wedgewood 2011). As always, the truth lies somewhere in the middle.

In this chapter, I hope to show that both cognitivism and discursivism are complementary 'takes' on human cognition and language and that each requires the other. One reason that cognitivist and discursivist paradigms must ultimately be complementary is that in practical terms, there is simply very little human cognition that is not at the same time linguistic. Thus, on the one hand, the cognitive traditions cannot escape addressing language because cognitive processes at some level are available only in language. That said, it remains the case that the language of the cognitivist is atomistic, componential, and systematic—ultimately a series of hierarchically organized, mental representations in the head of the individual. On the other hand, the discursive traditions cannot escape addressing cognition because linguistic processes are inexplicable without some recourse to mentation. But the architecture of cognition and the taxonomy of cognitive abilities, as derived from the experimental and psychometric disciplines, seem to account for only a small portion of the complex and interactive processes of shared meaning-making that are present in the linguist's transcripts. Given that the dementias, and particularly Alzheimer's disease as the most common form of dementia, are primarily understood as diseases of the brain and ultimately of cognition, and given that the most common manifestation of Alzheimer's disease is found in the everyday talk of persons with the disease (see Schrauf *in press*), Alzheimer's disease becomes a privileged site within which to think through issues of individual and social cognition.

In the first section of the chapter, I lay out the current, official articulation of Alzheimer's disease by the National Institute on Aging, the Alzheimer's Association, and the American Psychiatric Association: an unquestionably cognitivist account of compromised cognitive mechanisms with broad implications for behavior in general and language in particular. I pay particular attention to the 'cognitive architecture' that underlies this account. At the end of this section, I offer some reflections on how language is framed in the cognitivist vs. the discursivist accounts.

In the second section of the chapter, I take up the cognitive abilities as described in the official account and attempt to *read cognition into conversational data*. For this reading, I rely especially on Guendouzi's chapter in this volume in which she identifies the cognitive capacities that might be at work in turn-by-turn speaker implicature and listener inference and how the compromised cognition of the person with dementia might be explained in these terms (chapter 2). However, I take the liberty of departing from her reliance on Relevance Theory (Wilson and Sperber 2004), and I apply her insights to Bruno Bara's cognitive pragmatics (Bara 2010, 2011). In effect, this section suggests an interpretation of conversational data based on the standard cognitive architecture.

In the third section, I move in the opposite direction and attempt to *read cognition out of conversational data*. That is, I look at how one might move from the conversational data of persons with Alzheimer's disease to suggest candidate cognitive mechanisms that might undergird their actual talk. That is, I draw out the implications of the analysis for an alternative cognitive architecture. For this, I draw on four chapters in this volume in which the authors present transcribed data from their studies in clinical or ethnographic settings: Guendouzi (chapter 2), Pope (chapter 3), Davis, Maclagan, and Cook (chapter 4), and Lindholm (chapter 7). (This leaves aside the valuable Chapter 5 by Wray, which deals primarily with caregiver response to the use of formulaic language by persons with dementia, and Chapter 6 by Roberts and Orange, which is a much-needed review of the literature on discourse in Lewy Body Spectrum Disorder).

Alzheimer's Disease and Language Framed within Cognitive Science and Neuropsychology

In 2011, the National Institute on Aging and the Alzheimer's Association (NIA/AA) announced new diagnostic criteria of the disease for research purposes (McKhann et al. 2011), and in 2013, the American Psychiatric Association also announced new criteria in the fifth edition of the *Diagnostic and Statistical Manual of Mental Disorders* (APA 2013). Both sets of criteria are essentially concordant (see Müller and Schrauf *in press*), and given the cognitive bent of the NIA/AA guidelines, I work from those in this chapter.

A diagnosis of Alzheimer's disease requires that the patient's cognitive or behavioral impairment be manifest in at least two of five areas: (a) memory (specifically the ability to acquire new information); (b) reasoning, complex tasks and judgment; (c) visuospatial abilities (specifically face and recognition of familiar objects); (d) language; and (e) personality. Of these, the deficits in working memory, executive function, and lexicosemantic organization form the key elements of the cognitive architecture compromised in Alzheimer's disease.

Episodic/Working Memory

In contrast to previous diagnostic criteria (notably DSM-IV), the new guidelines note that nonamnestic presentations of the disease are possible, but that the "most common syndromic presentation of AD dementia" is amnestic (McKhann et al., 2011, 264). Specifically, the amnestic form is marked by the degeneration of working memory: that is, an "impaired ability to acquire and remember new information," or "impairment in learning and recall of recently learned information—symptoms include: repetitive questions or conversations, misplacing personal belongings, forgetting events or appointments, getting lost on a familiar route" (p. 264). Indeed, there is "a wealth of neuropsychological evidence showing that episodic memory impairment (i.e., amnesia) is usually the earliest and most salient aspect of the AD dementia syndrome" (Salmon and Bondi 2009). However, the ability to recall stored information is a complex process that intimately involves attention and executive functions as well, and as will be clear below, it is the interaction of these components that figures largely in the cognitive deficits seen in Alzheimer's disease.

Episodic memory or working memory is a critical feature of cognition in general. Although a number of models have emerged in the literature (see Miyake and Shah 1999), Baddeley's original, multicomponential model is considered foundational (1986, subsequently revised in Baddeley 2003). In this model, information is attended to and manipulated by an *executive function* while stored temporarily in either phonological or visuospatial formats (i.e. in either the *phonological loop* or the *visuospatial sketchpad)* or in multicoded format in the *episodic buffer.*

In a review of measures of working memory, Kemper (2009) notes that the majority of tests are derived from *Forward and Backward Digit Span* (Wechsler 1958) in which the testee hears or sees a series of digits and must recall them (either forward or backward). As the numbers of digits that a person is required to remember increases with each series, it becomes possible to quantify the 'span' of any one person's working memory. As is obvious, *Backwards Digits* differs from *Forward Digits* in that the former requires both holding the series in memory while performing manipulations on them. That is, whereas in *Forward Digits* a person might commit the numbers to memory by holding them in the visuospatial sketchpad or phonological loop and then repeating them when requested, in *Backward Digits* he or she must both hold the series in the visual sketchpad or phonological loop while simultaneously reporting them in reverse order—crucially involving the central executive.

Tests of working memory, like those described above, have been key components in the assessment of Alzheimer's disease. For instance, in the Folstein *Mini-Mental Status Exam* or *MMSE* (Folstein, Folstein, and McHugh 1975), the patient must commit to memory three common words and then repeat them several minutes later. Retrospective analysis of the CERAD database (Consortium to Establish a Registry for Alzheimer's Disease) showed that delayed recall (over immediate recall, intrusion errors, and recognition errors) provided the best early predictor of the disease (Welsh et al. 1991). In prospective research, measures of delayed recall and mental control were found to be the key predictors of which participants will eventually present with Alzheimer's disease (Tierney et al. 1996). Interestingly, decrements in delayed recall and executive function preceded impairments in perceptual (visuospatial) and language functions (Traykov et al. 2007).

Cognitive Architecture. In terms of cognitive architecture and functioning, the assumption is that these assessments draw on the foundational ability to encode information and retain it below awareness while engaged in another cognitive task. Clearly, this ability is a *sine qua non* of normal functioning. Thus, the clinical test is assumed to sample the same ability that undergirds the quotidian behaviors mentioned in the guidelines (McKhann et al. 2011, 264): "repetitive questions or conversations," (i.e. the inability to hold in mind the responses to recent questions or to keep hold of the thread of conversations in which I'm involved), "misplacing personal belongings," (i.e. the inability to remember where I put things or where I saw them last), "forgetting events or appointments," (i.e. the inability to recall my recent commitments), and "getting lost on a familiar route" (i.e. the inability to keep in mind where I'm at).

Executive Function

The new NIA/AA guidelines refer to deficits in executive function as follows: "Impaired reasoning and handling of complex tasks, poor judgment—symptoms include: poor understanding of safety risks, inability to manage finances, poor decision making ability, inability to plan complex or sequential activities" (McKhann et al. 2011, 264). However, these are molar effects of an underlying dysfunction that emerges quite early in the clinical syndrome and which has its effects primarily in difficulties with "the concurrent mental manipulation of information" (Salmon & Bondi, 2009, 259; see Perry and Hodges 1999), and "set shifting, self-monitoring, or sequencing" (Salmon & Bondi, 2009, 259; see Lefleche and Albert 1995).

Clinically, executive functions are often measured via non-lexical tasks such as the *Porteus Maze Test* (Porteus 1950), the *Trail Making Test- Part B* (Reitan 1955; Tombaugh 2004), and *Raven Progressive Matrices* (Raven, Raven, and Court 2000). The paper-and-pencil versions of the *Porteus Maze Test* requires the participant to trace a path through a maze (varying in complexity), and the *Trail Making Test* requires the participant to look at a random array of numbers and letters and to connect them in some order (e.g. 1-2-3-4, and so on, or 1-A-2-B-3-C, etc). *Raven's Matrices* requires that the participant consider successive series of patterns of shapes and symbols and then select the next likely shape or symbol.

Cognitive Architecture. In terms of cognitive architecture and functioning, the assumption in such testing is that the ability to detect patterns, abstract implicit rules, foresee obstacles, and plan sequences of action is an application of underlying cognitive, executive function. Further, although the tests involve inconsequential and artificial stimuli, performance on these clinical instruments is taken to be consistent with real world phenomena such as "poor understanding of safety risks, inability to manage finances, poor decision making ability, inability to plan complex or sequential activities" (McKhann et al. 2011, 264). The logic is that the clinical tests target a central processing mechanism that undergirds all cognitive behavior.

Lexicosemantic Organization of Long-Term Memory

The new diagnostic guidelines specify impairments in language as follows: "Impaired language functions (speaking, reading, writing)—symptoms include: difficulty thinking of common words while speaking, hesitations; speech, spelling, and writing errors" (McKhann et al. 2011, 264). Neuropsychological research on language in Alzheimer's disease has concentrated especially on the progressive degeneration of lexical retrieval and the related organization of semantic memory.

Impairments in lexical retrieval have long been associated with the early stages of Alzheimer's disease (Bayles and Kaszniak 1987; Bayles, Tomoeda, and Trosset 1992). In the neurocognitive literature, lexical retrieval is primarily assessed via confrontation naming and verbal fluency tasks. In confrontation naming, an individual is shown pictures and asked to name the objects or actions depicted. One of the most frequent such instruments is the 60-item *Boston Naming Test* (Kaplan, Goodglass, and Weintraub 1983). In other versions of the instrument, pictures are selected so that the corresponding names run from high to low familiarity, as in the *Graded Naming Test* (McKenna and Warrington 1983). The logic of these tests is that semantic referents stored in memory may be activated through the visual modality (seeing the picture), triggering a subsequent search in lexical memory for the appropriate label (finding the word). Verbal fluency tasks take either semantic or phonemic forms (Lezak 1995). In the semantic fluency task, the participant is asked to name as many exemplars in a specified category (e.g. animals) as possible within a limited time span. In the phonemic fluency test, participants are usually asked to name as many words beginning with F, A, or S as they can, again within a limited time span.

Research shows that semantic fluency is relatively more impaired than verbal fluency among patients with Alzheimer's disease versus normal controls (Henry, Crawford, and Phillips 2004). Later stages of the disease are marked by 'empty speech' in which vague substantives such as "thing" and "stuff" substitute for either superordinates or exemplars (Nicholas, Obler, and Albert 1985). Although there has been some debate whether loss of this knowledge is due to deficits in retrieval (impaired access) or storage (erasure of the mnemonic trace), it now seems clear that "AD results in a true loss of semantic knowledge rather than only an impaired ability to retrieve information from an intact semantic memory store (also see Salmon and Bondi 2009)".

Cognitive Architecture. The underlying assumption in terms of cognitive architecture and functioning is that the mental lexicon has a hierarchical superordinate-exemplar structure, and this structure deteriorates with the progression of the disease (Chenery, Murdoch, and Ingram 1996). Thus, performance on the semantic and verbal fluency tasks is thought to mirror at a clinical level the communicative deficits associated with the disease at a molar level: "difficulty thinking of common words while speaking, hesitations; speech, spelling, and writing errors" (McKhann et al. 2011, 264).

It is important to note that these three clinically and experimentally dissociable skills—working memory, executive function, and the hierarchical organization of long-term lexicosemantic memory—are in fact deeply interwoven. Clearly, working memory includes an important executive function vis-à-vis the encoding, retaining, and manipulation of information, and executive functions are implicated in the retrieval of information (lexical forms, semantic referents, underlying world-knowledge) from long-term memory.

Language in Cognitivist and Discursivist Approaches

Before considering how deficits in working memory, executive function, lexical retrieval, and semantic organization might be manifest in real-world conversation, it is important to articulate how language is operationalized in the cognitive tradition just described. Of course, tests of working memory and executive function do not target language *per se*. Rather their focus is on central mechanisms that undergird cognitive functions generally. Nevertheless, particularly in the case of tests of working memory, the majority of such tests employ semantically meaningful, lexically-encoded items that testees are required to process, remember and manipulate. On the face of it, the use of linguistic items justifies the generalization of these cognitive functions to more complex forms of language. At a deeper level, the near absolute necessity of employing *some* such linguistic items argues for the thoroughly linguistic nature of cognitive functioning. (Even a test employing non-linguistic stimuli, such as perhaps symbols or line drawings, will very probably require linguistic instruction!)

Those tests that *do* target language as their object are however a different matter because they necessarily involve covert assumptions about how language operates and how it is structured. Tests of lexical retrieval such as confrontation naming and verbal fluency are designed to trigger the production of individual words in response to simple stimuli. However, the stimuli are presented outside any meaningful context in which either the stimuli or the corresponding responses (i.e. words) might figure. Thus, whereas in actual talk the act of selecting a word is massively multidetermined by topic, setting, interlocutor, register, etc., the assumption in confrontation naming or verbal fluency is that semantic representations (concepts)—triggered by the visual processing of line drawings or pictures—have clean, one-to-one links with downstream phonological or orthographic representations that may be produced at will. Tests of verbal fluency make the same assumptions, except that the item-prompts themselves are single lexical forms, albeit categorical and perhaps prototypical. At the heart of this view lies a thoroughgoing representationalism according to which semantic concepts, their corresponding lexical (and phonological and/or orthographic) forms, are all mentally and neurally represented and manipulated (i.e. processed) in cognition (for a review of the development of this tradition in cognitive science, see Potter and Te Molder 2005). In sum, in the neuropsychological testing situation "language" is reduced to individual vocabulary items that are neurally and mentally represented inside individual minds.

From the perspective of applied and clinical linguistics, this view of language, and indeed of its cognitive representation, is strikingly one-dimensional. From the discursivist perspective, language is language-in-use—*talk-in-interaction*—with an emphasis on how people use talk to *do* things in social contexts: entertain, explain, illustrate, command, suggest, imply, report, query, parry, criticize, complain, deceive, prescribe, inform, etc. The underlying assumptions about the nature of language in this tradition are perhaps best characterized in the introduction to a related volume entitled *Conversation and Cognition*, Potter and te Molder (2005) summarize this approach as follows:

1. Talk is a medium of action
2. Talk is locally and situationally organized.
3. The point of view of the interactant is basic to understanding talk-in-interaction.
4. The primary analytic approach is empirical study of natural interaction.

In this tradition, research aims at capturing how people use language in real-world situations, and thus data collection focuses on audio- and video-taping in naturalistic settings and unstructured interviews. Analysis relies on the micro-analysis of fine-grained transcriptions representing all the verbal messiness of overlapping, interruptive, always partial, eminently quotidian and *co-constructed* conversation.

A review of the data sets gathered by the authors in this volume demonstrates precisely this method. Guendouzi (chapter 2) and Lindholm (chapter 7) carried out what might be termed 'linguistic ethnographies' in day care centers. As a participant observer, Guendouzi participated in conversations among persons with dementia, their caregivers, and herself in a rehabilitation day care center over a year and a half. Also as a participant-observer, Lindholm collected 30 hours of video-taped data during lunch periods and planned activities in an adult day care center among persons with mild- to mid-stage dementia. Other authors set up unstructured interviews with individuals in assisted living facilities. Pope (chapter 3) analyzed student-recorded conversations between Black and White university students who were paired with older Black and White persons with dementia in an assisted living facility. Davis, Maclagan and Cook (chapter 4) report on 25 audio- and video-taped conversations between the researchers (or university student volunteers) and one older woman, diagnosed with dementia, living in an assisted living residence.

Reading Cognitive Mechanisms *into* Conversational Data of Persons with Dementia

As noted above, the new diagnostic guidelines make clear connections between affected abilities and language functioning: from compromised working memory to 'impairment in learning and recall of recently learned information,' and 'repetitive questions or conversations;' from impaired executive function to 'inability to plan complex or sequential activities,' which would presumably include speaking and writing; and from degenerating lexico-semantic organization to 'difficulty thinking of common words while speaking, hesitations; speech, spelling, and writing errors.' While it is possible to draw these various links from specific mechanisms to specific language difficulties, it remains the case that any impairment likely involves a complex interplay of mechanisms. Thus, from the viewpoint of the contributors to this volume, it may be more interesting to zero in on how specifically pragmatic functions might be compromised by Alzheimer's disease.

As Guendouzi and Davis review in the opening chapter, two key concepts in the pragmatic approach to language are speaker implicature and listener inference. These notions are grounded in the observation that the intended sense of a message (speaker implicature) is often not deducible in any straightforward sense from the lexical meanings of the words themselves, but requires attention to a number of external factors (e.g. the setting and purpose of the conversation—the interactional frame, the conversational thread) and internal factors (e.g. shared schemata, scripts, world-knowledge, and the like). That is, a speaker utterance, in the form of a locutionary act, commonly involves the speaker's intention that the utterance *be understood* in a particular sense, and listeners who share the setting and purpose of the conversation, and the background knowledge and assumptions of the speaker may be relied upon to infer that meaning. Thus, from the cognitivist viewpoint, we ask, how do impaired working memory, executive function, and lexico-semantic organization affect the processes of speaker implicature and listener inference? More to the point: can we read such affected processes in conversational data?

As I noted above, Guendouzi addresses these issues in chapter 2 of this volume in terms of Relevance Theory. As a complement to her interpretation, and for purposes of reading the standard cognitive architecture into conversational data, I add Bruno Bara's cognitive pragmatics (2010, 2011) to the mix. I do this because, in his analysis of communication, Bara provides a micro-analytic, cognitive account of turn-by-turn implicature that relies regularly on the analysis of 'mental states' and 'mental representations,' and this way of framing the issues is clearly sympathetic with an analytics that emphasizes within-person cognition and the mental representationalism that marks cognitivist approaches. This in no way impugns his marked emphasis on the collaborative nature of meaning-making in conversation. Indeed in the opening paragraph of his summative article "Cognitive pragmatics: The mental processes of communication," Bara (2011) says,

> The basic idea behind this work is that communication is essentially a cooperative activity between two or more people in which the meanings of each transaction are constructed by all those actors together engaged in the shared task of reciprocally attending to the other communicant's words (2011, 443).

Nevertheless, if we are to move fairly seamlessly from the cognitivism of the neuropsychological framing of Alzheimer's to a tenable pragmatic and discursivist account, Bara offers a workable bridge.

Implicature in Cognitive Pragmatics

Speaker implicature and listener inference depend critically on both interlocutors having activated a common interactional frame and sharing the knowledge (cultural, group, or interpersonal) necessary to interpret one another's utterances and intended meanings. Bara discusses these notions in terms of mental states (e.g. shared beliefs) and behavior games: "A behavior game is that structure which enables actors to coordinate their interpersonal actions, and that actors employ to select the intended meaning of an utterance among the many meanings that utterance might in theory convey" (Bara 2011, 454). Further, as in any account of implicature, utterances involve 'communicative intent' (pp. 448-449).

At its most basic level, communication succeeds or fails at the turn-by-turn level, the smallest unit of which can be considered as an utterance by one interlocutor ('A') and uptake and response by another ('B'). Bara provides a useful five-step outline of the cognitive acts required in listener uptake (2011, 462; based on Airenti, Bara, and Colombetti 1993), which I have reproduced in the left-hand column of Table 1). Given a turn in which speaker A produces a concrete utterance, with a specified communicative intention, speaker B's comprehension involves two initial stages. In Stage One, B reconstructs A's mental state based on A's locutionary act, and in Stage Two, B reconstructs A's intended meaning. In Stage Three, actor B both forms a representation of A's mental states in intending the message and alters his or her own mental states as a result. Parsing these practically simultaneous acts amounts to accounting for B's comprehension of the message, crucially including listener inference. Finally, in Stages Four and Five, B formulates and delivers his or her response.

Table 1: Cognitive Analysis of Inference Turn-by-Turn

Bara (2011)	Guendouzi (Chapter 2; this volume)
Stage 1: Expression act. A's mental state is reconstructed by B starting from the locutionary act. *Stage 2: Speaker meaning*, where B reconstructs A's communicative intentions, including the case of indirect speech. *Stage 3: Communicative effect*, which consists of two processes, (a) *Attribution*, where B attributes to A private mental states such as beliefs and intentions, and (b) *Adjustment*, where B's mental states concerning the topic of the conversation may be altered as a result of A's utterance, *Stage 4: Reaction*, where B produces the intentions he will communicate in response, *Stage 5: Response*, in which B produces an overt communicative response.	(1) focusing attention on a speaker's utterance, (2) retaining their utterance in working memory, *Working memory: executive function, phonological loop, episodic buffer* (3) processing the propositional content, *Morphosyntactic processing, Lexical retrieval, retrieval from long-term memory, pattern matching* (4) considering the relevance of the utterance to the current situation, and (5) extracting any potential implicature that may be inherent in the utterance *Schema and script processing, heuristic thinking, metaphorical processing*

How might communication fail in this model? Bara defines a "communication failure as an abortive attempt to produce a given communicative effect on one's partner" (2011, 472). From this perspective, communication fails because B either *cannot* or *will not* capture the communicative intent (the implicature) of A's utterance. Bara discusses these three possibilities in terms of *noncomprehension*, *misunderstanding*, and *refusal*.

First, wespeak of *noncomprehension* if B cannot work out A's initial utterance or intended meaning (Stages One and Two). As an example, let's say that I enter a corner store, and I notice again that the graffiti on the front window has not been removed. I select a pack of paper towels and a bottle of milk as my purchases, place them on the counter, and say to the cashier, "Well, give a kid with too much time on his hands a can of spray paint, and what do you expect?" If the cashier is not thinking of graffiti on the storefront, and if my utterance does not trigger that activation, then he or she will very likely not comprehend my utterance or my meaning. This is because, at the cashier's counter, the expectable interactional frame or game to be played is something like: 'Paying for a Purchase,' and my comment about kids and spray paint doesn't fit that frame. Not surprisingly, the cashier may simply reply, "What?" Effectively, this 'what?' serves as an appeal that I establish a shared frame or game for our interaction.

Second, m*isunderstanding* results if the cashier captures the utterance (the locutionary act) but does not capture my intended meaning. Perhaps he hazards the guess that my buying paper towels has something to do with cleaning up paint at my house, and he laughs and says, "Were your kids helping you paint something?" This 'guess' is effectively the attempt to establish a frame within which my utterance might make sense.

Third, in a *refusal*, "B understands what A is saying but refuses to comply with A's orientation" (p. 472). The cashier might stay resolutely within the 'Paying for a Purchase' frame, and reply, "The paper towels are on sale two for a dollar."

In all three cases, the communication fails at both the levels of speaker implicature and listener inference: at the level of implicature, because A has not provided enough clues to establish a frame within which his comment might be interpreted, and at the level of listener inference, because B cannot make the appropriate inference and construct a response to keep the conversation going. Hence, B suspends the 'game,' and repair may take any number of forms. It is interesting to note in this example that the inferences required to process my comment about spray paint and kids require a rather complex embedding of schematic world-knowledge. First, my comment involves no lexical reference to graffiti, but rather the most potent cues are 'kids' and 'spray paint.' Second, in turn these links presuppose a simplified world in which graffiti is done by 'kids' and not adults and that kids use spray paint (and not, for example, paint brushes or felt-tipped markers). Third, there is the implication that kids painting graffiti is socially reprehensible ("what can you expect?"). These complexities notwithstanding, B's initial difficulty in capturing the implicature seems to stem from A's making the comment without announcing a different 'game' (e.g. "Complaining About Graffiti") within which it would make sense.

The Underlying (Standard) Cognitive Architecture

Given this understanding of turn-by-turn speaker implicature and listener inference, what might be the relevant cognitive abilities, from within the cognitivist tradition that undergird comprehension in a single turn? Although not working directly from Bara's model, Guendouzi (chapter 2) provides a brief outline of some of these abilities, and I have arranged this passage in a format parallel to Bara's in the right-hand column of Figure 1 (with my elaborations in italics). Where Bara notes that B must reconstruct A's utterance from its locutionary form and construct a representation of the intended meaning (Steps One and Two), we might locate Guendouzi's discussion of (1) attentional focus and (2) the retention of the utterance in working memory, both of which are clearly components of Baddeley's model of working memory. Her 'processing the propositional content' (3) can be unpacked to include the psycholinguistic acts of morphosyntactic comprehension and lexical retrieval, but these occur simultaneously and in conjunction with (4) recognition of the current interactional frame which requires acts of retrieval of information from long term memory and pattern matching, and (5) various acts of cognitively based, listener inference, including schematic processing, heuristic thinking, metaphorical processing, and the like.

In specific application to persons with dementia, Guendouzi describes how compromised abilities might have direct effects on listener inference: (a) the lack of attentional resources may result in partial intake of the interlocutor's utterance or information in the speech setting, (b) the necessity of re-attending to that utterance or information in the speech setting may interfere with, interrupt, or block ongoing processing, (c) incoming information may not link up to previously stored information (possibly due to cortical or sub-cortical damage), and (d) an inability to inhibit irrelevant information may result in overactivation of semantic networks, which again interferes with, interrupts, or blocks ongoing processing. Obviously, the effect of any one of these, and the multiplicative effect of the interaction of two or more, will result in deficient comprehension of the propositional content, the illocutionary force, and the communicative intent of the utterance. Since it is in the very nature of conversation to move along, the person with dementia may very quickly experience cognitive overload, drop out of the ongoing talk, and perhaps inappropriately re-engage downstream.

Given this analytic taxonomy of cognitive difficulties (lack of attentional resources, diminished temporary storage capacity in working memory, slowed executive manipulation of information, and deteriorating webs of lexical and semantic association), we might attempt a more or less straightforward interpretation of conversational data. Returning to Guendouzi's data chapter, consider the dialogue between Guendouzi (R) and Ms. A. (pp. 52).

WHAT'S YOUR NAME (source: Guendouzi, this volume)

1 Ms. A:	and what's your name again?
2 R:	ge [
3 Ms. A:	no let me read it (*leans over and peers at R's name-tag)* and how do you say that jendooza //dʒɛnduzə/ ?
4 R:	guendouzi /gɛ:ndu:zi□/
5 Ms. A:	so where are you from? You're not from around here are you?
6 R:	no I am from England.
7 Ms. A:	England mhm I thought you weren't from round here (.) so tell me again what's your name (.) and where are you from?
8 Ms. B:	they don't let us, do they? (*looking towards the care assistant and her cup)*
9 R:	do you want some more coffee (*looking at Ms. B)* or cookies?
10 Ms. B:	(*looking intently at author)* I know you oh you?
11 R:	yes, I came last week remember?
12 Ms. C:	that's a nice one (*looking at picture)*
13 R:	that's Italy (.) I think.
14 Ms. A:	now (*looks at author)* don't tell me you are from (0.5)
15 R:	England
16 Ms. A:	oh England no I haven't been there and so: what is your name again?

Ms. A asks for the researcher's name. When the researcher begins to say her name, Ms. A asks instead to read it (on the name-tag), and she asks Guendouzi how the name is pronounced. In cognitive terms, Ms. A seems to be strategically maximizing the input by insisting on reading the name herself (l.3 "No, let me read it") and then attempting to pronounce it (l.4). That Ms. A has captured the information is evident in her drawing an inference about the researcher's provenance, presumably based on her unfamiliarity with the orthographics and pronunciation of the name (l. 5 "You're not from around here, are you?"). In pragmatic terms, Ms. A's articulating this inference gives evidence that she is indeed engaged in the appropriate behavior game (Bara, 2011)—politely querying a person with a 'strange' last name about her ethnic origin during a 'mutual introduction sequence.' Nevertheless, despite this attention to, and multimodal processing of, the information, Ms. A seems to forget it by immediately asking again (l. 7 "What's your name and where are you from?"). Or *perhaps* her asking again is an adroit strategy to fix the information in her memory. In any case, a scant seven turns later, she seems to have lost the information, and she asks again for the researcher's name and provenance (ll. 14, 16).

Reading cognition into these few lines, we might say that Ms. A attended appropriately (and even effortfully) to the input, but that her almost immediate forgetting was due to the interactive factors of diminished working memory storage capacity and the effort of attending to additional but distracting interchanges by Ms. B, Ms. C., and the researcher (in lines 8-13). Of course, even this would remain highly interpretive, but the cognitive account is certainly plausible. Further, more involved 'readings' of cognition would be possible. As Guendouzi notes, her data set in fact includes numerous examples of Ms. A's engaging in precisely this behavior, and therefore it is hypothetically possible to test in other places whether Ms. A was capable of retaining this information in the absence of intervening turns by others. More ambitiously we might develop a coding system for 'depth of processing' by noting how persons with dementia give conversational evidence of having attended to, established linkages between (made associations), and manipulated information and then retained, re-expressed, used, or lost this information. That is, using conversational data we could reasonably operationalize cognitive abilities like attention, memory storage, semantic organization, etc. In sum, reading cognition into conversational data is certainly a tractable project.

Reading Cognitive Mechanisms *out of* Conversational Data of Persons with Dementia

Alternatively, there is the challenge of reading cognition *out of* conversational data. An especially ambitious version of this project would start purely from conversational data and attempt the task of developing from scratch the cognitive architecture that would seem to underlie the interactive achievement of conversation. Thus, whereas the cognitive sciences work from a kind of methodological individualism and cognition-in-the-head, this approach would renounce (as a working principle) the individual as the source of cognition and take talk-in-interaction as the unit of analysis. As mentioned in the introduction to this chapter, variants of this approach are favored by Arundale (2008) and Haugh (2008, 2009). Nevertheless, eliding over decades of work in cognitive psychology and neuropsychology runs counter to the spirit of rapprochement that drives this epilogue, and hence it may be more productive to accept the more tractable task of testing whether conversational data presuppose alternative cognitive mechanisms in addition to those in the standard armamentarium. Even this would be a herculean task, however, and in the following I do selective readings of some of the material in the chapters of this volume to find pointers, precursors, and potential candidates. This project is conditioned by the actual readings and theoretical commitments of the several authors who have provided transcribed data in their chapters: Relevance Theory in Guendouzi's chapter (Sperber and Wilson 1995; Wilson and Sperber 2004); Bourdieusian habitus in Pope's chapter (Bonilla-Silva, Goar, and Embrick 2006), Interactional Pragmatics in Davis, Maclagan, and Cook's chapter (Locher and Graham 2010), and Emergent Pragmatics in Lindholm's chapter (Perkins 2005, 2007, 2008).

Special Purpose Inferential Device: "What's Your Name Again?

Given the discussion of Guendouzi's data in the previous section, I will begin with her chapter, "So What's Your Name? Relevance in Dementia" (chapter 2). As I noted above, Guendouzi does not in fact work from Bara's cognitive pragmatics, but rather develops her analysis in terms of Sperber and Wilson's Relevance Theory (Sperber and Wilson 1995; Wilson and Sperber 2004). Without reviewing Relevance Theory itself, I note that Guendouzi argues that the innate tendency to infer communicative intent is indeed operative in persons with dementia, though importantly conditioned on their cognitive abilities. As noted above, she presents conversational data from residents in a day center with whom she interacted, and her analysis concerns how these individuals went about satisfying key parameters of Relevance Theory. Notably, these include, as the 'first default parameter of RT,' establishing the identity of their interlocutors:

> ...the identity of an interlocutor is a quickly established or given piece of information in a conversation that might dictate the appropriate degree of intimacy between the participants. Indeed, interlocutors need this

> information to frame their conversations and choose the appropriate communicative behaviors for the context. (p.53)

The data shown above give evidence of Ms. A's acting out this parameter.

A second parameter is the interlocutor's need to establish the degree of intimacy that is appropriate for the conversation. As Guendouzi notes, for the neurotypical individual this may well follow immediately from establishing interlocutor identity, but for persons with dementia, the search may be more explicit and indeed labored. Finally, individuals in conversation, including persons with dementia, seem to obey a third parameter, according to which they seek shared or common ground with interlocutors. The reader can return to Guendouzi's chapter to see how these parameters play out in the talk of persons with dementia, but the point is that, according to Relevance Theory, these behaviors would seem to be automatic and innately structured as instantiations of the Cognitive Principle of RT.

Cognitive Architecture. These observations open an interesting avenue for thinking about alternate architectures of cognition. Where the cognitivist paradigm emphasizes central processes of working memory and executive function, and a hierarchically organized lexico-semantic system, there may be reason to explore other cognitive faculties, perhaps more intimately tied to the specifics of conversational comprehension and production. Sperber and Wilson have advanced the view that "a relevance theoretic comprehension procedure might fit with more modular accounts of inference, particularly mind-reading" (Sperber & Wilson, 2004, 279). In accord with the key notion in Relevance Theory that every communicative expression carries the "presumption of its own optimal relevance," they argue that humans possess a "special purpose inferential comprehension device" that grounds the automatic propensity for extracting relevance. Put simply, speaker implicature and listener inference are sourced in a specialized cognitive module in the mind/brain. Although Guendouzi does not make specific reference to such a device, her observation that persons with dementia act fully in accord with the Cognitive and Communicative Principles of RT, even despite their deficits in attention and working memory, would seem to confirm both the existence of such a 'special purpose inferential communication device' and the idea that it remains unaffected by the Alzheimer's disease.

Embodied Cognition: Smile and Nod

Chapter 4 by Davis, Maclagan, and Cook is not ostensibly about cognition. Rather the authors frame their analyses in terms of interpersonal pragmatics (Locher and Graham 2010): an approach that "allows the examination of relational, affective, and emotional signaling in addition to informational content" (Chapter 4, p. 94). The chapter reports a multimodal analysis of the verbal and gestural narration of several stories by a woman with dementia named Maureen Littlejohn who lives in an assisted living facility. Ms. Littlejohn has an assembly of small stories which she introduces into her talk, and upon which she elaborates, depending on her interlocutor's expressed interest and engagement.

In a prior examination of the Littlejohn corpus, Davis and Maclagan (*in press*) analyzed Littlejohn's responses to interlocutors who showed an interest in her stories, by providing: (a) simple recipient responses such as "mmhmm" (she stayed on the same topic 73% of the time), (b) emotive or evaluative assessments, such as "that's good," or "that's beautiful" (she stayed on topic or picked up another thread 93% of the time), or (c) longer comments or informational summaries (she stayed on topic or picked up another thread 80% of the time). Littlejohn's continuation of her stories and elaborations of them suggest that she reads her interlocutor's responses as evidence of attunement and alignment with her stories, and affiliation with her person.

In Chapter 4 of this volume, Davis, Maclagan, and Cook turn their attention to Littlejohn's use of gesture and head nods during her storytelling. Since she repeats her series of stories, albeit differently according to context and interlocutor, the authors are able to track her patterned use of certain movements. For instance, in a series of stories about her mother and apples told to two listeners (one of whom was videotaping the conversations), the authors find that she punctuates her telling at the narrative high points, and she ends her narrations, by turning her gaze from the interlocutor to the videographer, smiling and then turning back to the interlocutor. Davis et al. interpret these actions as follows:

> The head turn and the smile signal the completion of her story and (a) show emphasis (b) show her awareness that JW is there, filming her, (c) identify boundaries of discourse chunks that may or may not include routines and small stories, and (d) keep the floor, although they can also show that she is getting ready to shift perspective (Maury-Rouan 2011) or start a new, frequently related story. (p. 109)

There is also in these movements a recognition and perhaps confirmation by Littlejohn that she is connecting with—aligning, attuning, affiliating with—her interlocutors. Not surprisingly then, with this awareness she shows herself a competent storyteller, attentive to her listeners and ensuring their engagement.

Cognitive Architecture. Are conversational alignment, attunement, and affiliation technically *cognitive* abilities? From a cognitivist perspective, with its emphasis on central processing mechanisms and mentation within individuals, these seem like emotional and interpersonal, but not strictly-speaking cognitive, abilities. Yet from a discursivist paradigm, where cognition is eminently (though not exclusively) socially sourced, the ability to detect, monitor, invite, deflect, and refuse alignment, attunement, and affiliation are without doubt key functions. Departing even further from the traditional cognitivist paradigm, one could reasonably argue that these behaviors give evidence of 'embodied cognition' of the sort that Taylor propounds: "Our understanding is itself embodied. That is, our bodily know-how, and the way we act and move, can encode components of our understanding of self and world… My sense of myself, of the footing I am on with others, is in large part also embodied" (Taylor 1995, 170-171). In direct application to persons with dementia, Kontos argues that persons with dementia can be seen to signal personhood and agency via semiotic practices rooted in bodily engagement with the world. (Kontos 2004). With regard to Littlejohn's gesturing, this is precisely the point that Davis, Maclagan, and Cook make in their conclusion.

> It is often assumed that persons with dementia are no longer able to take the perspective of another person in conversation. However, a closer look at Ms. Littlejohn's apple stories shows her using gesture to clarify for her listeners just how a lean-to was built to store apples in the winter, and verbally introducing different information into a story that was repeated within one interaction. This is one way she can retain personal agency in an institutional setting. (Chapter 4, p. 118-119).

As pragmatics opens to the semiotic significance of the non-verbal, perhaps more cognitive accounts of such signaling will gain traction. However, moving from signaling alignment, attunement, and affiliation to an 'embodied cognition' that might underlie these acts is a far greater challenge for the standard account of cognitive architecture with its emphasis on individualism and cognition-in-the-head (mental representations). These issues are not unlike those posed by the notion of habitus, as taken up by Pope in her chapter, and I turn to that chapter to extend this discussion.

Social Habitus as A Condition of Cognition: "Ain't Hittin' on Nothing"

In a fascinating intergenerational study in which older (85+), black and white persons with dementia were paired with young, cognitively unimpaired, black and white interviewers, Pope (Chapter3) addresses the discursive and pragmatic practices in both cross-race and same race interviews. Pope shows that in same race dyads the younger partners used "devices that signaled approval, desire for more information exchange that drew members closer, used speech practices that inferred group membership, demonstrated attention to speaker intentions, and clarified communications…" (p. 84). On the other hand, the individuals in cross-race dyads "seemed more likely to infer or express disbelief, to not recognize conversational cues as readily, or request person-based information in forms more difficult for PWD" (p. 85). Pope interprets her data in terms of *habitus* as developed by Bourdieu and extended to issues of race by Bonilla-Silva.

> The anthropologist Bourdieu proposed the concept of habitus as a set of predispositions or habituated practices shaped by our history and situated cultural positioning (Bourdieu 1977, 72-73), with potential effects on communication practices during social interaction between members of different social classes. Extending Bourdieu's observation, segregation may produce a tendency for behaviors beyond our conscious intention or the memory of their formation (Bonilla-Silva Goar & Embrick 2006), which may include tendencies for speech acts in interaction. (p. 65)

Thus, the discursive and pragmatic practices employed by Pope's conversation partners in dealing both explicitly and implicitly with race in their encounters may have been driven by the "deep cultural conditioning that reproduces and legitimates social formations" (Bonilla-Silva, Goar, and Embrick 2006, 233). However, in analytic terms, the evidence for such conditioning in participants' articulations is often deeply subtle and ambiguous.

For example, in a cross-race dyad consisting of an older black woman with dementia (Ms. W) and a young white female interviewer, the interviewer has introduced the topic by asking: "What time 'y'all eat?" As Pope points out, this formulation in which the verb ("do") is dropped may be heard either as a grammatical elision common among speakers in the American South, whether white or black, *or* it may be heard as a potentially inauthentic attempt at Black vernacular speech. Their dialogue continues as follows.

DINNER (source: Pope, this volume, p. 73)

192: Ms. W:	I wonder if it's worth going over there eating.
193: W-Int:	[-] I don't know.
194: Ms. W:	[?] eat them black eyed peas, [-] collard greens. I ate that salad [?]
195:	they have that old stuff over there.
196: W-Int:	[?huh] (Laughter)
197: Ms. W:	I'm tired of that. We used to get tired of chicken [?]….
198: W-Int:	What is in the paper today? [-] Ain't hitting on nothing [referring to the newspaper]

[Change of subject]

Lines 194-196 report Ms. W's listing of available foods in the facility dining room. As Pope comments, "In line 196 the White interviewer does not pick up the cue about common foods but laughs, though the laughter is not heard as shared." That is, there is no evidence in the transcript that Ms. W shared in the laughter. Rather, Ms. W continues her thought in line 197 by elaborating on the foods and expressing that 'we used to get tired of chicken', but the interviewer doesn't pick up on this. Instead, she changes the topic, asking about the newspaper and providing her own response, using nonstandard English ("Ain't") and slang ("hittin' on nothing"). Pope interprets this as follows: "The use of nonstandard English and slang by a White speaker in an interracial interaction as supposed dialect has been considered "styling," and inauthentic in the presentation of an identity when performed by Whites (Strausbaugh 2006)."

At root, given just these lines, we don't know quite how to interpret the unshared laughter. Did Ms. W. not join in the laughter because she heard it as customary for the interviewer, heard it as the interviewer's nervousness in her role as interviewer, heard it as the interviewer's nervousness at interviewing a Black woman, or just didn't hear it? If anything, given Ms. W's making a commentary ("I'm tired of that") and extending the list to include chicken ("We used to get tired of chicken"), we have to assume that Ms. W either chose to ignore the laughter or heard it as encouraging her to continue. Similarly, where the interviewer employs the slang "ain't hittin' on nothing," we don't actually know from the data that Ms. W heard the phrase (either consciously or unconsciously) as a form of inauthentic 'styling.'

In sum, we don't know for sure whether any race-based element was part of the communicative intent or listener inference on the part of either the older black woman or the young white interviewer. I make these notes, not for the purpose of challenging Pope's interpretation. Quite the contrary, I suspect that the evidence in the rest of the interview would provide cumulative and comparative evidence for the veracity of these very interpretations. Rather, I make these comments to show that the effects of social habitus on individual illocutionary acts is stunningly subtle and that listener inference is not only extremely hard to detect in a transcript but probably massively undetermined by immediate prior turns (except where the implicatures are unquestionably direct) in actual conversation.

At a cognitive level, these issues of subtle, habitus-driven implicature, plus ambiguous and (possibly) unconsciously strategic inference, raise the thorny issue of pre-conscious and unconscious motivation and knowledge. Further, once we see these phenomena operative in the cross-race data as unconscious dynamics of a socioculturally conditioned habitus, there is every reason to assume that similar dynamics are active in much of our conversational behavior in many other (non-ethnic) topics. From a methodological and theoretical standpoint, Pope's analyses pose the greatest challenge of all to the standard cognitivist account. Indeed, we seem to need something like *habitus* in a more complete account of human cognitive architecture, but it is by no means clear what kind of cognitive ontology will accommodate both mechanisms like 'working memory,' 'executive function,' *and* a socioculturally conditioned habitus. This remains a challenge for both cognitivism and discursivism alike.

Conversational Group as Cognitive Resource: "Wilson"

Lindholm analyzes her naturalistic, conversational data of persons with dementia in a day care center in terms of Emergent Pragmatics (Perkins 2005, 2007, 2008), and I leave it to the reader to review that theory in more detail in Chapter 7. Lindholm focuses especially on repair initiators in her data: those moments when an individual expresses some difficulty in comprehending and/or responding in the conversation. As a fairly straightforward example, I repeat a portion of her data extract #10. Ferdinand is an elderly person with dementia, and he is speaking of a farm that he knew as a boy. Anna has also been diagnosed with Alzheimer's, and Olga is an older, cognitively unimpaired, participant in the center.

WHAT WAS HER NAME? (Source: Lindholm, this volume, p. 230)

07 Ferdinand:	so it was owned owned by a (0.6)
	Mrs *Wil*son (0.2)
08	(mt) (0.8) her husband died
09	(1.7)
10 Anna:	**what did you say [her name was]**
11 Ferdinand:	[and his spouse] wife to[ok his place

12 Olga: [*Wil*son
13 Ferdinand: it was [now
14 Anna: [(Wilson)

In line 10, Anna executes a repair initiator with her question for clarification about the name of the owner of the farm. She doesn't interrupt Ferdinand with this question, but asks it approximately 2 seconds after the end of his turn. On the face of it, there is no immediate reason to assume that Anna's repair initiator has anything to do with her cognitive deficit. It may be the result of perfectly ordinary inattention to the details of Ferdinand's utterance. Perhaps she was momentarily distracted, or perhaps she is making a bid for the floor. On the other hand, even if her question does result from a cognitive difficulty, the usual cognitive mechanisms would easily suffice to explain it. That is, slowed processing of the incoming speech signal could result in her inability to register the information, and logically enough she might be asking that Ferdinand provide the name again.

Interestingly, however, the more holistic view of Emergent Pragmatics focuses our attention on both the *intra*personal processes (perhaps working memory and executive function) and the *inter*personal processes that in fact compose any conversational interaction. As Lindholm points out repeatedly in her data, this draws our attention to the group as linguistic and cognitive resource. She makes precisely this point in analyzing the extract above. In line 11, Ferdinand overlaps with the end of her question to continue his thought, and Olga overlaps with the end of his utterance in line 12 to give Anna the information for which she has asked: "Wilson." Without attending to Olga's interruption, Ferdinand continues his story in line 13, and in line 14 Anna confirms her reception of Olga's utterance by repeating the name: "Wilson." In effect, Olga compensates for Anna's missing the name of the farmer's wife provided by Ferdinand at the start of the extract. In one sense, we might say that the success of Anna's ongoing communicative participation (her 'cognition') is aided by Olga. (Olga keeps Anna involved). In another sense, Ferdinand's telling his story depends on the successful participation of his listeners, and without them there is no communicative event. Olga doesn't simply help Anna, her action in fact facilitates the progress of the entire communicative event. Cognition cannot reside simply in the individuals, rather cognition takes place in the group.

Cognitive Architecture. I urge the reader to review the many and more complex examples provided by Lindholm, but for the present, and from the viewpoint of the cognitive paradigm, I wish to highlight the significance of the almost seismic shift implied by sourcing cognition in the group rather than solely within the individual. Again, from the cognitivist perspective, language is largely a question of mental representations (lexical, semantic, and syntactic) that reside within the individual mind/brain and that are activated in phonological or orthographic form for the purpose of communicating. On this view, communication is about successfully exchanging these representations. However, the irreducibility of the social in conversational cognition derives (at least) from the critical dimensions of communicative intention, speaker implicature, and listener inference. In essence, decomposing a lexical utterance into its semantic referents will rarely result in successful comprehension of speaker meaning. Rather, interlocutors become resources for one another in collectively activating (and deactivating) shared knowledge, focusing attention on relevant features of the topic, collaborating on the direction of talk, and repairing misunderstandings.

As Lindholm's chapter makes clear, this has important implications for how we understand Alzheimer's disease. Where others in a group of interlocutors provide repair for missteps, malfunctions, or deficits of the person who is cognitively impaired, and where this in fact advances collective cognition (e.g. collaborative storytelling, shared problem-solving, joke-swapping, and a host of other common conversational events), we truly speak of social cognition.

Discussion and Conclusion

The aim of this chapter has been to think through issues of cognition in Alzheimer's disease via the analysis of conversational data. A brief articulation and analysis of the most recent criteria for diagnosing the disease (according to the National Institutes on Aging, the Alzheimer's Association, and the American Psychiatric Association) shows that the major symptoms of the disease are traced to impairments in three key cognitive mechanisms: working memory, executive function, and lexicosemantic memory. Given this cognitive point of departure, and drawing from selected transcripts in this volume, I have attempted, first, to read cognition *into* the conversational data of persons with Alzheimer's disease—by trying to explain pragmatic breakdown in terms of the standard cognitive architecture of working memory, executive function, and lexicosemantic organization, and then second, to read cognition *out of* conversational data—by considering the actual pragmatic functioning (problematic or not) of persons with Alzheimer's disease and then asking what cognitive architecture might account for that functioning. A synoptic summary of these secondary analyses includes the following:

- *Compromised Working Memory and Executive Function.* In her data chapter, Guendouzi provided an insightful cognitive analysis of pragmatic breakdown of listener-inference-of-speaker-implicature in terms of the standard architecture of attention, working memory, and executive function. I took the liberty of integrating her analysis with Bruno Bara's cognitive account of turn-by-turn implicature (Bara 2010, 2011), and re-analyzed one of her excerpts. That is, (excerpting from data in chapter 2) although Ms. A had been given the background information ("What's your name?") that she crucially needs to engage in ongoing acts of inference with her interlocutors, her slowed processing, diminishing working memory capacity, and diffuse attention make it impossible for her to retain that information while continuing to process incoming input. In sum, the standard account is clearly applicable to observed conversational data.
- *Preserved Drive-to-Inference.* Applying Sperber and Wilson's Relevance Theory (Sperber and Wilson 1995; Wilson and Sperber 2004), Guendouzi argues in her data chapter that the impulse of the person with dementia to establish fundamental parameters of conversational engagement are unimpaired by the disease (at least in the early to moderate stages). That is, the drive to establish the identity of the interlocutor, the drive to gauge the appropriate level of intimacy, and the drive to establish common ground: all are clearly of concern to persons with dementia. In essence, persons with dementia can be seen to spend considerable amounts of their limited cognitive resources on these obtaining and retaining this information. To the researcher in pragmatics, this makes eminent sense, because speaker implicature and listener inference are absolutely foundational in human conversation. In fact, at the level of cognitive architecture, this argues for the possibility of a *specialized inferential module.*
- *Intact Attention to Alignment.* Longitudinal research presented by Davis and Maclagan (*in press*) and Davis, Maclagan, and Cook (this volume) about a woman with dementia named Ms. Littlejohn shows that she remains exquisitely sensitive to *receiving* the interlocutor's signs of alignment, attunement, and affiliation and equally solicitous in *sending* signals of alignment, attunement, and affiliation. Although Ms. Littlejohn shows other evidence of the effects of Alzheimer's disease in her behavior, it is clear that the ability to attend to alignment is unaffected. The fact that the data

show her doing so non-verbally (and presumably below awareness) argues for a deeply *embodied form of cognition.*

- *Deep Cultural Conditioning.* In one of her analyzed excerpts, Pope shows that that Ms. W, a Black woman with dementia, and her interlocutor, a young and cognitively unimpaired White woman, may have been sensitive to subtle discursive signals concerning race and interracial relating. Arguably, these signals are very likely sent and processed at pre- and unconscious levels, and proceed from 'deep cultural conditioning,' perhaps best captured in the notion of *'social habitus.'* Current cognitivist accounts treat this kind of knowledge as a 'representation' within the mind/brain, but this seems a somewhat simplistic way of accounting for the agentive-prompting, restraint-setting, socially-sensitive and identity-defending mix of attitudes, knowledge, and emotional experiences that comprise a social habitus.
- *Social Cognition.* Lindholm analyzed repair initiators and the individual and group responses that repair initiators seem to occasion. Among a number of examples in her data, the one that I elected to repeat concerned a woman with dementia, Anna, who hadn't caught the name of a character in a story being told by Ferdinand (also cognitively impaired). Anna asks for the name of that character, but Ferdinand does not recognize her request. Rather he continues with his narration. Meanwhile, Olga (another interlocutor) repeats the information to Anna in the midst of Ferdinand's ongoing narration. Thus, a very ordinary and unremarkable occurrence, common in almost any conversation demonstrates how attention and working memory are effectively socialized—offloaded onto the conversational environment. In essence, the *group becomes the cognitive resource.*

In addition to the standard abilities of working memory, executive function, and long-term lexicosemantic memory, it would seem that a cognitive architecture adequate to actual conversation would require some versions of the above abilities—derived from the analysis of actual conversational data. One of the challenges that this volume sets for discursivism in general, and pragmatics in particular, is finding a way to integrate these empirically identified cognitive abilities with the standard account.

My arrangement of these chapters and the order of material has not been governed either by the table of contents, nor has it been haphazard. I began with the standard, cognitivist view because, on the one hand, it has 'official' status from clinical, public health, policy, and even research standpoints, and on the other hand, because it represents an undeniable wealth of biological, cognitive, and behavioral empirical data and analysis. The next four chapters represent a decidedly more social view of cognition, and these are anchored by the last chapter (Lindholm's) in which cognition is most obviously accomplished by the group. This ordering also facilitates a discussion of the key tensions explored by this epilogue: (a) the marked differences in cognitivist vs. discursivist views of language, (b) the contrasts between cognitive defects and preserved abilities, and (c) the emphasis on individual vs. social cognition. Despite these apparent dichotomies, the overall goal of the chapter is to emphasize mutual enrichments.

Cognitivist vs. Discursive Views of Language. Throughout this chapter I have painted the cognitivist and neuropsychological view of language as a set of representations (semantic, lexical, morphosyntactic) in individual minds—a view that lends itself to understanding the effects of Alzheimer's disease as essentially a breakdown in both the mechanisms that process these representations (working memory, executive function) as well a breakdown in the mechanisms themselves (degeneration of lexicosemantic organization). What is left out of such a view is the *situatedness* of actual talk, its purpose, the abilities and motivations of the interlocutors, and their emotional states and nonverbal signals, etc. Also missing is the messiness of actual talk: the false starts, interruptions, overlaps, repetitions, repairs, etc. To the discursivist, these are not reducible to noise in the otherwise clean and underlying exchange of propositional content. Rather, as research in the discursive disciplines repeatedly shows, all of these factors ('situation' and 'mess') have palpable effects on the progress of talk, the intentions of speakers, and ultimately their very meanings. In effect, these conversational phenomena have implications for individual cognition, and it has been one of the aims of this chapter to begin to think about how conversational data might be mined to redraw the map of cognitive architecture.

Cognitive Deficits vs. Preserved Abilities. A second tension in cognitive vs. discursive research on Alzheimer's disease concerns the opposition between a 'defectological' view of the disease vs. a 'preserved abilities' view. The former generally starts with the mind/brain and emphasizes what an individual *cannot* do, and in fact this view can lead to what Kitwood has called 'malignant social psychology' (Kitwood 1997) and Sabat has called 'malignant positioning' (Sabat 2006). That is, the very assumption that an individual is impaired can lead to lower expectations on the part of caregivers and others—and a consequent impoverishment of social environment. The preserved abilities view, on the other hand generally starts with the 'person' (see Leibing 2006) and emphasizes what a person *can* do—with adjustment and social support—and, from the discursivist view, leads to a more careful analysis of how to scaffold the participation of a person with dementia, beginning perhaps at the level of individual turns (see Schrauf and Müller, *in press*). The work in this volume clearly shows a preference for finding and identifying preserved abilities over cognitive defects, and it may be one of the signal strengths of discursivist work on Alzheimer's disease to contribute to this badly needed corrective. From a scientific viewpoint, however, it is important that we integrate a careful understanding of the actual nature of cognitive compromise with an equally careful understanding of preserved abilities.

Individual vs. Social Cognition. A final tension that drives our continued research on Alzheimer's disease is that between individualist vs. social views of cognition. Although there are debates about this issue in the literature, research and treatment of linguistic (read: *conversational*) impairments in Alzheimer's disease may perhaps best be approached from a perspective that thoroughly interweaves the individual and social. Summarizing Perkins, Lindholm says,

> Pragmatic behavior is viewed as a result of complex interactions among semiotic, cognitive, and sensorimotor elements in the intrapersonal and the interpersonal domain. The elements interacting may constrain or facilitate one another, and any malfunctioning capacity in one domain can create a state of interactional imbalance both within the domain and across domains. This will result in a redistribution of resources, compensatory adaptation, in an attempt to maintain equilibrium. (Chapter 7, p. 216)

Hence, a truly adequate account of the architecture of cognition will necessarily include a sophisticated articulation of social cognition—not as an occasional, optional, second-order activity, but rather as a defining element of what it means to 'cognize.' Given this expanded view of cognition as social and an emphasis on identifying and fostering preserved abilities, discursivists make important and decisive contributions to the quality of life of individuals with dementia, and the chapters in this volume forge new links in an ongoing chain of such contributions.

References

Airenti, G., B. G. Bara, and M. Colombetti. 1993. Conversation and behavior games in the pragmatics of dialogue. *Cognitive Science* 17:197-256.

Arundale, R.B. 2008. Against (Gricean) intentions at the heart of human interaction. *Intercultural Pragmatics* 5 (2):229-258.

APA- American Psychiatric Association. 2013. *Diagnostic and statistical manual of mental disorders (5th edition).* Arlington, VA: American Psychiatric Publishing.

Baddeley, A. 2003. Working memory and language: An overview. *Journal of Communication Disorders* 36:189-208.

Baddeley, A.D. 1986. *Working Memory*. Oxford: Clarendon Press.

Bara, B. G. 2010. *Cognitve pragmatics: The mental processes of communication.* Translated by J. Douthwaite. Cambridge, MA: MIT Press.

. 2011. Cognitive pragmatics: The mental processes of communication. *Intercultural Pragmatics* 8 (3):443-485.

Bayles, K.A., and A. Kaszniak. 1987. *Communication and cognition in normal aging and dementia.* Boston: Little, Brown, and Company.

Bayles, Kathryn A., Cheryl K. Tomoeda, and Michael W. Trosset. 1992. Relation of linguistic communication abilities of Alzheimer's patients to stages of disease. *Brain and Language* 42:454-472.

Bonilla-Silva, E., C. Goar, and D. Embrick. 2006. When whites flock together: The social psychology of white habitus. *Critical Sociology* 32:229-253.

Bourdieu, Pierre. Outline of a Theory of Practice. Translated by Richard Nice. Cambridge: Cambridge University Press, 1977.

Chenery, H., B.E. Murdoch, and J.C.L. Ingram. 1996. An investigation of confrontation naming performance in Alzheimer's dementia as a function of disease severity. *Aphasiology* 10 (5):423-441.

Davis, B., and M. Maclagan, *in press*. "Talking with Maureen: Extenders and Formulatic Language in Small Stories and Canonical Narratives." In *Dialogue and Dementia: Resources for Cognitive and Communicative Engagement*, edited by R.W. Schrauf and N. Muller: Psychology Press.

Folstein, M.F., S.E. Folstein, and P.R. McHugh. 1975. Mini-Mental State: A practical method for grading the cognitive state of patients for the clinician. *Journal of Psychiatric Research* 12:189-198.

Haugh, M. 2008. The place of intention in the interactional achievement of implicature. In *Intention, Common Ground, and the Egocentric*

Speaker-Hearer, edited by I. Kecskes and J. Mey. Berlin: Mouton de Gruyter.

—. 2009. Intention(ality) and the conceptualization of communication in pragmatics. *Australian Journal of Linguistics* 29 (1):91-113.

Henry, J.D., J.R. Crawford, and L.H. Phillips. 2004. Verbal fluency performance in dementia of the Alzheimer's type: A meta-analysis. *Neuropsychologia* 42:1212-1222.

Kaplan, E., H. Goodglass, and S. Weintraub. 1983. *Boston Naming Test.* Philadelphia: Lee & Febiger.

Kemper, S. 2009. The role of working memory and language development over the lifespan. In *Language development over the lifespan*, edited by K. de Bot and R. W. Schrauf. New York: Routledge.

Kitwood, T. 1997. *Dementia reconsidered: The person comes first*: Open University Press.

Kontos, P.C. 2004. Ethnographic reflections on selfhood, embodiment, and Alzheimer's disease. *Ageing and Society* 24:829-849.

Lefleche, G., and M.S. Albert. 1995. Executive function deficits in mild Alzheimer's disease. *Neuropsychology* 9:313-320.

Leibing, A. 2006. Divided gazes: Alzheimer's disease, the person within, and death in life. In *Thinking about dementia: Culture, loss, and the anthropology of senility*, edited by A. Leibing and L. Cohen. New Brunswick, New Jersey: Rutgers.

Lezak, M.D. 1995. *Neuropsychological assessment.* 3rd ed. New York: Oxford University Press.

Locher, M., and S. Graham, eds. 2010. *Interpersonal pragmatics*: Mouton.

Maury-Rouan, C. *Do listener's facial expressions influence speaker's discourse?* 2011 [cited. Available from http://www.gesturestudies.com/Contributions/Maury-Rouan/Maury-Rouan.html.

McKenna, P., and E. Warrington. 1983. *The Graded Naming Test.* Windsor, UK: Nelson.

McKhann, G.M., D.S. Knopman, H. Chertkow, B.T. Hyman, C.R. Jack Jr., C.H. Kawas, W.E. Klunk, W.J. Koroshetz, J.J. Manly, R. Mayeux, R.C. Mohs, J.C. Morris, M.N. Rossor, P. Scheltens, M.C. Carrillo, B. Thies, S. Weintraub, and C.H. Phelps. 2011. The diagnosis of dementia due to Alzheimer's disease: Recommendations from the National Institute on Aging-Alzheimer's disease workgroups on diagnostic guidelines for Alzheimer's disease. *Alzheimer's and Dementia* 7 (3):263-269.

Miyake, A., and R. Shah, eds. 1999. Models of Working Memory: Mechanisms of Active Maintenance and Executive Control. New York: Cambridge.

Müller, N., and R.W. Schrauf. in press. Conversation as cognition: Reframing cognition in dementia. In *Dialogue and dementia: Cognitive and communicative resources for engagement*, edited by R. W. Schrauf and N. Müller.

Nicholas, M., L.K. Obler, and M.L. Albert. 1985. Empty speech in Alzheimer's disease and fluent aphasia. *Journal of Speech and Hearing Research* 28:405-410.

Perkins, M. 2005. Pragmatic ability and disability as emergent phenomena. *Clinical Linguistics and Phonetics* 19 (5):367-377.

—. 2007. *Pragmatic impairment*. Cambridge, UK: Cambridge University Press.

—. 2008. Pragmatic impairment as an emergent phenomenon, edited by N. Muller.

Perry, R.J., and J.R. Hodges. 1999. Attention and executive deficits in Alzheimer's disease: A critical review. *Brain* 122:383-404.

Porteus, S. 1950. *The Porteus maze test and intelligence*. Palo Alto, CA: Pacific Books.

Potter, J., and H. Te Molder. 2005. Talking cognition: Mapping and making the terrain. In *Conversation and cognition*, edited by H. Te Molder and J. Potter. New York: Cambridge.

Raven, J., J.C. Raven, and J.H. Court. 2000. *Manual for Raven's Progressive Matrices and Vocabulary Scales*. Oxford: Oxford Psychologists Press.

Reitan, R.M. 1955. The relation of the trail making test to organic brain damage. *Journal of Consulting Psychology* 19:393-394.

Sabat, S.R. 2006. Mind, meaning, and personhood in dementia: The effects of positioning. In *Dementia: Mind, meaning, and the person*, edited by J. C. Hughes, S. J. Louw and S. R. Sabat. Oxford: Oxford University Press.

Salmon, D.P., and M.W. Bondi. 1999. Neuropsychology of Alzheimer's disease. In *Alzheimer's disease 2E*, edited by R. D. Terry, R. Katzman, K. L. Bick and S. S. Sisodia. Philadelphia, PA: Lippincott Williams & Wilkens.

—. 2009. Neuropsychological assessment of dementia. *Annual Review of Psychology* 60:257-282.

Sanders, R.E. 2005. Validating 'observations' in discourse studies: A methodological reason for attention to cognition. In *Conversation and*

Cognition, edited by H. Te Molder and J. Potter. New York: Cambridge.

Schrauf, R.W., in press. "'What They're Said to Say': The Discursive Construction of Alzheimer's Disease by Older Adults." In *Dialogue and Dementia: Cognitive and Communicative Resources for Engagement*, edited by R.W. Schrauf and N. Müller. Psychology Press.

Schrauf, R.W., and N. Müller, eds., in press. *Dialogue and Dementia: Cognitive and Communicative Resources for Engagment.* Psychology Press.

Sperber, D., and D. Wilson. 1995. *Relevance: Communication and cognition (2nd edition).* Oxford: Blackwell.

Strausbaugh, J. 2006. *Black like you: Blackface, whiteface, insult & imitation in American popular culture.* New York: Penguin Books.

Taylor, C. 1995. *Philosophical arguments.* Cambridge, MA: Harvard University Press.

Te Molder, H., and J. Potter, eds. 2005. *Conversation and cognition.* New York: Cambridge.

Tierney, M.C., J.P. Szalai, W.G. Snow, R.H. Fisher, A. Nores, G. Nadon, E Dunn, and P.H. George-Hyslop. 1996. Prediction of probable Alzheimer's disease in memory-impaired patients: A prospective longitudinal study. *Neurology* 46 (3):661-665.

Tombaugh, T.N. . 2004. Trail Making test A and B: Normative data stratified by age and education. *Archives of Clinical Neuropsychology* 19 (2):203-214.

Traykov, L., A.S. Rigaud, P. Cesaro, and F. Boller. 2007. Neuropsychological impairment in early Alzheimer's disease. *Encephale* 33 (3):310-316.

Wechsler, D. 1958. *The measurement and appraisal of adult intelligence, 4th edition. (Baltimore: Williams & Wilkins; Spanish Translation).* Madrid: TEA Ediciones S.A.

Wedgewood, D. 2011. The individual in interaction: Why cognitive and discourse-level pragmatics need not conflict. *Intercultural Pragmatics* 8 (4):517-542.

Welsh, K., N. Butters, J.C. Hughes, R.C. Mohs, and A. Heyman. 1991. Detection of abnormal memory decline in mild cases of Alzheimer's disease using CERAD neuropsychological measures. *Archives of Neurology* 48 (3):278-281.

Wilson, D., and D. Sperber. 2004. Relevance theory. In *The Handbook of Pragmatics*, edited by L. R. Horn and G. Ward. Malden MA: Blackwell.

CONTRIBUTORS

Boyd Davis (editor)
Applied Linguistics/English, UNC Charlotte, Charlotte NC 28212, USA
bdavis@uncc.edu

Dr. Boyd H. Davis is Bonnie E. Cone Professor of Teaching in Applied Linguistics/English and Professor of Gerontology at University of North Carolina – Charlotte. Her areas of interest include narrative, pragmatics and stance in sociohistorical linguistics; Alzheimer's speech; and digital collections of speech. Her most recent books are *Alzheimer talk, text and context* (Palgrave 2009; 2005) and *Fillers, Pauses and Placeholders* (Benjamins 2010, co-edited with N. Amiridze, M. Maclagan). Her fifteen-year longitudinal collection of conversational interviews with persons with Alzheimer's disease is one cohort in the online digital *Carolinas Conversations Collection*, sponsored by the National Libraries of Medicine. She is co-Principal Investigator for this portal, available at Medical University of South Carolina. Recent articles appear in *Language Policy*, *Corpus Linguistics and Linguistic Theory, Topics in Geriatric Rehabilitation,* and *American Journal of Alzheimer's Disease and Other Dementias.*

Jacqueline Guendouzi (co-editor)
Communication Sciences & Disorders, Southeastern Louisiana U, Hammond LA, USA
jguendouzi@selu.edu

Dr. Jacqueline Guendouzi (co-editor) is the Knights of Babylon Professor of Communication Sciences and Disorders and Interim Department Head of Health & Human Sciences at Southeastern Louisiana University. Her areas of research include discourse analysis, pragmatics, and psycholinguistics in the context of communication disorders. In particular she is interested in how language processing is affected by cognitive deficits caused by dementia. She co-authored the text *Discourse Approaches to Dementia* (Lawrence Erlbaum, 2006) with Nicole Mueller, and recently co-edited the *Handbook in Psycholinguists and Cognitive Processing: Perspectives in Communication Disorders* (Psychology Press, 2011). She has published in the area of communication and gender considering the social causes of stylistic differences in men's and women's talk.

Julie Cook
First Year Writing Program, UNC Charlotte, Charlotte NC USA
jamick2@student.uncc.edu

Julie Cook recently completed her M.A. in English from the University of North Carolina at Charlotte, with an emphasis in Applied Linguistics, where she received the 2010 Blair Rudes Award for Excellence in Linguistics. Julie is currently a Lecturer in the First-Year Writing program at UNC Charlotte. Her studies are primarily grounded within cognitive pragmatics and sociolinguistics. Her latest research addresses metalinguistic scaffolding in children's literature (*Southern Journal of Linguistics*, 2012); pragmatics and performance in computer-mediated communication; and multimodal communication.

Camilla Lindholm
Scandinavian Studies, U. Helsinki, Helsinki, Finland
Camilla.Lindholm@helsinki.fi

Dr. Camilla Lindholm is an academy research fellow in Scandinavian Studies at the University of Helsinki. Lindholm uses the methods of conversation analysis and interactional linguistics to investigate interaction in institutional settings and conversations involving participants with communication difficulties. Her current research interests involve communication interventions and multilingual encounters in elderly care. Recent articles appear in *Communication & Medicine, Dementia* and *Journal of Pragmatics*.

Margaret Maclagan
Communication disorders, U. Canterbury, Christchurch, New Zealand
Margaret.Maclagan@canterbury.ac.nz

Dr. Margaret Maclagan is a linguist who has recently retired from the University of Canterbury in New Zealand where she taught speech-language pathologists. Her teaching areas involved language acquisition and language analysis, including phonetics and acoustic analysis. Her research areas are sound change over time in New Zealand English and in Maori and language change over time in people with Alzheimer's disease. She is a co-author of two books on New Zealand English, Gordon et al. (2004) *New Zealand English: its origins and evolution* and Jennifer Hay, Margaret Maclagan, Elizabeth Gordon (2008) *New Zealand English* and co-editor, with Boyd Davis and Nino Amiridze of *Fillers, Pauses and Placeholders*

J. B. Orange
Communication Sciences and Disorders, Western U at London, Ontario, Canada
jborange@uwo.ca

Dr. J.B. Orange is a Professor in and the Director of the School of Communication Sciences and Disorders at Western University at London Canada. He is an Associate Scientist with the Lawson Health Research Institute in the Aging, Rehabilitation & Geriatric Care Centre at St. Joseph's Health Care - Parkwood Hospital, London. He also is a Research Associate with the Canadian Centre for Activity and Aging at Western. His peer-reviewed publications and funded research address language and cognitive-communication disorders of adults and older adults. His research has special emphasis on discourse and communication of individuals with various forms of dementia and their family caregivers. Current research projects include the analyses of language and discourse of individuals with Alzheimer's disease, frontotemporal lobe dementia, Parkinson's disease, and amyotrophic lateral sclerosis. Other on-going studies include developing and assessing communication enhancement education and training programs for family caregivers of individuals with dementia.

Charlene Pope
College of Nursing, Medical U of South Carolina, Charleston SC USA
popec@musc.edu

Dr. Charlene Pope, PhD, MPH, RN, FAAN, is Chief Nurse for Research and a Core Coordinator for the *Center for Disease Prevention and Health Interventions for Diverse Populations* (REAP) at the Ralph H. Johnson VA Medical Center and Associate Professor at the Medical University of South Carolina (MUSC) College of Nursing in Charleston, South Carolina. Dr. Pope has a PhD from the University of Rochester with a concentration in sociolinguistics and did a post-doctoral fellowship in preventive cardiology to apply communication methodology to health service research. With Dr. Boyd Davis, Dr. Pope is Co-principal investigator (PI) of the NIH/NLM funded, MUSC-based *Carolinas Conversations Collection*, a Web-based archive of recordings of people over 65 from diverse ethnic and linguistic groups. Other studies include VA-funded studies of racial disparities in communication, decision-making, and diabetes care (HSR&D), nurse communication in home telehealth monitoring of heart failure (QUERI), and interprofessional communication in care transition handovers

Angela Roberts-South
Communications Sciences & Disorders, U Western Ontario, London, Ontario, Canada
asouth4@uwo.ca

Angela Roberts-South is Clinical Supervisor at H.A. Leeper Hearing and Speech Clinic, University of Western Ontario, Faculty Lecturer at University of Western Ontario and Consulting Speech Language Pathologist/Research at National Parkinson Foundation Centre of Excellence. A PhD student at U. Western Ontario, she has just been awarded (first in her competition) a Canadian Institute of Health Research Fellowship Award and the Prize in Aging for two years. Angie's interest is in the area of language and discourse performances in individuals with movement disorders (e.g, her specialty is Parkinson's disease) and who may exhibit cognitive impairment.

Robert W. Schrauf
Applied Linguistics, The Pennsylvania State University, University Park, PA 16802
rws23@psu.edu

Dr. Robert W. Schrauf is Professor and Head of The Department of Applied Linguistics at Penn State University. His areas of interest include cross-cultural gerontology, narrative gerontology, Alzheimer's disease, experimental and longitudinal approaches to multilingualism, and bilingual autobiographical memory. He is a fellow of the Gerontological Society of America and on the editorial boards of the *Journal of Cross-Cultural Research* and *Cross-Cultural Research.* He is co-editor with Kees de Bot of *Language Development over the Lifespan* (Routledge, 2009) and co-editor with Nicole Müller of *Dialogue and Dementia: Cognitive and Communicative Resources for Engagement* (Taylor and Francis, 2014).

Alison Wray
Language and Communication, Cardiff University, UK
wrayA@cardiff.ac.uk

Dr. Alison Wray is a Research Professor in Language and Communication at Cardiff University, UK. Her doctorate, from the University of York, examined the role of the right hemisphere in language processing. Her research specialism is formulaic language, on which topic she has written two monographs, *Formulaic language and the Lexicon* (CUP, 2002) which won the 2003 book prize of the British Association for Applied Linguistics, and *Formulaic Language: Pushing the Boundaries* (OUP,

2008). This research examines the psycholinguistic and sociolinguistic motivations for learning, storing and using multiword expressions, and offers an explanation for their resilience in acquired language disorders. In her recent research she has explored the role of formulaic language in people with Alzheimer's and also how it is used by their carers. In 2013 she joined the Grant Advisory Board (care, services and public health funding stream) of the Alzheimer's Society. She has also published two successful student textbooks, *Projects in Linguistics and Language Studies* (with Bloomer, Hodder, 3rd ed. 2012) and *Critical Reading and Writing for Postgraduates* (with Wallace, Sage, 2nd ed. 2011).

SUBJECT INDEX